Speech
and
Language
Problems

a guide for the classroom teacher

George O. Egland

Department of Speech Pathology and Audiology
Western Michigan University

Prentice-Hall, Inc.
Englewood Cliffs, New Jersey

13-827402-9

Library of Congress Catalog
Card Number 72–102289

Printed in the United States of America

Current Printing (last number):
10 9 8 7 6 5 4 3 2 1

Prentice-Hall International, Inc., *London*
Prentice-Hall of Australia, Pty. Ltd., *Sydney*
Prentice-Hall of Canada, Ltd., *Toronto*
Prentice-Hall of India Private Limited, *New Delhi*
Prentice-Hall of Japan, Inc., *Tokyo*

Preface

This text on speech correction defines various speech and language problems at the elementary and the secondary levels. Methods are suggested for the analysis, prevention, and correction of these problems in everyday classroom situations, where the assistance of teachers may enable speech therapists to give more attention to pupils needing special help.

Sharp lines of distinction have been avoided among symptoms, causes, needs, and methods classified under separate labels as for specific disorders of speech and language. For example, the treatment of a child with cerebral palsy recognizes the possibility of combined problems of hearing, language, misarticulation, fluency, voice, and emotional maladjustment. His treatment is considered in each chapter which applies to a facet of his complex involvement.

The author wishes to acknowledge the encouragement and counsel of Dr. Charles Van Riper and other staff associates in the Department of Speech Pathology and Audiology at Western Michigan University. Special appreciation goes to his sister, Carol M. Turner, whose experience as a high school teacher of English and Speech provided useful suggestions in correlating speech correction with language instruction in the classroom. The author also acknowledges the assistance of Susan L. Roon in research on infant speech and language development.

G.O.E.

Contents

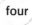

four

five

Problems of Speech
Output in the Classroom   82

six

Helping the Child who Misarticulates   98

seven

Helping the Child with a Language Problem   142

eight

Helping the Nonfluent Child   171

one

Speech, Language, and the Classroom Teacher

We can still only theorize on how language originated in the human race and how an infant actually achieves the ability to vocalize his needs and desires into sounds that communicate meaning. But as we study the foundations, characteristics, and factors which appear to affect language and its most universal form, speech, we increasingly appreciate this wonderful social tool that distinguishes humans from other living beings.

While there are similarities among the one thousand five hundred different languages spoken by man, there are also great differences in their elements, structures, and mechanics. Most language codes rely upon the production of sound and its auditory perception; in some, the system of sounds may be produced by drumbeat or whistle-pattern, rather than by the speech articulators. Other languages require a greater reliance upon visual or tactile cues. Linguistic analysis has also shown that some of the language systems adopted by "uncivilized" tribes are actually far more intricate in their design than is English, for instance. Each language functions effectively only because certain of its features have been arbitrarily selected and fixed through convention to symbolize certain meanings for its main purpose, communication.

Finally, in this chapter we shall briefly consider why and how the classroom teacher should share in this task of improving a child's communicative ability through regular language, not only in speaking, reading, and writing, but in listening, thinking, and all the other facets which enter into the functions of language.

The Importance of Speech and Language for Pupils and Teachers

Because our speech grew so gradually from its hazy origins in our infancy, because it is so familiar and seems so natural and operates so effortlessly and automatically, we tend to overlook the miracle and magic of it all. Speech and other forms of language enable minds to function and to meet with others;

feelings to be expressed, resolved, and adjusted to; and records of knowledge to be stated, transmitted, and preserved for the benefit of others. Through language we acquire aspirations, formulate our goals, procure aid in solving our problems, and evaluate our performances. Through language we gain self-satisfaction from tooting our verbal horns over success and find solace in our laments over failure. Through language we find recreation and enjoyment, and maintain or regain mental health.

The importance of speech and language for self-satisfactions through social acceptance, control, and as an outlet for self-expression is meaningfully expressed by school children of different ages when they are asked such a question as "Why do you want to talk?" Kindergarteners give such replies as: "Because I can tell you something"; "I talk and I get things I want"; "I want children to play with me"; "So I can play cowboy-and-Indians"; "It's fun to talk"; "I like to bring things to show-and-tell."

Third-graders give these reasons for talking: "I like to read and recite"; "I have to read and recite"; "Because I like to have friends and it's fun to talk with them"; "I can tell kids what I want them to do"; "I can tell about things"; "I can answer my teacher's questions"; "I can go shopping for Mother"; "I can answer the phone and talk with my friends on the phone."

Pupils at the junior-high level become aware of extended, social, and sophisticatedly mature reasons for talking: "If I recite and talk in class, I get better grades"; "The teacher asks questions and I answer"; "I like to talk with my friends and tell them things"; "I have to give oral reports"; "I'd like to be in a play"; "Sometimes I talk Dad and Mom into giving me things"; "I talk with my friends about our problems"; "It's fun to tell jokes."

When a group of teachers were asked to list their professional uses of speech, they replied: "To give pupils clear instruction, information, and directions; to talk effectively with parents; to discuss matters with other teachers, principals, and other school personnel; to give talks before groups, such as at P.T.A.; and to talk over problems with fellow teachers—at times, I'm afraid, we gossip and share our school problems too much in the lounge, or enjoy light-hearted talk. But it makes us feel better, I guess."

The foregoing reasons for speaking suggest that teachers exercise speech in both professional and nonprofessional ways—to serve their teaching roles as well as to fulfill their ordinary human needs. Studies show that the verbal behaviors of teachers and of their pupils become remarkably similar, from influences which may be either constructive or destructive from the standpoint of teaching and learning in the classroom. Consequently, by analyzing classroom talk by teachers and pupils, through their "Verbal Interaction Category System," Amidon and Hunter[1] have outlined and suggested some realistic ways to improve teaching. They give practical guidelines and illustrations to help teachers to analyze and to evaluate various verbal interactions which either help or hinder teaching and learning in the classroom situation. For example, a teacher may profit from a self-inventory in which she takes stock of her self-initiated talk: giving information or opinions, giving directions, asking narrow questions which call for predictable answers, or asking broad ones which require unpredictable answers. Every teacher can profit from analyzing the nature and effects of her verbal responses to pupils; whether she *accepts* their ideas, behavior, and feelings through reflecting, clarifying, encouraging, summarizing, or commenting on them; or whether she *rejects* their ideas, behavior, and feelings through talk which criticizes, ignores, discourages, rejects, etc. Likewise, it would be well for a teacher to check and govern pupils' responses to herself and to fellow pupils, so that their talk might facilitate their education rather than detract from it. These same needs and policies are also important for therapists, parents, and others who are in positions to influence children through spoken as well as written instruction.

Definitions of Speech and Language

What is language and what is speech? How do we learn language and how do we learn to speak? These are difficult questions.

We normally learn to speak without ever having to define and analyze the act. We are inclined to consider learning to talk in a class with learning to walk—something that just emerges like a mushroom "when the time is right." However, if parents were to look for pamphlets and books designed to instruct laymen on matters of children's speech and language development, they would find relatively little in comparison with materials on other subjects. Even the most widely circulated books on child care usually give only brief consideration to speech and language. Why is this?

Parents frequently look upon speaking as an entirely hereditary function. They explain their children's functional speech disorders by such conclusive statements as: "Well, we've been told that he had an uncle who spoke that way"; "My husband says that he was slow in talking, too, but he came out of it"; "I guess that some people are just born that way"; and "It's his God-given cross to bear, I s'pose."

However, despite the fact that so many children learn to talk as well as they do without much direct parental attention to the process, it is difficult to define what language and speech entail. We shall borrow terminology from the field of linguistics, the scientific and philosophic study of language. We shall seek what the linguists are exploring—the nature and mechanics of language and speech.

As Whatmough[2] states, language may be defined from several aspects. It is a form of systematic symbolism, a grouping of characters which are arbitrarily set by agreement or convention to signify meaning for purposes of communication. A language *symbol*, unlike a *sign*, usually has no direct relation to the object or the event which it represents; there is nothing in the nature of things that gives a symbol its prescribed meaning. Speech uses a system of symbols commonly called *words*, which are arranged in a certain order, termed *syntax*. The meanings from words and their orderly arrangements in sentences are governed by the law called the *probability of occurrence*. From a social standpoint, language is a form of group behavior, a means of transmitting information in an economical and powerful way. On the mental plane, language has been theorized to be the essential vehicle by which we think.

Therefore, if we combine its piecemeal linguistic attributes, language may be defined as a human, culturally established, and voluntarily acquired means of communicating our information, ideas, emotions, and desires by means of conventionalized symbol systems. These verbal symbol systems may depend upon any of our perceptual senses—auditory, visual, or tactile— singly or in combinations.

Speech, or oral language, is ordinarily dependent upon the listener's auditory perception of the sounds produced by speech organs. But when the recipient cannot hear, the postures and movements of our oral speech may be "lip-read" as visible speech. Or, as Helen Keller has so admirably demonstrated, if one can neither hear nor see spoken language, its patterns of vibrations, postures, and movements can be felt, interpreted, and exchanged communicatively. Speech, the oral form of language, is the most universal form of language on earth. Most of the world's languages are only spoken; they have no written form. Speech is also the first and basic form usually to be learned and used in the life of an individual. In speech, as in written forms of language, its symbolic features closely adhere to convention. The code of speech symbols, designed for a particular language, follows a statistical regularity; otherwise it would not be reliable for interpretation or communication. Effective speech consists of verbal symbols of physical events which convey information because the sender and the receiver similarly interpret the meaning of the symbols and their syntactical arrangement. This implies that each language must have its own certain rules, established and learned—rules which are based upon the probability of occurrence.

Normally we learn to understand speech and to speak before we read, and to read before we write. Every teacher of reading knows that a child will not have an adequate foundation for reading unless he has attained an adequate speech foundation.

Factors of Speech and Language Development

Language depends upon an interwoven combination of factors. In the first place, if the child is to acquire a language, he must belong to the social group in which that language has been adopted and used. As a member of this group, the child gradually learns speech, first to understand and then to speak it. Gradually and by cumulative stages he learns the meaningful patterning of verbal symbols, the grammatical rules of word order, word classes, function-grouping of words, accent, inflection—all conveyed by articulated sound. In order to achieve this sequence of marvelous feats needed for understanding speech, for speaking, and later for reading and writing a language, the child ordinarily needs certain basic equipment, conditions, and skills. However, it is difficult to specify the essentials for speech, because occasionally individuals prove that there can be exceptions to the requirements for speech. Persons have fooled the experts by learning speech articulation without even a vestige of tongue, or with serious involvement from cerebral palsy, or from aphasia. It is important not to lose faith in a speech-handicapped person because he lacks one or more of the ordinary requisites for speech. A person may understand speech but may not be able to speak it. Or the reverse may be true: a mentally retarded child, for instance, may be overly trained to "mouth" or to "parrot" words without being taught their meaning.

Many forces, some instinctive and some modifiable, are associated with speech and language. Our search for the causes of speech and language problems has given us a long list of overlapping factors which are usually considered necessary. In education we have debated the issue of nature versus nurture, that is, whether factors are inborn or whether they are primarily environmental and acquired from experience and learning. But when we are confronted with this nature-nurture issue in our diagnosis and treatment and have no valid evidence to blame nature rather than nurture, it is more practical to give nurture the benefit of the doubt and to work from that standpoint. We can do more about nurture than about our heredity once we are born.

In all professions there have been tendencies at times to follow fads and the "latest" instead of relying on impartial observation, testing, and judgment. Since speech therapy is still in the exploratory stage, there appears to be a need and a temptation to coin the words of our working vocabulary in terms as abstruse as the subject. Often in reports of investigations of speech and language development, we find puzzling, elaborate, or overworked terms, such as *educable*, *peripheral*, *perceptual readiness*, *disadvantaged*, *brain-damaged*, *central*, etc.

These terms lack meaning and value unless they are clarified and substantiated by details. These vague but impressive labels may reflect a waste-basket classification of disorders. They are used to hide ignorance, to avoid the harshness of being specific and truthful, or to excuse further search, work, and possible failure. A tag like *brain-damaged* attempts to describe the cause and symptomatology of many perplexing cases of speech and language problems. In general, it is more productive of success merely to make an honest survey of a problem with clear-cut observations rather than to attempt a premature classification of the problem and an overconfident and superficial prognosis.

Later chapters will indicate how the five overlapping spheres of a child's background operate in the complex dynamics of his speech and language development: the perceptual, intellectual, organic, social, and emotional areas. But we introduce the following categories of background causes early in order to orient us to the various areas to be kept in mind.

In speaking we must learn to perceive, to identify, and to discriminate correctly and rapidly from hearing, seeing, and feeling kinesthetically the postures and movements which enter into speaking. We need our ears and eyes to receive speech; we need our self-hearing and kinesthetic feel to monitor and thereby to control our speech production. Yet, some of the perceptual difficulties may be corrected through retraining, compensation, and aid from artificial devices.

Perceptual factors are mentioned first in this series of speech requisites because of their importance in the early diagnosis and treatment of speech and language problems. Perceptual problems are often closely associated with other problems, emotional, social, and psychological, the symptoms of which may lead us to overlook the perceptual causes. At times, the perceptual cause is primarily social or psychological in nature. For example, a child who has perfectly normal ears, eyes, and tactile sense may not have acquired the necessary perceptual skills through maturation and use. Listening, for instance, is a complex acquired ability, so important that it has been listed as one of the essential communicative skills to be taught along with speaking, reading, and writing. Every teacher depends upon listening in her classroom activities; every good teacher works to encourage, train, and utilize her pupils' listening abilities. A teacher often has listening and related perceptual skills in mind when she refers to a child's "social maturity," "attention span," "distractibility," "listlessness," "interest level," "erratic behavior," "nonconformity," "autism," "aloofness," "apathy," "laziness," "cooperativeness," etc. Terms like these should remind us that perceptual development is primarily related to many facets of a child's behavior: his organic make-up, his physical and mental health, his social environment, and his mentality.

Mental abilities are obviously important for the acquisition of speech and language, which requires complex learning, judgment, and creativity. Because of the high correlation between intelligence and language ability, we sometimes measure intelligence too narrowly in terms of language skills. Furthermore, because so many of our tests of intelligence depend upon verbal language ability, it is difficult to determine a valid IQ for the person who cannot comprehend speech or talk. Nonverbal tests of intelligence may be difficult to administer and to interpret in the light of related factors other than the client's intelligence. We may be relatively certain that a person's IQ score is correct, but we must be careful not to assume that it takes a certain level of IQ to learn language and to speak in a worthwhile sense. Although subnormal intelligence ordinarily slows up and limits the language learning process, we have a tendency to overrate the "gray matter" required for speech and to overlook the fact that subnormal intelligence may be compensated for and perhaps raised by sympathetic teaching or improving the general health. Our treatment of a person may go astray and create further complications and handicaps for him when we assume that he who is slow to talk, or who does not talk well, must be stupid.

ORGANIC

Our meaning of the term *organic* in this list of factors upon which speech and language depend refers to all the physical structures and their motor functions used for speech and language reception and expression. We say "used for speech" instead of "needed for speech" because physically subnormal persons keep reminding us that speech may be achieved even though their regular speech organs of articulation, breathing, vocalization, etc., are faulty. Organic factors are often related to factors in other categories. Organic problems, such as blindness and deafness, often lead also to social and emotional problems, and these, too, affect speech. A cleft palate may interfere with speech vocalization and articulation; in addition, it may increase susceptibility to ear infections which, if not treated, might lead to problems in speech reception and production. A child who cannot walk, who must endure a limited life in a wheelchair, thereby may be subjected to an array of social and psychological factors which handicap his speech and language development. But here again we should remember that many of the complications of a handicapped person may be prevented, reduced, or corrected.

Because the *organic* concept includes the motor function of physiology as well as anatomy, we should also include neurological factors in this category. Even though we have relatively little understanding of how the brain functions for speech, we know that it somehow has governing control over the whole wonderful network of processes. There are theories which credit the human brain with having a built-in patterning which predisposes a child to communicate and to deal with speech sounds symbolically, even without training to do so. But, as cautioned earlier in this chapter, we should not let the mystery of the brain and our awe for its role in our behavior lead us into making it our scapegoat when we fail in diagnosis and treatment of speech and language problems. We resort too often and too readily to the terms "brain-damaged," "aphasic," "cerebral dysfunction," etc., without justifiable evidence to do so. The indiscriminate use of these broad and commanding diagnostic terms can falsely create hopelessness in others; it can block further search and treatment of causes which may be remediable. When we enter the realm of neurology, we are reminded more than ever that our teamwork with the best of specialists is required.

The social-personal needs which relate to a child's speech and language development start at his birth and continue as a social response acquired in group settings to make speech the most important channel for learning and living with other members of his group. Vygotsky[3] believes that speech begins as a social act (a "pre-intellectual stage") learned from others and for social purposes, and that later it becomes internalized as a self-directed thought process (a "pre-linguistic stage") continuing to be used socially, too. At first, these two processes are rather separate, but eventually thought becomes verbal; speech becomes rational. Word meaning becomes the unit of verbal thought, referring to a class of objects, a generalization *as well as* a unit of language for social interchange. Therefore, Vygotsky theorizes that thought is neither "speech minus sound" nor a function that is "pure" and unrelated to language. Rather, words and thoughts are related as a living process, not preformed and constant, but in an emerging, evolving, developmental way.

Parents, too, often indicate that social matters are related to speech problems when they offer such explanations for speech problems as: "The older children talk for him"; "He gets what he wants without talking"; "I think he gets more attention from not talking"; "We've tried to force him to talk, but that doesn't work—it makes him clam up more than ever"; "He'd talk if he wanted to; he's just stubborn"; "He's shy like this, the way his father was. He doesn't talk much yet."

When we consider how emotional factors influence speech and language development, we realize more clearly how much overlapping there is in the foregoing classification of causes. For instance, should we class speechlessness in a pupil as being fundamentally an emotional, physical, intellectual, or social disorder? Should we categorize "negativism" as a social phenomenon or as a personal emotional maladjustment? When the negativistic child becomes mute, hyperactive, and unruly and is given medical tranquilizers to lower his emotionality, we tend to look upon the problem as emotional and organic. But when we treat his social behavior by manipulating his social environment, then we are inclined to classify the problem as social. Are "social maturity" and "emotional security" synonymous? May they be separated? Or may they correspond to the two sides of a postage stamp: the social side to that of the human figure, the symbols, and directives; the emotional to the gummed side, which adds affective flavor, and which insures permanence to the stamp?

In education and in therapy we are told over and over to "consider and treat the whole child," until we become bored or impatient with the trite expression. But, as we learn more about speech and language processes and the correction of their problems, we should have renewed respect for the genuine substance of this threadbare advice. On the other hand, we may well beware of meaningless definitions in the area of emotions and in neurology. These terminologies pigeonhole our thoughts without much consequence in such foggy terms as "emotional security," "emotional stability," "emotionally hyperactive," "emotionally disturbed," "emotionally maladjusted," "an emotional child," etc. If we actually do have facts to communicate about emotion, we should try to convey them clearly.

Linguistic Elements and Characteristics

Having defined speech and language and their requisites, let us attempt to analyze their elements. In speech correction it is necessary to know as much as possible about linguistics, the study of the structure and functionings which constitute the warp and woof of language and its most universal form, speech. Unless we keep abreast of linguistic knowledge, our principles in teaching and in correcting speech may violate the natural principles by which we learn and modify speech. We must not forget that *speech*, after all, *is language*, for language purposes. Teaching and correcting speech without due regard to its language aspects is like teaching a pianist to be a musician merely by teaching him the parts and mechanics of the piano—its keyboard scale of notes, whether or not it is in tune, and, perhaps, how to tune it—without much attention to its real function, the total art of playing music. McDonald,[4] for example, has specifically tried to correlate modern linguistic principles with the testing and treatment of misarticulation. We should similarly try to work more closely within the framework of language when we deal with speech-voice problems, stuttering, delayed speech, and aphasia.

The following discussion of the elements and characteristics of language and speech is a mere introduction to these linguistic features. Books by Fries,[5] Sapir,[6] and Whatmough[2] will give detailed discussions of general linguistic subjects. Fodor and Katz[7] provide views on the philosophy and structure of language. Moses[8] and Miller[9] discuss language from its phonetic, phonemic, and prosodic standpoints. Cofer and Musgrave[10] analyze the problems and linguistic processes in verbal learning; Myklebust[11] focuses upon the development and disorders of written language.

ELEMENTS OF SPEECH

Is speech composed of elements? If so, what are they? May these elements or units within the construction of speech be identified and measured? Do these elements of speech have significance in the development of speech, in its functioning, and in our teaching and correction of it? If so, do speech elements exist in steps or hierarchies? If speech elements do follow an operational sequence, at what "step" and in what order should we proceed in therapy, for instance?

We find divergent views on the definitions of the atoms, molecules, and formulas that constitute speech. Much of our disagreement comes from our differences in orientation—like the situation portrayed in the old fable about the three blind men inspecting an elephant. If we view speech physiologically, acoustically, or phonetically, we are likely to reduce it to different levels and into smaller units than if we are linguistically oriented. Carrell and Tiffany,[12] for example, consider the *syllable* to be the basic physiological and acoustic unit of speech, while they regard the *phoneme* as the basic unit of language. In this context, a *phoneme* is a linguistic unit consisting of a family of sounds which are similar but not identical and which may be used interchangeably within words without changing their language meaning. Thus, in words like *to, stutter, it,* and *little,* the four different pronunciations of *t* vary considerably, even though we class all of them as the *t* sound—one of the approximately forty speech sounds (phonemes) which we count in English. These phonemic variations, called *allophones,* tend to be heard and judged as similar, although they actually differ physiologically or acoustically. Scientists like Fairbanks[13] and others have shown that when we speak a word or a sentence, we articulate and modify a relatively *continuous flow* of sounds that move by transition from one series of acoustic events to another. Our articulations thereby mutually affect each other because of physiological necessity and economy.

However, some linguists, who regard speech primarily from the standpoint of spoken *language,* place the smallest unit of meaningful language at a higher level than the phoneme. They believe that meaning begins with the *morpheme,* instead of the phoneme, and that meaning extends with the *word* and the *sentence.* They define the morpheme as the smallest division of speech-sound or sound-sequence which can still represent language-meaning. The morpheme, therefore, may consist either of a single phoneme, such as the *s* which signifies plurality in the word *cats,* or a minimal sequence of phonemes, such as *c, a,* and *t,* which symbolize the concept of the animal.

Other linguists judge that the *word* is the smallest functional unit of speech and that the sentence is the major functional unit. In this framework of thought, a *word,* differentiated from a *morpheme,* represents the smallest pattern of speech sounds that may be isolated and yet have complete meaning; while a *sentence* is a linguistic expression which combines a subject of discourse with a statement in regard to this subject. A few words, like *oh, ah,* and *a,* consist of single phonemes. But the word *lips,* for instance, has two morphemes, *lip* and *s,* and according to our previous definition, the word *lips* has four speech sounds, termed *phonemes.*

Backus and Beasley[14] and Zedler[15] believe that the starting point in the correction of speech misarticulation should be analytic rather than synthetic; that correction should start with the *thought* unit, and not with the phonetic sounds which are isolated from their language meaning. Zedler, for example, states that the synthetic process, which follows a reverse order of procedure from that of the analytical approach and which begins with meaningless sounds and words and works toward syllables and finally meaningful words and sentences, violates a fundamental principle of learning: that we should proceed from the known to the unknown. Modern teachers of language, too, are likely to favor the analytical approach, correlating speech with the meaningful aspects of language, especially the basic and serviceable language which the child has learned or should learn. Otherwise, a child's work upon speech elements may become dull and meaningless drill; training will be piecemeal, lacking correlation with language, and consequently without carry-over into the child's everyday established language.

Van Riper[16] clearly discusses another design for articulation therapy, one followed by many speech therapists who are more phonetically than linguistically oriented. Users of this method employ the synthetic approach, starting and working for mastery at the isolated sound level, then proceeding by successive steps up through the levels of the syllable, the word, the sentence, and finally to spontaneous language usage. In this therapeutic approach, therapists often develop a greater emphasis upon the *phonetics* of the faulty speech sounds than upon the phonemic and morphemic characteristics, and their contexts. In the early stages of this synthetic method, the child tends to work upon his faulty "speech sounds" separated from his language framework. A child with a lisp on the *s* sound, for example, may be taught to identify and to produce this sound as "the snake sound," "the tea-kettle sound," or "the flat-tire sound." Furthermore, after the child masters this prescribed sound in isolation, his work may extend to include this sound in "nonsense syllables" or later in "monkey words"—before introducing this sound in contexts associated with his established and meaningful language patterns.

Therapists who follow these steps believe that a faulty sound is more easily corrected when it is first dissociated from the child's established language framework. But therapists who are more linguistically oriented believe that this approach is narrow and artificial. They point out that the phonetics (acoustics) of the isolated "tea-kettle sound," for instance, do not correspond to the features of the variable *s* as it occurs in speech contexts of our language. Although a child may learn rather quickly to articulate a given "tea-kettle sound," he still finds that this particular sound does not substitute well for the family of *s* allophones as they interweave into the elaborate designs of his language. Therapists who do not adhere to linguistic principles usually have more difficulty in teaching a child to "reenforce" and to "transfer" his "tea-kettle" sound into his everyday language usage. They ignore the fact that speech sounds do not occur in isolation and also that they cannot be truly articulated in isolation. Carrell and Tiffany[12] and McDonald,[4] who has applied linguistic principles to articulation testing and therapy, point out that speech is much more than a series of separable sounds and that speech sounds lose their features and significance with language when they are isolated. We distort speech sounds when we attempt to isolate them apart from their necessary connections with speech sounds which precede and follow them in the flow of speech.

We may take practical advantage of the fact that our articulations of speech sounds may be helped as well as hindered by the articulatory influences from sounds which precede or follow them. This principle may explain why a child who has failed to learn a sound as a fixed articulated posture sometimes will correctly articulate this sound when it is connected with other helping sounds in syllables, in "key words," or in sentences. Later, in our chapter on articulation, we shall discuss how these "key words," exceptions to a child's misarticulations of a speech sound, may be used to good advantage in diagnosis and treatment.

Besides the physiological, phonetic, and acoustic features required for the production and reception of the many speech forms, careful concept formation and reasoning underlie words and grammatical structures. It is important to remember that these forms are learned through correct social patterning and reward—that they signify only what we teach and learn. For instance, a speech sound may have different meanings in different languages. Each child must discover the make-up of speech; each child must learn the creative art of using it in accordance with the arbitrary meanings and standards concerning words, their grammatical structures, and the inevitable change that appears in living speech.

SPEECH STANDARDS AND VARIATIONS

We recognize that speech depends upon standardization, which is conveyed as a part of our social heritage and usage, for reliable communication. However, a child learns language not only by direct imitation but also through his creative process of generalization and analogy. Meaningful rules of grammar and word order, for example, are learned and extended so that the child can become more than a limited echo. In the many speech situations of life, the child must use language creatively, far beyond the narrow bounds of direct imitation. Teachers especially appreciate the need for standardization, because the meaningful perception of language depends upon the ability to discriminate contrasts within the language forms, and because the meaningful expression of language depends upon the speaker's ability to express these contrastive elements in agreement with our standards. But our standards are variable too. They are evolving and ever changing with needs and usage.

PRONUNCIATION AND ARTICULATION

Dictionaries show that our pronunciations vary and that we must be careful in judging what is a "cultured" and what is an "uncultured" usage; what is correct and what is incorrect; what is standard and what is substandard. But we must be cautious in judging standards of speech even from our dictionaries. Most dictionaries focus upon lexical pronunciations—the forms of words spoken in careful, single-word fashion—instead of the conversational connected speech, the "natural" colloquial speech of our everyday usage. Moreover, most of our American dictionaries are based upon British pronunciations. In *A Pronouncing Dictionary of American English*, by Kenyon and Knott,[17] we are advised to judge correctness and incorrectness of pronunciation standards on the basis of actual cultivated usage. Under this rule, it would be misleading to say that a word is "almost universally mispronounced." This basis for judgment requires us to consider our obligations to regional standards as well as our adaptations to speaking the word formally or informally. For example, a classroom teacher who is dictating a list of separate spelling words to her pupils is not likely to pronounce many words in the same way that she would if she were using them in sentences, either in reading or in casual conversation.

The way in which our pronunciations vary with different speech usages explains why we sometimes disagree in our phonetic and phonic analyses of spoken words. For example, when the majority of us speak the word *Mary* in everyday connected reading or in conversation, do we pronounce the final phoneme of the word as a "short *i*" or as a "long *e*"? When we use this word in sentences, most of us pronounce the *y* as an unstressed "short *i*" sound, although we may perceive and firmly contend this phoneme to be a "long *e*" —as we pronounce the stressed final sound in *Marie*. We tend to hear what we are "set," inclined, and accustomed to hear—just as magicians make use of the fact that we fail to see what we do not expect to see. Some of the difficulties in retraining speech stem from these false mirages in our perceptions arising from narrow usage or prejudices trained into us by undependable rules from our school days. If we overlook these idiomatic exceptions, we shall of course have faults in our standards for judging speech.

STANDARDS OF FLUENCY

Speakers vary in their fluency. At one extreme of this fluency-nonfluency continuum, we find severe stutterers who may be practically speechless from their frequent and long hesitations, prolongations, repetitions, and allied reactions which break up the flow or sequential unity of their speech patterns. As Van Riper[16] points out, stuttering may be described from many angles, but it is difficult to define. Johnson and others[18] have studied the incidence and variability of nonfluency among speakers, as well as within an individual's speech. Its features are elusive and our standards for judging nonfluency are not standardized. Our judgments are indefinite and depend upon many factors, such as our cultural standards, the age of the speaker who is being judged, and the nature of his communicative situation. As listeners, we usually base our judgments of a speaker's fluency upon a combination of factors: the way he sounds in comparison to the rhythm patterns which we have learned to adopt, the degree to which the speaker's fluency interferes with his communication with us, and the extent to which the speaker appears to be otherwise troubled by his nonfluency. Our judgments of fluency are often more subjective than objective. We cannot agree on what constitutes fluency, on how to measure fluency or nonfluency, or on the relative importance which nonfluencies have in spoiling the flow of speech. Nevertheless, in America we highly value speech fluency, perhaps even to the extent of voting for Presidents largely on the contribution of our candidate's fluency to his personal image.

Our chapter on stuttering will emphasize that from the practical standpoint in speech correction we must examine and deal with the particular standards by which parents and others may be judging and handling a child's fluency. Causal factors of stuttering and our counseling and treatment in fluency problems are often related to misconceived fluency ratings which a child is expected to have, consequently inducing inappropriate standards which the child expects of himself.

STANDARDS OF VOCABULARY AND
GRAMMAR

School teachers learn that it is difficult to judge a child's vocabulary. It is often not clear to parents when a child utters his first true word. That first word may be hard to distinguish from jabber which does not fit our definition of a word. Our vocabulary tests are subject to error all along the child's developmental age scale. We get different estimates of a child's vocabulary whether we survey the number of words which he can recall or whether we sample the words he uses in conversation. Of course, we cannot test for and determine all the words that a child knows; we cannot expect that he will spontaneously use for us his full repertoire of "spoken vocabulary." Johnson[19] points out some of the difficulty in determining the extent of a person's vocabulary. Only a few words, like *and*, *the*, *a*, *to*, and *I*, make up a relatively large percentage of our written and spoken vocabulary.

The reliability of language tests and of intelligence tests which depend upon language skills is limited by the selection of the word samples used in the test, as well as by the method of conducting the tests. Teachers of reading are especially aware of the variables which complicate our testing of a child's vocabulary and other language potentials. A child's vocabulary is usually far greater than it appears—especially if he has lived in an environment different from that which we and our "standard" children have known. His vocabulary may have little overlap with ours or with his reading textbooks. Therefore, a child's difficulty in reading, writing, and spelling may result from ignorance of the vocabulary used in his textbooks. One supervisor of elementary education explained this difficulty as follows:

> In our large consolidated school, we get first-graders directly from the farm, from the fruit-orchards, from suburbia, from isolated and decaying sections of our city. Most of them are middle-class but some are from the lower socioeconomic levels. Most are white but some are Mexican and other nationalities which form pockets in our population.
>
> All of the differences in the backgrounds of these children may be seen when they

talk and learn to read. One trouble arises from the fact that our primers are made for middle-class children.We should have at least some primers which would *begin* with the past experience and vocabulary which each child already has, and which is meaningful to him in his social, cultural group. In other words, I feel that we should begin by meeting a young child at the levels where his home and environment have left him when he enters school and we take over—even though the language at some of these levels is not very clean or desirable by our middle-class standards.

When you overhear children speaking their everyday language on the playground, for instance, you realize why the language of their classroom and their textbooks is like foreign language to them—full of new words and grammar construction, and with meanings they have never experienced. If our textbooks were tailored only around experiences of their lives, and were fitted to their language, we and our middle-class pupils would be the ones who would flounder, get discouraged with reading, and appear deficient. We must operate on the basis of double standards until these outsiders have a reasonable chance to learn ours as well as their own.

A good share of a classroom teacher's efforts in teaching language is spent in the broad and tricky area of grammar: teaching the classes of words; their inflections, functions, and relationships in the sentence; their features which indicate tense, number, gender, etc. As one English teacher has stated:

At times I feel that teaching correct grammar is a losing, thankless battle. There's so much faulty grammar being used around a child—at home, heard on TV, and often used by their most influential and admired speakers—that we teachers are really working against tough and seemingly hopeless odds. And if our standards are to be judged on the basis of most common usage, I wonder at times about the correctness of my personal standards, the ones I'm inclined to teach. I've become less arbitrary and more compromising in teaching grammar. I try to do more than to brand things as "correct" or "incorrect," to reject the former and to hammer at the latter. I devise projects to teach awareness and the reasons for the different structures and functions in the grammar of English. In this way, the pupils are more relaxed and free to adopt a choice of standards in this or in that situation. I believe that more pupils are adopting higher standards than they otherwise would or could.

Why should teachers and speech therapists be concerned with the complexities of linguistics, the analysis of speech, language structure, and the functional processes that make up speech? Unless we are informed about these areas, we shall be unable to make a differential diagnosis of problems, and our treatment will lack focus and direction. We must diagnose beyond the immediate speech symptoms that appear to be faulty. A therapist, like a car mechanic, needs to be more than a "parts man"; he must consider the elements and relationships that cause malfunctions. Furthermore, experience will recommend that we follow the most likely and economical procedures in our diagnoses and corrections of ills. Otherwise, time and efforts and costs will be wasted.

References

1. Edmund Amidon and Elizabeth Hunter, *Improved Teaching, The Analysis of Classroom Verbal Interaction*. New York: Holt, Rinehart and Winston, Inc., 1966.

2. Joshua Whatmough, *Language*. New York: The New American Library of World Literature, Inc., 1960.

3. L. S. Vygotsky, *Thought and Language*. Cambridge, Mass.: The M.I.T. Press, 1962.

4. E. McDonald, *Articulation Testing and Treatment, A Sensory-Motor Approach*. Pittsburgh: Stanwix House, Inc., 1964.

5. C. C. Fries, *The Structure of English*. New York: Harcourt, Brace & World, Inc., 1952.

6. E. Sapir, *Language*. New York: Harcourt, Brace & World, Inc., 1921.

7. Jerry A. Fodor and Jerrold J. Katz, *The Structure of Language, Readings in the Philosophy of Language*. Englewood Cliffs, N.J.: Prentice-Hall, Inc., 1964.

8. Elbert R. Moses, Jr., *Phonetics, History and Interpretation*. Englewood Cliffs, N. J.: Prentice-Hall, Inc., 1964.

9. George A. Miller, *Language and Communication*. New York: McGraw-Hill Book Company, Inc., 1951.

10. Charles N. Cofer and Barbara S. Musgrave, *Verbal Behavior and Learning: Problems and Processes*. New York: McGraw-Hill Book Company, Inc., 1963.

11. Helmer R. Myklebust, *Development and Disorders of Written Language*. New York: Grune and Stratton, 1965.

12. James Carrell and William R. Tiffany, *Phonetics: Theory and Application to Speech Improvement*. New York: McGraw-Hill Book Company, Inc., 1960.

13. Grant Fairbanks, *Voice and Articulation Drillbook*. New York: Harper & Row, Inc., 1960.

14. Ollie Backus and Jane Beasley, *Speech Therapy with Children*. Boston: Houghton Mifflin Company, 1951.

15. Empress Y. Zedler, *Listening for Speech Sounds*. Garden City, N.Y.: Doubleday and Co. Inc., 1955.

16. C. Van Riper, *Speech Correction: Principles and Methods*. (4th ed.). Englewood Cliffs, N.J.: Prentice-Hall, Inc., 1963.

17. John S. Kenyon and Thomas A. Knott, *A Pronouncing Dictionary of American English*. Springfield, Mass.: G. C. Merriam Co., 1953.

18. W. Johnson, S. F. Brown, J. F. Curtis, C. W. Edney, and J. Keaster, *Speech Handicapped School Children*. New York: Harper & Row, Inc., 1967.

19. Wendell Johnson, *Verbal Man: The Enchantment of Words*. New York: Collier Books, 1965.

Questions

1. Discuss variations of human language systems. Illustrate by specific native types.
2. How does speech benefit various age groups?
3. In what ways will self-analysis improve the teacher's own use of speech in the classroom?
4. What is language, and what is speech?
5. How do we learn language? How do we learn to speak?
6. Discuss the correlation between intelligence and language.
7. What are the perceptual requirements of speech?
8. What organic factors affect speech?
9. Is speech a purely social development?
10. What is the role of emotions in speech development?
11. Why must the speech therapist correlate linguistics and speech correction?
12. Discuss the relationship of syllable, phoneme, allophone, morpheme, word, sentence.
13. How does the analytic method of speech correction differ from the synthetic?
14. Is speech a series of separable sounds? Explain.
15. What is the creative process of generalization and analogy in speech education?
16. May we rely upon the dictionary exclusively in judging standards of pronunciation and articulation?
17. Is it possible to establish standards for judging fluency?
18. What are the difficulties in judging a child's vocabulary?

Suggested Subjects for Term Papers

1. On the basis of Amidon and Hunter's Verbal Interaction Category, analyze the class work of a favorite professor for a month.
2. Write a character sketch of a person you know who is a fluent and impressive formal and informal speaker.
3. Consider other members of a class you attend. What is the correlation between their recitation and their social development, revealed in class, preclass and postclass behavior?

4. If you learned a foreign language in college or in high school, compare that process with your acquisition of English.

5. Tape-record, if permissible, a lecture or a TV or radio speech. Analyze the speech, phrase by phrase, for the speech sound connections with sounds preceding and following them.

6. Does history indicate that language variations are the prime barrier against international cooperation and peace?

7. Robert Louis Stevenson wrote the following in *An Inland Voyage*: "No disgrace is attached in France to saying a thing neatly; whereas in England to talk like a book is to give in one's resignation to society." Do you and your friends downgrade your speaking ability to conform to current concepts of American speech? If so, what will the pressure mean for you as a teacher?

8. Ask the help of eight or ten friends for a pioneering study to record your method of thinking. Do you "hear" yourselves using words for the thinking process? Is there a difference between thinking alone, calmly, and when under stress in a group?

9. Information often goes in through the ears and comes out through the mouth in changed form because of lack of attention, poor hearing, malice, or humor. Because of this discrepancy, what are the difficulties for: (1) newspaper men; (2) historians; (3) politicians; (4) teachers; (5) pupils?

10. Listen to radio forum programs for several hours and rate the callers on phonetic and phonemic pronunciations. Can you classify them by geographical regions? Were the speakers aware of their mispronunciations? How did speech variations handicap communication?

two

Normal Development
of Speech and Language

This chapter will trace the sequences and processes by which speech and language normally develop throughout their most important stages of the preschool period. Parents, teachers, and therapists who respectfully appreciate the rather orderly timetable of events which appear in normal speech development will be better able to distinguish normality from abnormality, to insure normality, and to correct abnormalities when problems of development occur.

Sequence and Stages

Speech is not learned in distinct and separate stages. Stages overlap; they usually do not stop when others begin. For instance, a child continues to babble and to play vocally beyond the time when he begins to speak words. Although normal children appear to follow a similar sequence in their speech development, there are individual variations in the onset and duration of a stage. For example, although we sometimes set one year as the milestone when children normally say their first words, it would be more realistic to forecast the period as a range of time, such as the age of ten to eighteen months. This latitude is advisable because often we cannot be sure if a child's first "word" is a true word or merely a combination of meaningless syllables.

Moreover, children who are judged as normal in their speech and language areas do not remain at any given level for the same length of time. The stage of saying only single words may last from four to seventeen months. Knowledge of a child's early speech and language development depends largely upon observations of what the child overtly expresses through speech. Therefore, our discussion will be mostly in terms of outward speech behavior, rather than of the development of the still more remarkable processes that involve learning, memory, comprehension, motivation, and creative application of language and other intangibles which are more difficult to observe, measure, and understand.

Early vocalization of grunts, coos, sighs, gurgles, and other indescribable sounds are not as random and useless as they may seem. Even the birth cry, a vital reflexive action, stimulated by anoxia and other physical stimuli when air passes through the vocal chords as air replaces the amniotic fluid in the lungs and starts the breathing process, has been found to be diagnostic and as individualized as a fingerprint. Photographs and tests have shown that there are speech-related functions occurring even while the infant is in the uterus—in movements of thumb-sucking, breathing action, vocalization, and hearing. Perhaps this prenatal speech requisite may partly explain why prematurely born infants are more likely to lag in their motor development, including speech and language achievements.

Babies mean noise. At times fathers especially fail to appreciate the rhyme and reason for all the infant's crying, grunting, whimpering, sighing, and hiccupping. Far from being concerned, even fond mothers often take pride in giving their babies the compliment, "Such a good baby—hardly ever cries." Important physical, psychological, and social foundations are being prepared even during the first month or so, when the infant's cries are mostly reflexive and seemingly meaningless speech sounds. Research by Irwin[1] and others has shown that an infant's early vocalizations are stimulated by such physical and environmental conditions as noise, light, temperature, postural changes, instability, restraint of movement, touch, pain, and hunger. By learning to associate the infant's crying with some of these causes, and by identifying certain cry patterns with particular stimuli, parents influence the child beyond his immediate needs. The child is thereby taught that parents are a source of comfort, that his crying brings self-satisfactions, and that his vocal behavior may be relied upon in the future to bring these rewards.

The characteristics of prespeech vocalizations appear to have definite pattern and sequence. It has been shown that the pattern and developmental stages which characterize infant crying may be another criterion of whether or not a child is brain-injured or mentally retarded. For instance, a brain-injured infant's early reflexive cries may be lacking in normal rhythm, inflectional patterns, vigor, duration, and response to stimulation.

During the first month or so of life, infants cry on both inhalation and exhalation, action sometimes termed "cry breathing," in which there is vocalization on a short inhalation followed by a gradual and longer exhalation. Most of the sounds in crying are vowel-like. In the comfort sounds of coos, grunts, and later babblings, there are semblances of such consonant-like sounds as the *k*, *g*, *n*, and *m*. A mother describes the vocalizations of her six-week-old child as follows:

> My baby has three distinct cries: a hard, sobbing scream when she has been
> suddenly frightened; an insistent "naaaa" with whimpers between, which means

that she's hungry; and a softer, stop-and-start series of "aaaaa" when she's bored with lying down or is tired.

While drinking her bottle of milk, Jill makes "one-toned" sighs with *m* or *n* sounds. After eating, and while lying contentedly and watching objects around her, she makes "oooo" or "eh" sounds, or takes a deep breath and releases it with a "ka" sound—almost as if she is doing vocal practice. She also coos with "oooo," "ahoooo," and "ehoooo" sounds while she watches a swinging mobile hanging near her crib.

From approximately the second month and continuing for a year or more, the infant's vocalizations show a progressive gain in variations of sounds and inflections, in vocal control, in their "mouthings," and in the differentiation of their patterns. Parents learn to identify certain cry-patterns and comfort sounds with their causes, and to react to them in ways that teach the child that his vocalizations have social significance. The mother describes the child's developmental changes at the age of eight weeks:

> Her vocal practice sessions are more frequent and are longer in duration, perhaps partly because she is awake more. I notice more variation in the length and inflection of her sounds. Her vocal sessions occur after eating, while lying alone, and less often when someone stimulates her by talking to her. Jill makes word-like sounds of one or two consonants followed by a vowel, tongue noises, various intake breaths and sighs, along with her cooing sounds. These syllable sounds begin with consonants but never end in a consonant. The vowels are becoming more tuneful, either with rising or falling inflections.

Between four and five months of age, self-stimulated vocal behavior appears:

> Jill frequently lies alone entertaining herself by watching things around her and calling out various sounds. Although her favorite entertainment is watching, mimicking, and chuckling in response to people's voices and facial expressions, she frequently "talks" when she is alone or not being amused by others. In this solo vocal play she delights in making loud squeals, raucous "ahhhh" sounds, and "vowel songs."

In the first year of life, the normal infant spends a great proportion of time in pleasurable babbling and in vocal play, much of which occurs while the child is alone. But there is need for some pleasurable, social joining-in by others to serve as an occasional impetus and reinforcement. Socializing the vocal practice and, especially, generating in the child the process of imitativeness may make speech learning a satisfying game of following the leader as well as being the leader. At around three or four months of age, an infant usually begins this practice of repeating sounds which he hears, sees, and feels. Descriptions of this imitative practice are found in the excerpt from Jill's diary when she was eleven weeks old:

When I talk to Jill, she watches my expressions and mouth movements very intently, smiles when I talk to her, and then tries sounds of her own after I pause. Sometimes she interrupts me. Today, in our play with funny sounds, she laughed for the first time. She also seems to enjoy "working" on one sound for a prolonged period of time, such as on "la" or "whoo." Her new sound this morning was "omo." She now "talks" readily to her stuffed rabbit, to herself, or to one person who is holding her attention in playful fondling and vocalization. But if several faces are stimulating her, she will watch expressions rather than make sounds.

These noncrying sounds, which begin early in an infant's life, are partly the products of the family's social stimulation and reinforcement from facial expressions, fondlings, and presenting of objects and pictures. They are also kindled, fanned, and self-consumed by the infant's self-stimulation through self-satisfaction and the necessary information from his personal acts. It is evident that these self-feedbacks are critical in the case of children who are born blind or deaf. A blind child misses some of the meaning, the inner and outer stimulations, and the directional cues which come visually from the speech act and its situational setting. Consequently, some blind children have special difficulty in learning how to use the lips and tongue in speech articulation. A deaf child, who misses auditory stimulation and cues, becomes handicapped not only in later speech but also in the early stages of vocal play, babbling, and imitative lalling—activities which lay the groundwork for speech motivation and learning.

An infant's repertoire of apparently random prespeech sounds appears to approximate the diversity of sounds produced by man for speech purposes in the world's one thousand five hundred languages. However, as Church[2] reports, recent phonetic analyses of early babblings indicate that their patterns and repertoire are more narrow, stereotyped, and different from later speech sounds than we have thought. Some linguists believe that in the second half of the first year, an infant develops his own unique, exotic language, a "quasi-symbolic" system of communication created from concrete gestures, cries, shrieks, and other behavioral actions. Some of the infant's sounds are physiologically built-in; some appear to be randomly made; some are discovered and molded either through vocal self-play or from imitation of outside patterns. During this first year or so of life, an infant plays and practices with a much wider variety of sounds than he will need in his later spoken language. Therefore, besides learning to adopt and to refine the particular sounds (phonemes) of his language, an infant is obliged to discard and to forget all the other exotic sounds and patterns which he has pleasurably sampled and played with during this period of prespeech vocalization.

FIRST WORD STAGE

When words emerge from a background of prespeech vocalizations and babblings, they continue for about a year to be intermingled with further babblings and jargon—vocalizations which are more speech-like than the sounds of earlier stages but which hardly fulfill definitions for true language. We should understand and respect the requisites which must precede the "first word" period—factors of physical and mental maturations, incentives for communication, experience, comprehension, models for his stimulation and learning, and sufficient practice for the acquisition of motor skills of speech.

A child's first word implies that he has learned the meaning and production of a vocal symbol within the realm of our conventional language system. Thus, a child who may have learned the meaning of a concept, but who may be expressing it first by a vocal symbol of his own invention or his approximation of its pronunciation, would not satisfy our adult definition of his mastery of a word.

During the latter part of an infant's babbling period, at about seven to ten months of age, he shows the beginnings of definite understanding and recognition of symbols in the form of gestures, voice inflections, words, and phrases. Before a child articulates his first words, he appears to lay the important vocal framework for speech and communication by learning the stress and intonation patterns for certain speech expressions so that often he can communicate effectively on this basis alone. The tunes and tempos in speech are as important as they are in song; without them, the carrier patterns of language are stripped of much of their meaning.

Recognition and understanding of signs and symbols were apparent in the following child at seven months of age: "My baby recognizes her bottle as a symbol for food, and her bathtub for water play. She has also recently learned the gleeful meaning of a particular trill sound made by her grandfather before playing with her."

From ten to eighteen months, a baby normally uses words of double syllables, similar to those found in babbling, such as "mama," "dada" for "daddy," and "bye bye," from the most easily produced vowels with the consonants *m*, *n*, *d*, and *g*. At one year, Jill spoke discriminatively and consistently in sound patterns which approximated the English pronunciations of words like "kaka" for "cracker"; "bye bye" for "bye bye"; "dada" for "daddy"; "baba" for "baby"; "juju" for "juice"; "ka" for "cat"; "eeow" also for "cat"; "fsh" for "fish."

It is important to point out that these words tend to be associated with experiences which are interesting and pleasurable for the child. Some of an infant's first words are associated and expressed with meaningful actions and gestures, such as waving with "bye bye," shaking the head with "no no," or reaching up to be lifted while saying "up."

An infant's first word often appears to be in the nature of a "word sentence," implying language concepts which will later be expressed in fuller sentence form. A child's first words appear to be learned and uttered in a global fashion, not pieced together from their phonetic elements. One might compare the growth of a child's language to his embryological growth—a trend toward more differentiated structures and their specific functions. Furthermore, an infant's first word, such as *daddy*, may begin with concepts which are broad and undifferentiated, later becoming more specific—for example, to mean *father*, apart from other men. On the other hand, an infant's use of *mama* may start as a particular name and develop into a class name, representing other mothers, even of animals or birds.

In our language concepts and their symbols, we generalize and categorize on the bases of perceptual similarities which we recognize between objects and events. Two types of categorization have been differentiated by linguists: "downward" and "upward" categorization. The child first categorizes in the "downward" way—subdividing poorly defined categories into more precise ones. For example, at first "car" may signify the common characteristics of cars, trucks, buses, and even tractors. Later, the child learns specific significant differences and terminology which specify these related objects. "Upward" categorization usually requires a greater degree of abstraction, since the distinguishing factor of similarity may depend upon a *single* and more subtle property of the thing categorized. For example, until a person learns that a mammal must have milk glands and that whales have these mammary glands, he would be inclined to categorize a whale as a fish, because of a whale's more obvious similarities to fish.

Most of the first words in a child's vocabulary are nouns, the result of our tendency mainly to teach infants the names of objects in his material environment. Verbs, associated with activities, are also frequent. Prepositions, such as *up* and *out*, may be used at first as verbs. The use of adverbs and adjectives usually follows, as maturation and more differentiated learning advance. At first, "big dog" may mean a single word, a noun-like word without the concept of bigness.

FIRST SENTENCE STAGE

While the infant is picking up his first words and before he expresses grammatically true sentences, his speech and language development may appear to lag. Outwardly, from about twelve to eighteen months, speech development does slow up. However, parents should neither be deceived and alarmed by this plateau in the child's speech growth at this time nor lose their interest in teaching speech when they may feel that they have fulfilled their satisfaction by helping him to reach his first and most dramatic milestone—his "first words."

The child may be using parts of speech in a grammatical framework different from what adults would expect and use at the moment. For example, the sixteenth-month-old boy who calls a snake "kioo" may be actually approximating the action-verb, *kill*, heard and prominently associated with a snake-killing act. A child's first words, such as *hot* for *stove*, *ouch* for *pin*, *bow wow* for *dog*, may be confusing because they are in a different grammatical context.

The child is engaged in other new developmental activities during this period, in expanding areas for all sorts of exploration and discovery, as mobility increases his independence and subjects him to new social contacts, behavioral adjustments, and communicative demands. From now on, he is confronted with more speech stimulation on the sentence and conversational levels as his life becomes socially more complicated and dependent upon language.

At about eighteen months, in addition to the continuing babbling, vocal imitation, and single words, the average child includes a period of practice called *jargon*, a rehearsal of sentence-like vocalizations which appear to be backed with meaning and which carry the prosody of speech—the framework of rhythms and intonations into which words of sentences will later fit. This stage of talking reveals important development:

> For the past month, Jill has gone through a stage of pretending to talk in sentences, to herself, her toys, and sometimes to people. Very few of the words resemble English, but her inflections and accents make this gibberish seem like real talking. Some of her sentence-length vocalizations indicate scolding, while other styles of expression suggest motherly warmth or sympathy with appropriate physical actions. I know that she has these thoughts in mind.

The transitory period of jargon has important linguistic and physiological values for the child as he learns to assemble the parts into the chassis of speech, to integrate and establish the speech patterns into a unified framework to fit the flow of connected speech. It is evident that speech is much more than a succession of words spoken as one would say each word in isolation. Words get a good share of their meaning from other words in their situational and sentence context, affected by their neighboring words, just as sounds of a word are influenced by their adjacent sounds. To be normal speakers, we must learn to think and speak in terms of larger units, by sentences rather than word-by-word. Furthermore, the meaningful patterns of tonal inflections, tempo, and accent can be learned and expressed only when speech is spoken in a connected and unified manner. Unless these elements of speech are learned and integrated within the flow of speech, the speech will lack fluency. Therefore, in a sense the child who is practicing jargon is like a singer who is learning the tune and tempo of a song having words of a foreign language before being obliged to learn and fill in with the words. A child has many skills to master, mentally and physically, before he can speak.

Usually at around the age of two a child is replacing the jargon with more genuine talking in the form of simple or compound sentences. Obviously, the grammatical construction of his sentences is not complete or correct, but the skeletal framework of his word functions and their order in sentences suggest that the child is learning and using some of the fundamental grammatical rules of his mother tongue. We stress the point that a child appears to learn the *rules* of syntax and grammar rather than learning each and every language construction by direct imitation.

At nineteen months Jill's types of sentences show the early stages of developing grammar and syntax.

"Read the book." "Bear ride the bike with Jill." "Heavy rock on blankie." "Sit down, sleeping monkey, sit down." "Monkey walk, monkey walking." "Apple back." "Go to sleep."

Although Jill's articulation was faulty in the above sentences, her statements and commands were easily understood. Her vowels and consonants, except *s*, *l*, *r*, and *j*, and her tonal patterns were relatively normal. Many of these words were spoken in the double fashion of noun-and-adjective or verb-and-object, or as single words, such as "more oranges," "big boy," "wash hands," "big truck," "more candy," "boy sleeping." Frequently occurring word groups, such as the above, tend to be heard and learned by a child as single words.

Two months later, her sentences have increased in complexity, with added articles, prepositions, and the possessive and plural forms:

"Roo climbed a tree." (In answer to a question about Roo.) "Read the book on ABC, Granddad." "Andy read the book." "Read the book about Santa Claus." "Oh, thank you." "There's a shepherd boy." "Two Marys and two Josephs." "Fix cow's head."

Jill's timetable at this and later stages of her speech and language development was advancing beyond that of the average child because of her enriched background of stimulation, learning, and practice. This case of Jill was purposely selected to illustrate some of the safe influences and practices which facilitate speech and language growth. Most children's speech and language development may be safely accelerated. No one ever fulfills his entire language potentials. We must be more willing to test existing norms and to revise the limits which we ascribe to mediocrity and precocity.

SPEECH FROM TWO TO FIVE

In the critical stage from two to five years, the child's expanding social roles and needs for communication demand a greater fund of vocabulary, a more adequate grammatical system, more refined articulation to suit the language patterns imposed by his society, and a greater fluency in the flow of connected speech. Dated in terms of language development, this critical period covers the child's first several years as a speaker of connected words or sentences. It is often stated that more new learning and adjustment per year are packed into these formative years of a child's preschool life than are likely ever to occur thereafter. This flood of learning and adjustments, which began at birth, continues not only in the development of language, but also in the meanings and the mechanics of a complex system of language devices. Under normal circumstances, the average child accomplishes this prodigious amount of learning with eagerness, pleasure, and seemingly with amazing ease—in contrast to the average adult's usual fretting struggle to learn a new language. But hazards may arise to disrupt a child's delightful interest and efficiency in learning to speak. Difficulties may arise when parents expect too much, or too little, of a child's abilities and attainments at certain ages. In later sections of this book we shall consider the problems and limitations in speech development. At present we shall continue consideration of what a child must yet accomplish in the interdependent and integrated learning and skills of language in the few years following his second birthday.

It has been estimated that a child must have a vocabulary of at least 150 to 200 words before he can speak in true sentences. Grammatically, he must learn two categories of vocabulary: a "closed category" of contentless words, which can serve in language as structural markers, sometimes called "function words" or "pivot words"; second, an "open category" of "class words", such as nouns, verbs, and other content words, to fill in the slots which are marked by function words. By learning these function words and their rules, the speaker can fill in with class words and thereby create the great variety of phrases and sentences which are required in language. For example, the child must learn the meanings and rules of using such function words as *a, my, the, to, in, at, that, there, what, why, not, both,* etc. In the sentence "*The* teddy bear fell *on the* floor *and* hurt *both of his* legs," the italicized function words contribute with the remaining class words to express some of the specific meanings of this sentence.

While a child is learning to refine the phonemes (sounds) in his speech, he should also be learning the meanings of language. In teaching a child to speak, we should not forget that speech is language, too. The failure to appreciate the wide range of factors and the need to integrate them in speech and language development is reflected in the following statements which parents and others have been known to make about their roles in helping children to speak better. One parent complained: "With a family of six to manage and a house to keep up, I'm too busy to take time out to give Peter speech lessons. Besides, he won't sit still long enough for me to teach him how to talk. That's why I want him enrolled in speech class." This parent evidently did not realize that a child can best learn speech in everyday situations, and that even the busiest parent who shares these commonplace experiences is in a good position to teach language and speech skills.

Another parent explained, while referring her three-year-old for help at a speech clinic: "If you could first teach him to make his sounds right, I think I could teach him the rest. As it is, I can't even understand him." She had the mistaken notion that articulation is learned as a preliminary and isolated skill, before one learns to talk.

In a Head Start program for four-year-olds who lacked many of the experiences, interests, knowledge, and skills needed for meeting middle-class school standards, one teacher stated: "So long as a child will talk and can be understood at all, I don't make any efforts to improve his speech or language.

Later, when he starts school, he will get that training. In our program, we work to socialize the children, to build their confidence, to teach them to share and to get along with others, and to introduce them to some experiences they have lacked." It is obvious that this teacher did not recognize the many opportunities for teaching speech and language while her pupils were experiencing and learning other values as well.

The average two-year-old child begins to connect two or three words in a sentence-like fashion and expresses the first rules of grammar: word order or syntax—the ways in which words and meaningful units of language are functionally arranged relative to each other and to the morphology—the rules for inflection, accent, functional uses of words. It is amazing how the young child learns the complexities of grammar, for instance, without being taught them in a systematic or deliberate way.

By three years of age, the average child normally uses about three or four words per sentence; at four years he has progressed to four or five words; and in another year to five or six words in an average sentence. We recognize that these figures are statistical averages of average children; they do not reveal the wide variations even among children grouped as normal. A three-year-old, who speaks usually with about three words per sentence, may sometimes speak with six, seven, or more words. But when we examine the progressive lengthening of sentences in two-, three-, and four-year-olds, we see that sentence length corresponds to the child's cumulative growth in the grammatical areas of word order, word meaning, word articulation, speech rhythm, and the meaningful patterns of inflection and accent. Therefore, moving from the stage of saying three-word sentences to the stage of saying four-word ones, for instance, entails much more development than simply tacking on an extra word.

Estimates of the average two-year-old's usable vocabulary have ranged from one hundred to four hundred words. But along this route of speech development, the child understands many more words than he uses. By two years of age, a child's stage of playfully talking in jargon, of make-believe talking in sentences, has been mostly replaced by talk with real words in real sentence context—although words and sentences are still crude and incomplete in several ways. Estimates of the average number of words in normal children's spoken vocabularies have ranged from four hundred to nine hundred words at three years; from nine hundred to ne thousand five hundred words at four years; from one thousand five hundred to two thousand five hundred at five years. Of course, the extent of a child's actual or usable vocabulary may be only roughly estimated, and the potential vocabulary which that child ideally could have learned under the best of conditions is still more conjectural, since the acquisition of vocabulary depends upon many factors.

Intelligibility ratings of the average child at two years of age have reported his articulation at about 65 per cent; at three years his connected speech at 70 to 80 per cent; and by four years his speech in context at 90 to 100 per cent, even though some sounds are still misarticulated. Yet, when we consider the statistical data which have been computed for the "average" child, we should be aware that this "average" child is a statistical creation that often fails to disclose the range and variability of the attributes which have been averaged. Generally, the growth in articulation is greater during the period from two and one-half years to four and one-half years than from four and one-half to eight. Analyzed from the standpoint of language phonemes, the "average" child at three years correctly produces 90 per cent of his vowels and diphthongs; by seven he masters 90 per cent of his consonants.

Studies have shown the usual order in which the child correctly adopts the various phonemes of English. By two or three years of age, the "average" child makes intelligible use of the vowels and consonants *m*, *b*, *t*, *d*, *k*, *g*, *w*, *h*, and *n*. However, these and other consonants are usually inconsistent, with faults in the form of substitutions, distortions, or omissions, especially when the consonant is at the end of a word. Between the ages of three and seven, the "average" child continues to refine and to add to the repertoire of phonemes which his language demands of him. As pointed out in Chapter 1, this process is complex, involving physical maturation, perceptual training, learning through trial and error, forgetting, approximation, and reinforcement. A child's articulatory course is rather irregular; it often has plateaus or even stages of decline. Six or seven years of learning, forgetting, and practice are usually required by the "average" child to master the speech phonemes and their clusters of allophones needed for speech in context. Ordinarily, the last sounds to be perfected are those of *r*, *l*, *s*, *z*, *ch*, *sh*, and blends of these sounds with other speech sounds; yet some children learn these sounds as readily as they learn the "easier" ones. In these ages, the child's speech sounds undergo errors of omission, substitution, and distortion—often in this sequence of misuse. Yet, it may well be that some of the child's difficulty in adopting some phonemes stems not from his physical inability to articulate them, but from the possibility that he has first learned a rather unique sound-language of his own—one that does not call for those particular phonemes until later when he is prevailed upon to add them to his language system. If this theory is correct, the usual methods in teaching and correcting articulation would need revision, placing emphasis upon phonemic instead of upon phonetic aspects.

Beginning at the age of two and continuing for the next several years, the child is confronted with variable demands for speech fluency. Fluency refers to the melodic and rhythmic flow of spoken language. *Spoken language* is used in this definition, instead of *speech*, because fluency is expressed, perceived, and judged within the framework of language patterns, not merely on a phonetic or articulatory basis. There is reason to believe that nonfluency and stuttering can also invade the language system, so that in one sense a speaker may become a "fluent" stutterer, an able speaker of a stuttering-like language. However, in the ordinary nonfluencies, found in varying degrees in all normal speakers and in beginning stutterers, fluency or nonfluency seems to depend partly upon speech and language variables, such as organization or disorganization of thought; adequate or inadequate vocabulary; adequate or inadequate system of grammar; weak or established patterns of speech melody and tempo to carry and to integrate the language units of speech; and immature or sufficiently fixed and automatic articulatory skills. As we analyze nonfluencies and their correlation with language, we realize, as Bluemel[3] points out, that linguists, too, have a stake in solving the riddle of stuttering.

In the period of about two to four years of age, the child's needs for fluency mount: as he begins to speak in connected words, as he learns the components and rules of sentence structure, as he acquires a wider fund and choice of words, and as his society places more demands and hazards upon the functions which speech fulfills. If we imagine what a two-year-old must learn and integrate for spoken language when he begins to speak and converse in sentences, we can better appreciate why this age from two to four is usually characterized by nonfluencies which too often grow into the problem of stuttering. Johnson and others,[4] who have studied the types and ranges of nonfluencies found in preschool children, point out that nonfluencies are normal and reasonable during this period of speech development, and that the hope for improving fluency and for preventing stuttering is greatest in these formative years, which fix the growth of attitudes, associated learnings, and habits. Yet, we may find that some of the basic roots which determine fluency or nonfluency in a child are set even earlier than at two years. In the chapter on stuttering, we shall discuss these points in detail; meanwhile, in our consideration of every child's speech development, it should be remembered that every two-year-old child faces the forks of an indistinct and unmarked road, one fork of which may lead to stuttering.

Between two and four years the development of speech skills may be irregular and marked with reversals which are usually temporary:

> Since Jill has begun to talk more in sentences, we have noticed that her articulation of some speech sounds has become more faulty. While she was speaking only with single words and short phrases, her speech was more clear and correct. Before she started to talk in sentences, she could say even the sounds that are difficult such as *s*, *r*, and *th*, in words like *ice cream*, *lettuce*, and *toothbrush*. Now, when some of these same words are spoken in sentences, they are said rather sloppily, as in the sentence, "I have fum ife kweam." But these mistakes are inconsistent. Her incorrectness or correctness of sounds seems to depend upon how fast she is talking, or upon how much she is attending to what she is saying, or how she is saying it, as if she is trying to say whole sentences as single big, unclear words.

As pointed out in Chapter 1, differences in articulation of speech sounds are necessitated by differences in the contexts of those sounds. Suppose that a child had learned first to articulate correctly the short expression "some more"; later uttering the long expression "I have fum mo foup; I like soup," he may be showing the effects which adjacent sounds have upon each other. *F* for *s* in *foup*, while *s* is correct in the second *soup*, may be due to the influence of the word *have* upon *fum*. A child tends to adopt short-cuts and economies in the face of the mounting demands which connected speech places upon his immature articulatory skills, especially when these economies, like the substitution of *f* for *s* in the above context, sufficiently approximate each other in sound, look, and feel. The fact that the second *soup* in the foregoing statement was spoken correctly, while the first was pronounced "foup," may be partly explained by the different influence which the preceding *k* sound has upon the *s*, an influence which reduces the lip involvement and which prepares the tongue to move closer toward the posture needed for *s*. Articulatory errors of children, even in these stages of speech immaturity, are not as haphazard as they may appear to be. However, by the time the average child is six or seven years old, his speech sounds are usually correct.

While the average child's language should be complete in structure and form at about five or six years of age, there is a wide range in this achievement, even among children who are otherwise judged normal. Much depends upon the child's speech environment.

Normal children of three years too often remain at infantile speech levels through lack of opportunity and practice. Jill's advanced speech and language development at the age of three suggested that her speech fluency was related to vocabulary and grammatical ability, with more expressive vocal inflection, with speech used for other purposes than for communication, and with a "readiness" to read visual symbols of language. Children often use pertinent vocabularies that show more alertness and attention to detail than adults would use in evaluating and reporting their experience. Children converse with toys and pets to dramatize situations of familiar experience. Children invent words for names of objects and actions and begin to associate printed trademarks and brand names with specific packaged foods and other products.

It is difficult to predict when the steps in speech development may be expected to occur, because the timetable of their occurrence and the extent of development depend largely upon each child's opportunities for favorable language stimulation and learning. In the case of a favorable speech climate, the timetable is compressed and growth in speech and language learning is accelerated, largely because parents have provided the child a warm, secure, and enriched environment, but safeguarded by their knowledge and respect for the limits and hazards. For "culturally-deprived" children with delayed speech and language, environmental conditions do not fulfill these developmental requisites. Later this chapter will discuss in more detail the role of parents and teachers in speech development.

SPEECH GROWTH DURING SCHOOL

Although the form or structure of a child's language is essentially complete when he enters kindergarten or first grade, every teacher realizes that there are wide and unfulfilled needs for continued speech and language development throughout school life. Reading and writing, which depend upon speech and its translation into visual symbols, require an increasing foundation of speech, backed by adequate vocabulary, refinement of grammar, and correct pronunciation. In turn, the learning and use of reading lead to a further development of speech. Reading skills make use of a variety of methods, including structural and phonetic analysis, which improve speech skills.

The following first grade teacher expresses the fact that the knowledge and skills required for reading rest upon a previous foundation of skills from speech:

> I can usually tell by listening to a child's speech whether or not he will have an easy or difficult time in learning to read. If he speaks words and sentences with a reasonable degree of correctness, if he has a good vocabulary and shows that experiences have provided him with interests and information, I can be pretty sure that he will be a good reader. If he lacks these basics, his reading will be handicapped.

An elementary school supervisor holds the following views concerning speech growth during school ages:

> Language achievements become the means as well as the goal in much of the schoolchild's curriculum. Behind his academic achievements in language lie the resources of his everyday speech achievements. As teachers of reading, we must also be teachers of speech; our speech therapists, too, must realize that they are improving speech for language purposes. We must not let the school's teaching of reading and speech become separated from the spoken language of a child's personal life—especially not when he is beginning to read. Some of our primers fail to recognize this need; they use language and dwell on topics that are foreign to some of the children. In such cases, we should have primers that will more closely correlate the child's speech with his reading, so that he can start with meaning, interest, security, and a reliance upon skills which he already has. Furthermore, if he has learned language standards which are different from ours, he will need extra help in order to learn our standards together with his own. At times, a teacher of beginning reading may need to compose an individualized primer, based upon the child's vocabulary, comprehensions, and interests— resources which a particular child already has acquired. An alert teacher will detect these special needs in a child if she conducts oral class discussions as a part of reading exercises.

It is not unusual to find articulatory errors in a child's speech when he enters kindergarten, first grade, or even third grade. The consonants *r*, *l*, *s*, *ch*, *sh*, and *j* and their blends with other consonants are likely to be the ones which remain troublesome. But these articulatory errors are usually corrected by the time the child reaches the second or third grade.

But, as a child continues in school, he usually learns far more than how to improve the mechanics of his speech, reading, and written language. From the uses which these forms of language afford, he must gain the social, emotional, and cognitive purposes of speech. One third grade teacher has stated the need for a proper balance between speech skills and their functions:

> I believe that most of us with our large classes are obliged to work on improving pupils' tools or skills without giving enough attention to putting them to use. In language, for example, we teach and test on lists of vocabulary, rules of grammar, spelling, reading, and writing skills, but lacking time we often fall short in teaching how these skills and resources can be put to worthwhile use. They must learn to use speech in other ways: to seek information, to seek opinions, to give opinions, to elaborate, to clarify, to evaluate, to doubt, to compromise, to harmonize, to encourage, to criticize, to hypothesize, to joke, and to speak for sheer enjoyment. But in the classroom we usually ride too tight rein on most of these justifiable functions of speech—later complaining that our high school and college students have become too apathetic, lacking in originality, leadership, initiative, security, poise, etc. I think that we make them deficient by restricting their rightful freedoms of speech in school.

Even though a child enters first grade with a superior speech foundation, he must continue to add to it if he is to progress in reading. Normally he does. In the course of learning to read and in his uses of reading, a child's speech and language should improve. Every effective teacher of reading works on speech while she teaches reading. Consequently, most children, especially in kindergarten, first, and second grades, usually show progress in their articulation and uses of language as they learn the phonics and other attributes of language, presented through the reading program. Certainly, every subject and activity in school can and should in some way contribute to a pupil's growth in language and speech, whether the subject is reading, English, art, music, shop, physical education, or extracurricular activities. A child's progress through school is generally measured in terms of his language achievements, and when a pupil does not meet these language standards and uses, we find that he often becomes frustrated and is variously labeled as "emotionally disturbed," a "low achiever," a "behavior problem," a "delinquent," and eventually a "school dropout." Later, this chapter will outline ways in which parents and teachers can help in speech and language development.

Parents' Role in Speech Development

Ordinarily, no one has a more important position in a child's speech and language development than have his parents. Most parents realize this fact, but many do not. Yet many parents who are not acutely aware of their responsibilities are still fulfilling their roles effectively on an intuitive basis. Fortunately, a mother tends "naturally" to be a good influence and teacher of childhood speech if she has normal maternal instincts and love for her child and if she makes a habit of using appropriate and perceptible symbols of language expression in rewarding interactions with her child. There are parents, however, who possess these personal qualities and yet, because of external circumstances, may be unable to fulfill their roles in influencing and teaching language. In the case of twins, for example, a loving and alert parent may find that the twins' influences upon each other are canceling some of the influences which that conscientious parent is trying to give. But teachers and therapists should understand parental roles in speech development in order both to arouse their responsibilities and interest and to give support and counseling in the areas of their deficiencies. A therapist who works in an extensive program to prevent speech and language problems discovered that parent education is not easy:

> Our main function is to prevent speech problems before they develop. Prevention requires that we contact parents-to-be and parents of preschool children, that we arouse parental interest and sense of responsibility for speech, give them information on the essential stages of speech and language development, and suggest how parents can help their children to reach these steps. Our greatest trouble, however, is to spark enough initial interest in parents to get them to come and to take advantage of our educational program. The ones who come are mostly parents who are already concerned because they have children with speech and language problems. Since our program is rather unique in that it aims at prevention rather than cure, we want to get at parents whose children have not yet developed problems. But how can we arouse their interest and get our foot in the door, so to speak?

The following list of policies for parents is a suggested guide not only in diagnosing the parental factors underlying speech and language problems but also in counseling parents to be more helpful, especially in the preschool stages of speech.

"T.L.C."

Trite as this expression has become, "tender loving care" continues to be as essential to a child's all-around growth as it ever was. Myklebust[5] states that the first specifically human act in the language-learning sequence appears to be the infant's babbling and that this babbling may rest upon an infant's need for identification with the talking human with whom he associates pleasure and babbling. Neglected, orphaned, mistreated, and rejected children who fail to get enough loving care and personal security are often delayed in language and in other ways also. It is partly for this reason of insuring early personalized "T.L.C." that some pediatricians advise that infants be breast-fed instead of bottle-fed. Bottle-feeding may be done with warmth, personal contact, etc., but too often it leads to self-feeding for the sake of feeding, without the psychological and social rewards from the mother and mothering.

A child's natural parents are not the only ones with the capacity for this "T.L.C." Neither is it likely that a child will be spoiled by getting too much of this important attention. If a child is orphaned or if his parents cannot give him the many benefits which come from love, trust, and intimate relationships, others may adequately substitute for the child's natural parents. This fact has been proved by many adoptive parents, foster parents, the child's relatives, his peers, institutional attendants, baby-sitters, and various professionals—including teachers, who may substitute for inadequate parents. At times, even professionals must work through others who are in better positions to provide these human essentials; sometimes "amateurs" and laymen can supply these needs better than ones who are specifically trained to do so. For instance, in one program for young, neglected, and emotionally disturbed children, it was found that elderly people, men and women, voluntarily serving as loving "foster grandparents," were most effective in giving these children the close and satisfying companionship they needed.

A superintendent of a state hospital has maintained that the most basic psychiatric need of his mental patients is still the old-fashioned one of daily "T.L.C." and that this need is administered best by his regular hospital attendants rather than by his psychiatrists. Another psychiatrist who has studied disturbed communication in children found that serene mothers gave their children the gift of their serenity and that disturbed mothers injected disturbances into their children's behavioral patterns, including speech. Parents should be especially careful to provide affectionate attention for a child during his first year of life, since this is the most plastic period of human development.

SPEECH MOTIVATION BY PARENTS

Parental encouragement and reward for a child's efforts at speech should begin with his earliest cries. Motivation should continue throughout the preschool vocalizations of babbling, echolalia, jargon, and the real speech of words and sentences. Just as the slap-stimulated birth cry gives the satisfaction of knowing that a baby is alive and breathing, so should the following months of crying be received by parents with tolerance, discrimination, cheerfulness, appropriately rewarding responses. When a baby cries for purposes of hunger, discomfort, and other physical needs, he should learn that his vocal behavior has communicative power and that it may be relied upon to bring happy and beneficial results from parents. Stunting effects on later speech development may occur if crying is overly ignored, discouraged, or punished.

When a baby reaches the stage of smiling, of making body gestures, of cooing and giggling, parents should participate with him in making the acts playful, pleasurable social interactions. When the child begins to babble, social stimulation and participation by others should be on a limited basis. Much of the child's babbling will be done, and should be allowed, while the child is alone—usually in a state of comfort, solitary play, and practice. However, parents should do some imitative babbling with the child in order to stimulate, socialize, and establish in him the pleasurable game of imitating vocal patterns in others. Most parents enjoy this period of babbling in their child, some to the point of participating so much that they monopolize the practice, forcing the child to become a silent spectator and denying him his important share in the fun of practice. Other parents, either intentionally or not, may habitually silence his mouth with pacifiers; some parents surround the child and the crib with too many entertaining and distracting visual trinkets which encourage him to be a visual but silent manipulator. As a general policy in the areas of stimulation and motivation, it is important for a child to explore and discover himself as well as his social environment.

When a child is in the stage of speaking his first words, parental encouragement and teaching of his speech continue to be important. First words, crude and faulty as they usually are, should be respectfully attended to, gladly acknowledged, and rewarded with appropriate response. In this interaction process, the responding parties have good opportunities to offer constructive remodeling of the child's approximated words.

Again, during the second year of life, parental motivation of speech sometimes goes astray when the child is passing through the jargon stage of practicing imitative sentences. During this stage of jargon, as in the babbling stage, the child needs some time for this partly private practice, often in conversation with himself, with toys, dolls, etc. Although the child's sentence-like jabber in this jargon stage may make it appear that his speech is in a decline or at a standstill, parents should look upon it as another important step, a stage which deserves respect and interest. Later, the child will learn to replace these prosodic strings of gibberish with words learned from others and strung according to the rules of grammar. However, if parents become critical and if they interfere with his playful practice with jargon, he may not only become wary of speaking but may also fail to learn its important patterns of rhythm and inflection.

Understanding parents are careful of their stimulation of a child's speech in that critical age between two and four years of age, when he must talk in family conversations with immature sentences and under numerous pressures. During this period, the child's fluency may be taxed by parents and others who inject too much excitement, eagerness, and insistence on correctness into speech; while, on the other hand, a child's motivation to talk may be dampened or confused if parents fail to provide him with enough satisfying speech incentives. His urge to speak may become weakened by doubts if he must speak too often to "deaf ears" or to critical or unappreciative listeners.

PARENTAL MODELS FOR SPEECH

In speech, the child learns what he hears, sees, and sometimes must feel, in the speech models which are most prominent and frequent in his experience.

Normally this modeling is the responsibility of parents who knowingly set the examples which their children adopt. But at times the main setting of examples is done by others—siblings, neighbors, and baby-sitters—who may or may not set good examples.

If a child were born and reared entirely in the presence of deaf parents who uttered only fragments of language, spoken in a monotone and communicated mainly through their manual language of gestural signs, that child would learn to communicate in similar fashion, even though he could hear normally and would learn to speak correctly if predominantly correct speech patterns could be modeled for him. Studies have shown that "first" or "only" children tend to have better speech in childhood than do twins. In their more self-contained relationship, twins sometimes learn from poorer examples set by each other, while singletons tend to have the advantage of wider learning opportunities in the more correct adult models of speech.

Early infant crying, being reflexive and caused by physiological and physical stimuli, is not taught through example. Later, as the child becomes more sophisticated and learns to use cry-patterns for other purposes, his parents may start to mock his cries, with a punishing effect, perhaps, to shame him for being a "cry-baby" or a "sissy" in that cry situation. In this case, the parents would be imitating the child in a negative sense, setting an example of what not to do. This discipline may cause a child to repress his crying and to substitute uncontrolled sobbing, pouting, or other reactions. Such parental punishment of a child's crying in one situation may cause a generalized repression of his crying. In our dual cultural standards, which distinguish manliness from femininity, we portray verbally and in other ways how boys should follow the model of masculinity by not crying. The higher incidence of stuttering among boys may partly stem from such curbs imposed upon the naturally human and wholesome expressions of emotions.

When the stage of babbling begins, the need for some parental imitation of that babbling arises. However, when parents imitate babbling, they should be judicious in their timing and degree of that imitation. One understanding mother explained in this way how she babbled with her five-month-old infant son:

> Timmy has been babbling for about two months now. He does a lot of it by himself and seems to enjoy it. So, for the most part, I just listen to it, enjoy it, and do not interrupt it. But sometimes we "talk" back and forth in our babble. He seems to get a kick from it—watching and listening to my babble too. At times, when I imitate his sounds, he'll smile and continue to do more of the same. We're not conversing in words yet, but we surely have fun pretending. After we have had a spirited exchange of babbling with a sound like "ahgah," I'll sometimes overhear him playing by himself with that same sound. Several times he has greeted me with that sound or has made it to attract my attention to him.

When a child is in the stage of speaking "first words," parental speech models serve more to lead and to teach. We might think of this stage as being the first recognizable milepost of a new road, a course which reroutes him from his "language" of babbling to a new conventional road which must be paved with meaningful and intelligible words, constructed and marked by grammar, all in accordance with the standards of form and function which his culture maps out for him to learn. This, of course, calls for much learning through example.

Opinions differ about whether or not parents should imitate "baby talk." Most authorities believe that a young child's crude and faulty words and sentences should never be imitated, but that he should always be spoken to in correct forms of articulation and grammar. Others believe that some imitation of the child's immature pronunciations may be helpful to the child if the imitation is done sparingly and at opportune times and not in a way to suggest criticism or teasing of the child. However, all authorities agree that a child needs a preponderance of correct examples if he is to learn to speak correctly.

If a child has a good relationship with his parents and has not become inhibited by their tactful efforts to correct his mistakes, imitation and effective correction of the child's error may often be done more directly. For example, one four-year-old who substituted *h* for *s* in many words, such as *hitting* for *sitting* and *hoeing* for *sewing*, but who had proved his ability to say the *s* in many other words, was given some direct reminding through imitation by his speech-therapist mother, who described her approach as follows:

> David was using *h* for *s* in about one-third of his words beginning with *s*. So, I hit upon an idea of using some pairs of words, different in meaning but similar in pronunciation except for their beginning sounds of *s* or *h*. For example, I showed David a picture of a boy sitting on a chair and asked whether the boy was "sitting" or "standing." He replied, "Hitting." I answered, "No, he's not *hitting* anything. He's *sitting*. He's *sitting* on the chair, isn't he?" After making several responses with *hitting*, he began to reply with *sitting*. In the same way, I showed him a picture of a lady sewing and asked: "Is that lady *hoeing*, as Daddy does when he is hoeing in the garden?" Here, too, he immediately recognized the differences in meaning, but it took several of our pleasant exchanges before he replaced *hoeing* with *sewing*.

Beyond the "first word" stage, a speaker normally builds his speech from the continuing patterns which are spoken in his environment. When a person is born deaf, he is greatly handicapped in lacking the chance to hear and learn speech models from parents or others; when a person loses hearing after having learned speech, his speech deteriorates when external models of it can no longer guide him in articulation, rhythm, intonation, etc. Words, grammar, and vocal patterns in language must be learned by example because they are arbitrary and illogical. We are impressed by this arbitrary nature of language when we compare foreign languages in terms of their structure and rules governing gender, syntax, and accent.

A parent who models the various aspects of oral language for a child has the same responsibilities that are needed by a teacher of a foreign language. In addition, because of a young child's shorter span of attention and other immaturities, the patterns to be imitated and learned must have the following attributes:

Personal appeal
Perceptual clarity
Brevity, simplicity, and attainability of models
Sufficient experience and practice
Good parental speech habits
Speech etiquette

Personal appeal. Unless a child is favorably disposed toward a parent and that parent's speech patterns, he will not imitate and adopt those examples as his own. The child who finds pleasure and security in his identification with parents will readily imitate their speech in the process of that identification.

Perceptual clarity. When parents speak to children, especially for purposes of teaching them to speak, they should speak loudly enough, slowly enough, and within view. It follows that parents have a responsibility to control noise or to counteract noise and other home conditions which distract and interfere with listening, looking, and general attention. The brief attention of young children is often the fault of others, not of their innate deficiency. When a child is deaf or blind, a parent must provide him with models which emphasize his remaining intact avenues of perception. For every child, speech models should be sufficiently perceived in a foreground sense, not as an indistinct part of a background in which other events overshadow the speech act. A social worker once gave the following reason that young children living under crowded and noisy tenement conditions are often delayed in their speech:

> It is no wonder that children in slums often have speech problems. They don't hear much speech, and many are not spoken to very often. When a large family is obliged to live together in one room, with a hubbub of noise from the inside and the outside, with the continual blare from TV and physical turmoil around them, children lose interest in talking. They may wall themselves off from this excess and irrelevant noise.

Brevity, simplicity, and attainability of models. When a child is in the babbling stage, parents should do some stimulation with babbling; when he nears and enters the first-word period, their predominant examples should be on the single-word level; when he approaches the sentence stage, they should feature short sentences, with a gradual increase in the length and complexity of the sentences as the child progressively follows in the wake of learning. However, the correctness of sentences should not be sacrificed for the sake of brevity and simplicity. Neither should parents radically shorten sentences by omitting function words needed for building phrase and sentence structure. The average three-year-old would not be getting adequate patterns for his language learning if a parent who burned a finger on a hot stove were to comment to the child: "Ouch! Mommy finger hurt! Hot stove!" Instead, these words and thoughts would be placed in a better and more intact grammatical form by saying: "Ouch! I hurt my finger. The stove is hot!" Or, "Ouch! My finger hurts! That's a hot stove." As Lee[6] points out from her study of syntactical development, the grammatical structures of phrases, clauses, and sentences must be learned as cohesive grammatical units, expanding from important "pivot" words and "kernel" sentences. If parents abbreviate speech to the point of omitting basic parts of the language framework, a child will fail to learn the correct structure and rules of grammar.

Sufficient experience and practice. Parental speech patterns will be ineffective and useless unless they are backed by meaningful experience and fixed by practice. For example, the word *ouch* and its meaning are best learned in the act of experiencing some pain. Words and language expressions which are abstract and difficult to demonstrate and to conceive will need more experiencing before they are clarified and fixed in usage. If learning and practice are done under favorable conditions, the child will often "outlast" the parent in his fresh eagerness to learn and enjoy the uses of language.

Good parental speech habits. A child will talk as his parents do if they are his main source of speech influence and learning. However, if other speakers in the family, or elsewhere, are more influential than his parents, he will adopt those models which have the most impact and reinforcement. Three important speech characteristics which parents often neglect, and which detract from the examples set for a child, concern rate of speaking, distinctness in articulation, and attitudes toward speech and conversation with the child. In addition to a moderate pace, good speech models should be free from mumbling, slurring, and other mannerisms which obscure the parts of words, phrases, and sentences. If a child must learn from speech which is rattled off carelessly while he is still in the stages when he must use more attention and deliberation in his reception and production of speech, he may catch and learn only the high spots of what is said. He may understand the gist of our indistinct utterances, but he will miss important details of how to speak these meanings.

Speech etiquette. In the conventional observance of social rules or personal speech rights, which give proper respect, dignity, decency, and honor to young and adult speakers, we have double standards expressed and enforced in many ways, some of them subtly and some openly. We hear this discrimination against children in such remarks as "A child should be seen but not heard"; "Let us talk; run along and play; don't bother us"; "You're not old enough to talk about this—you're not dry behind the ears yet"; "Oh, cut out your chatter, and let us talk." Often adults violate the personal dignity and privacy of young children by publicly talking about them in their presence when they peddle, exploit, and make fun of what young children say. We prevail upon young children to put on a show to please and entertain us, our visitors, and others by their recitations, songs, and "cute" talk. We make open demands upon children: "Say *thank you*"; "Tell the lady *good-bye*"; "What do you say when you walk in front of someone?"; "Tell the man your name! Has the cat got your tongue?" We allow older siblings to monopolize family conversation and let the youngest child, perhaps, contribute only the conversational dregs or nothing at all. Adults often fail to acknowledge and to give credit to the young child for his faltering but sincere offerings in family conversations. When a young child is fumbling with words and grammar, we may fail to give him time and audience until he works through his difficulty in expression. And if we help him in these difficulties, are we really helping *him*, or are we mainly relieving our own impatience? As Johnson[4] advises in *An Open Letter to the Mother of A "Stuttering" Child*, parents should be as friendly and considerate toward their speaking children as they are toward house guests. An experienced kindergarten teacher cautions parents on the following practice, which is likely to boomerang and to cause children to fear speaking with the teacher:

> I have uncovered several damaging plots in which parents have threatened speech by making teachers into "bogie men" by such preschool threats as "You'd better not talk like that at school or you'll catch it from the teacher" or "If the teacher hears you use that word, she'll give you heck!" I've known several children who dared not speak in school at all, because of scare tactics used by parents.

Impact of School and Teacher

In addition to physical adequacy and emotional adjustment, speech is one of the most obviously important assets a child can bring to school. Without an adequate understanding of speech and the ability to speak, a young child enters school with handicaps and frustration, alone and surrounded by strangers with whom he cannot communicate. It is important to remember, too, that stuttering may be precipitated when added pressures and adjustments cause conflicts during this critical transition into school. From that first eventful day of school, the child must depend upon speech and language to serve him socially and academically in this new major sphere of his life. In the classroom his verbal interactions supply him with information, guidelines for discipline, motivation and direction in learning, and evaluation. On the bus, in the playground, and at lunchtime he learns and employs the various social uses of speech: exciting attention, relating, disputing, explaining, and expressing enjoyment as well as inner tension. Meanwhile, his speech life continues at home, where standards are sometimes at odds with those imposed by his school.

We are generally correct in assuming that school influences and learning have favorable effects upon a child's speech and language. Speech progress is most noticeable in kindergarten, first, and second grades. The school ordinarily deserves much credit for this progress, but a high degree of the speech and language growth comes from normal maturation and the experiences and improved skills which continue in the home and other areas of the child's expanding life. For some children, however, school becomes their first and most important opportunity to learn normal speech. An elementary supervisor describes children who enter school with the capacities for speech but without previous opportunities to develop them:

> Seriously inadequate speech is the most pathetic handicap I see in some children when they come to school. Of course, some of these children are mentally retarded and, in that case, no one can be blamed for that innate cause of their retardation. But when a child comes to school with evidences of adequate physical and mental abilities but speaking unintelligibly in a language of gestures, grunts, and the barest use of English sounds, I wonder what could have been missing or wrong in his environment and training. We teachers sometimes find it difficult to assume responsibility for such a speech-retarded child, recommending that he either be kept at home until he "matures," that he be placed in "special education" classes, or that a speech clinic provide him with adequate speech before admitting him to school. Well, we know that such a child should be admitted to the regular kindergarten, where the teacher, aided by guidance from the school's speech therapist and other educational specialists, can offer that child the regular educational opportunities of the kindergarten program, plus other services which the speech therapist, school nurse, and school diagnostician may contribute.
>
> We believe that the mentally retarded child, lacking in speech and language, needs speech therapy which is integrated and conducted within the special education teacher's classroom program. If additional speech therapy is needed for this child, he may get that aid from the school's speech therapist; if no speech therapist is available at school, it may be possible to send him to a speech clinic for this special training. But in all of these alternatives, I believe that the child's kindergarten program should be the focal hub of his learning and rehabilitation. If we reject him and "pass the buck" by sending him home for another inadequate year, that added year of neglect may do him more harm than good. Or, he may not get any help if he is sent from pillar to post to get disjointed examinations and token bits of therapy without follow-up and integration with his up-to-date life. Of course, it means extra work for us kindergarten teachers to admit such a handicapped child into our programs and to make our classrooms his "home room." But by so doing, our kindergarten programs perhaps will not only give him what he needs but will also be a source of information, a vehicle for implementing and transferring his gains. From experience we learn that we cannot afford to dump a problem child upon educational specialists and expect them to put him in shape for us, to work out all solutions to his problems from positions outside our regular educational programs. No, a pupil needs our help as much as he needs theirs, while specialists need our help as much as we need theirs.

Because school has this strong impact upon a child's speech, it is important that parents and teachers make special preparations for his school entrance.

The chairman of a school's parent-education program recognized this problem:

A popular topic on our P.T.A. agenda each year centers around helping youngsters to make a better transition from home to school. Teachers and parents share interest in this topic because both know that a child's approach to school determines whether he will like or dislike school, whether his attitudes will foster learning or will prejudice him toward teachers and school generally. We know the importance of those first impressions a child gets from that first day or week of school, but parents sometimes forget that a child's attitudes toward school and teacher begin to form long before he enters the schoolroom. Parents usually try to make their children eager for school by suggesting some of the interests and rewards which education and school activities will bring. But some of these parents who try to build eager anticipations of school may unwittingly plant fears instead. Teachers, too, may make the mistake of thinking more about the law and well-oiled machinery of their classrooms than they do of the need to welcome children into school.

There are various ways by which parents and teachers can cushion the impact which teacher and school have upon a child. If the child has learned the basic social adjustments at home, his transition to the many formal and informal group adjustments at school will not be abrupt and difficult. The perceptive teacher will realize that her new pupils will not bring equal degrees of these skills and securities to school. She will be ready to meet them at the particular developmental points where their homes have left them. She will be patient with the children who are shy, insecure, weak, fearful, and who show signs of being socially and culturally deprived. She will use the well-adjusted children as helpful bellwethers to lead and reassure the timid ones along the strange routes. The following teacher tells how she prepares her room for the opening scene which greets kindergartners when they enter her classroom on the first day of school:

I generally have an interesting exhibit set up in the rear of my classroom to capture their fancies on that first day. Sometimes it's a cage of hamsters, an aquarium with fish, a turtle, a frog, or a jar of bugs or butterflies. Once I brought a parrot, an active talker and comical acrobat. I place these attractions where the children can informally get together and satisfy their natural interests for a while before I begin the first moves to regiment them as a group. But I use their common current interests, which had drawn them together at the attraction table, to keep them absorbed and unified at their seats. I may then invite the children to tell about similar personal experiences. Some of the pupils will be eager to tell, and I let them do so. I may supplement their verbal contributions by showing them some pictures which are related to the topics being discussed. Even though a few pupils appear too shy to do any talking, I usually find that they will become sufficiently involved to raise their hands or respond in some other nonverbal way. As soon as possible I try to find some avenue whereby each child can feel that he is being appreciated as a participating and contributing member of the class. I believe that if the shy and silent child can be thawed out early, he will not become fixed in behavioral habits which chain him personally and publicly to his timidity.

Schools have other ways to prepare preschool children for their satisfactory entrance into school. An elementary school principal paved a smoother way for entering kindergartners by using the following method:

> We have four projects which give preschoolers a positive picture of what to expect in school. In May of each year, we invite parents and their kindergartners-to-be to visit our school and enjoy a special one-hour program prepared for the orientation. We demonstrate some samples of interesting kindergarten activities, the young visitors may share seats with the regulars, and the teacher may tell an interesting story with illustrations projected on a screen from a strip film.
>
> Another project which prepares preschoolers for school is aimed at culturally deprived children who are enrolled in our Head Start programs. The children are introduced to some of the kindergarten activities, visit other parts of the school, enjoy the playground equipment, and generally finish the term with the feeling that they would like to return to school.
>
> Another dual project is carried out through a Mother Study group, which sponsors a panel discussion on the subject of preparing children for school and presents its information to one of the year's P.T.A. meetings.
>
> Finally, our school system conducts a spring preschool clinic in which all children who are slated for enrollment in kindergarten come with their parents for a free examination, which includes brief medical, visual, dental, and speech checks. We often find that children's attitudes toward school will be favorable if we can allay the parents' anxieties about their children and school.

Teacher-Pupil Relationship and Speech Climate. As teachers and parents, we see many signs which indicate that a child transfers many of his ideals, models, and identifications from home to school—in the areas not only of speech and language but also in other behavior. One parent described the change in her first-grader as follows:

> I'm gladly amused and a little put-out by the way Mary places her teacher ahead of Daddy and me when it comes to anything connected with her school. She idolizes her teacher and thinks that everything she says and does is entirely right and proper. I even suspect that she is adopting some of the teacher's mannerisms. Mary insists that she will be a "teacher like my teacher when I grow up."

A principal of an elementary school made this appraisal of the divided allegiance which pupils generally must reconcile when their school lives are added to their home lives:

> When I see the adulation and unquestioned trust which most young children give their teachers, I am reminded more than ever that we should have our very best teachers in the earliest grades of school. The school version of the old saying

"Like mother, like daughter" is just as surely "Like teacher, like pupil." Our dedicated and capable teachers realize this professional charge too. For some neglected children, who come from broken and inferior homes, the teachers may be substitute parents, to provide the love, respect, encouragement, and guidance which their homes have failed to provide. For kindergarten, first, and second grades, where the foundations and initial skills of recitation, reading, writing, and arithmetic are first exercised, I believe that we should be most careful and critical in our training, selection, and evaluation of teachers. Unfortunately, the public, the governing boards of education, and even the teacher-training institutions do not always adhere to this view. If they did, the qualifications, standards, salaries, and prestige for "lower el" teachers would not tend to be lower than they are for secondary and college teachers.

School programs are meant to serve the pupil, not the teachers or therapists. Our pupil, not we, must accomplish his learning and growth in speech and language. We may go through the motions of inspiring, leading, and helping him in these learning processes, but unless our pupil is inspired and willing to follow and work under our leadership, the goals of teaching or therapy will fail.

A pupil coming to school should find his teacher continuing in the role of a parent-away-from-home. If a child has been neglected at home, if his parents have not given him sufficient support, care, and training, then the teacher, the therapist, and other school personnel have an obligation to make up for this parental lack. It follows, therefore, that every teacher and speech therapist must understand parents' roles in speech development. There is little fundamental difference between the roles of the teacher and of the parents in helping children in speech and language development.

A pupil should like school, his teacher, and therapist, and should feel that he is treated without condescension. Furthermore, he should have no reasonable cause to develop chronic dislikes for other school personnel: the bus drivers, custodians, principals, school nurses, other teachers, office clerks, cooks, etc. He should learn to regard his school's personnel as a source of help, justice, security, and pleasure. The rules and standards for a pupil's conduct should be fair, clear, and consistent. When he is punished, he should understand that he is being punished because of his acts of misbehavior, and not because he, as a person, is being rejected.

The teacher-pupil relationship demands trust and unbroken faith on the part of the teacher. This means that whatever the child tells in private to his teacher or therapist will be kept for confidential professional consideration— not peddled in teachers' lounges, recorded in open files, or reported to parents or to anyone who is not rightfully concerned. One teacher expresses her views on this matter of acceptance as follows:

I find that it's rather trying to treat some of my pupils with warmth and respect when they are unruly, dirty, and have obnoxious habits. But when I remind myself that these children need me more than the adequate children need me, I treat them more objectively, and they become more willing and confident to change and to meet my standards.

A teacher should prove that she is tolerant of mistakes and failures, that she respects the child's intent and efforts and views failures constructively. A teacher who can help a child develop a realistic philosophy toward mistakes and failures will find, for instance, that a speech defective child will be willing to speak and to expose his defects and to work unashamedly to correct his flaws. Not all children look to their teachers as a source of encouragement and necessary help. Not all teachers, in turn, know how much to help, when to help, and in what area help is needed.

The speech climate of a classroom is generally improved by any influence which will add to pupils' satisfactions from successes and rewards. Speech tends to flourish if the air of a classroom is charged with worthy motivations which end in real satisfactions. However, in our highly competitive society we sometimes exploit the bare motivating force which comes from simply injecting uncontrolled raw competition into a task situation, without allowing a child a fair chance to win or gain satisfaction from the competition we imposed upon him. At times, after competition has been used to goad a child through a successful task, he may be offered phony rewards which do not satisfy except that they relieve the pressures from more competition. It is not difficult to find children who dislike certain tasks, including speaking, because of the fierce, cutthroat competition which teachers permit or encourage around those tasks. There are also children who no longer feel it worth the effort to have another star stuck after their names.

Nowadays a child may learn that his teacher is a person who can unbend from seriousness, autocracy, and rigidity. A male principal of a large consolidated school gave his reason for regularly eating school lunch with the children:

> I enjoy going through the cafeteria line with the children and eating with them. I think that they appreciate my company, too, from the first grade on up through high school. We have interesting chats; I mix in some fun and kidding; and they learn that a principal is not such an ogre or "square" after all.

Tendencies to restrict classroom recitation were emphasized by a speaker at an educational conference when she said:

> In our classroom teaching we tend to talk *at* our pupils, instead of *with* them. We treat pupils like little blotters to absorb knowledge, direction, and opinions. Although pupils usually get opportunities to answer our verbal questions, we merely solicit faithful translations of what we have told them, without giving them enough encouragement and chance to initiate and express original thoughts of their own. As teachers, we freely exercise our rights to judge and evaluate what they say, but we seldom encourage or allow them to evaluate what we say.

A teacher learns that other conditions affect the child's speech climate in school. They may arise from home conditions, such as worries about suitable clothing, or physical factors like inadequate diet, which may either sap vitality, morale, and interest, or create hypertension. Experiences outside the classroom, but associated with school, may cast a foreboding shadow over the entire speech picture at school. Demoralizing influence may come from conflicts on the playground or from troubles on the school bus. A first-grade teacher explains how children's moods and morale may be affected by problems on the school bus:

> There are times when one must search far afield for the causes of children's corrosive worries in the classroom. I've had kindergartners who were gnawed by adult worries, adopted from their parents' concerns over family finances, threats of marital separation, death of relatives, racial discriminations, etc. Last year two young pupils spent two miserable weeks in a gloomy stew which clouded their interests and recitations in class before I discovered the cause and solved the problem for them when I learned that a sixth-grade bully was forcing several young children on her school bus to save and give her their choicest portions of their pail-lunches. When this racket was unearthed and stopped, my young pupils again joined us in spirit and action.
>
> I find that some of the younger children who ride long distances and for long periods on the school bus arrive at school physically tired and emotionally wrought up. Some are also prone to carsickness. They may land at school green with nausea or having shamefully vomited on the bus or at school. In one of our consolidated schools, some of the children who arrive on early bus runs are obliged to remain outdoors for forty minutes before they can enter the building to start classes, unless the weather is bad. Some of the bus drivers have extremely difficult jobs, carrying sixty pupils of assorted ages for three hours each day, with the double task of keeping children in order and transporting them safely. If there is any area in our educational programs that is underpaid and neglected, it's our system of school busing. I believe that each bus driver should have an educationally oriented attendant who would free the driver to attend strictly to driving and who could convert those long miles and wasteful daily hours into enriching ones for the children. We haul those children as if they were livestock. It doesn't take much imagination or consideration to see how those buses could become mobile classrooms, equipped with loudspeakers to provide music, talks on nature along the route, taped stories, and various other activities for enjoyment and learning. If we reduced the fatigue and made bus trips constructive, we teachers in the classrooms would be better able to continue in like vein with the children when they land at school. Parents are often aware of these problems too.

There are other conditions within the classroom that affect speech climate for the pupil. Noisy classrooms, disorganized and lacking in discipline, tend to discourage recitation and make communication difficult. Strict time-limits on speaking may put damaging pressure on a pupil. He may also be thwarted if the policy is too critical and arbitrary, perhaps where grading is too strictly based upon speech performance.

A child's speech climate in school is also revealed by his attitudes toward speaking in the classroom, his willingness to talk with teachers, classmates, and other school personnel. This climate also correlates with his teacher's degree of respect and appreciation for what he says, an indication of whether or not she is a good listener. A child needs an atmosphere in which a teacher and classmates show respect and patience, do not interrupt his speaking, try to understand him, and acknowledge in a constructive way what he says. As a general rule, if a teacher sets a good example in this kind of listening, her pupils will be inclined to do so, too.

References

1. Orvis C. Irwin, "Speech Development in the Young Child: 2. Some Factors related to the Speech Development of the Infant and Young Child." *Journal of Speech and Hearing Disorders*, 17, No. 3 (September 1952), 269–79.

2. Joseph Church, *Language and the Discovery of Reality*. New York: Vintage Books, 1961.

3. C. S. Bluemel, *The Riddle of Stuttering*. Danville, Ill.: The Interstate Publishing Co., 1957.

4. W. Johnson, S. F. Brown, J. F. Curtis, C. W. Edney, and J. Keaster, *Speech Handicapped School Children*. New York: Harper & Row, Inc., 1967.

5. H. R. Myklebust, "Babbling and Echolalia in Language Theory," *Journal of Speech and Hearing Disorders*, 22, No. 3 (September 1957), 356–60.

6. Laura Lee, "Developmental Sentence Types: A Method for Comparing Normal and Deviant Syntactic Development," *Journal of Speech and Hearing Disorders*, 31 (November 1966), 311–30.

Questions

1. Discuss the sequence and stages by which the child learns speech and language.

2. Describe the role of prespeech vocalization.

3. How important are social influences in prespeech vocalizations?

4. What is the value of self-feedback in prespeech vocalization?

5. What are the requisites for the "first-word" period?

6. How effective are stress and intonation patterns in the child's speech expressions?

7. How do body actions assist speech?

8. Explain "downward" and "upward" categorization.

9. Describe the "jargon" stage of speech.

10. How does the child learn grammar?

11. In speech development what period of a child's life is most critical?

12. Define "closed" and "open" categories of words.

13. Why should we avoid segmentation in teaching speech and language skills?

14. When does the child learn grammar fundamentals?

15. Describe the course of the child's mastery of articulation.

16. What must the child achieve to attain speech fluency?

17. Describe a primer best suited to develop reading skill.

18. Are language and speech best taught as an end in themselves?

19. What school subjects should develop speech and language?

20. How would you appeal to parents for cooperation in preventing speech problems?

21. Discuss the effect of lack of "T.L.C." on speech growth.

22. How may parents motivate speech development?

23. Why should babbling be encouraged when the child is alone?

24. Discuss the importance of parental speech models.

25. Should parents use baby talk to the child?

26. Why must a speech model be personally acceptable to the child?

27. Discuss conditions which block the child's avenues of perception.

28. How must parents adjust sentence models to the child's needs?

29. What are the guidelines for experience and repetition in speech practice?

30. What speech faults must parents and teachers avoid as poor examples?

31. What double standards in speech etiquette harm young children's efforts to learn speech?

32. Do adults tend to expect too much of a child's speech as he begins school?

33. Do you agree with this teacher: "For me, the first several days of each school year are always the most challenging days of teaching"?

34. How does the teacher-pupil relationship affect the speech climate?

Suggested Subjects for
Term Papers

1. In view of the fact that at age two a child usually begins the use of simple or compound sentences, do our common primers influence speech patterns to best advantage? Make a survey of a number used in kindergarten and in grades one and two.
2. Observe a child of two years for six weeks for evidence of his growing command of grammar in that time.
3. Make a survey of the opinions of speech authorities on the development of stress and intonation in primitive human speech and any similarity to animal vocalizing.
4. On buses, in shops, and elsewhere, observe patterns of parental interruption of children's speech and the reactions of the children.
5. At a school for the blind, report your discussions with teachers and pupils on how persons blind from birth learn to speak.
6. Write an autobiography of your tongue. When was it first conscious that it was being made to talk? How did it learn to speak the language up to age six?
7. In "The Strange Case of James Joyce" (*The Bookman*, September 1928, page 16) Rebecca West wrote: "Your baby has no words, but it will use sentences for hours together, sometimes pausing for thought and adding a pungent dependent clause, till it builds up a kind of argument-like mass. Indeed the chief difficulty of teaching a child to talk is to persuade it to abandon the wordless sentence, which perfectly conveys all the emotional communication it wishes to make, and to go through the labor of memorizing words for the purpose of making the intellectual communications it will feel no need to make for some years to come." Is this statement valid in today's understanding of the psychology of speech?
8. Audit five classes from any grades one to twelve. Make intelligibility ratings of pupils' recitations on a scale of 25 to 100 per cent and analyze the speech traits which hamper intelligibility.
9. If for several years you have known an "A" student who has been over-stimulated by parents to excel in school, describe the pressures and their effects on the child.
10. Introduce your rogues' gallery of the kinds of parents whose influence thwarts normal development of their children's speech.
11. How early does the child learn the politics of living, in appearing to please those in authority, such as parents and teachers? What obligations fall on adults? Give examples.

three

The Teacher as a Team Member

A teacher who taught first in an isolated country school and later in a modern consolidated system compares her teaching roles in these different situations:

> In my first eight years of teaching in one-room schools, I had to be just about everything to my pupils. My teaching of twenty-five children, ranging from first to sixth grade, was a continual challenge which demanded adaptability, flexibility, ingenuity, and endless work. Nevertheless, I believe that we gained some priceless values in those one-room schools. Pupils of all ages learned to share responsibilities and to sense their personal worth in all sorts of ways.
>
> When I recollect my old one-room teaching days and compare them with my present modern regimen, I find myself in sympathy with many of these child complaints about schools and teachers. Of course, we have gained in many ways from specialization and its teamwork, but we also see an over-focus upon the teaching of subject matter and the treatment of ills, not persons.
>
> But there are hopeful signs that we are meeting these deficiencies in education. We are seeing more team-teaching at all levels in education, both in the regular school subjects and in the special ones of art, music, foreign language, speech correction, health education, sex education, religion, physical education, etc. In the matter of cooperativeness, the spirit of the old one-room schoolroom is returning, but now we have specially trained coworking adults in our corps, and our resources for helping are far greater than when twenty-five children could rely only on themselves and me.

Who Belongs on a Speech Therapy Team?

Speech correction and other branches of special education show evidences of the same conflicting trends which the foregoing teacher has pointed out in general education. In the past, speech correction has suffered from the youthful insecurity of a new profession—struggling to establish its respected identity within the halls of education and medicine and yet attempting to maintain sufficient autonomy. Certification standards and training requirements have reflected the different needs and philosophies to be found in the different work settings of speech correction.

At present in many states, speech therapists who work in public schools are required by state law to qualify for regular teaching certificates. Many speech therapists who work in public schools are also required to join the regular educational associations. Because the great majority of speech therapists in the United States work in public schools, they must come under the general jurisdiction of those schools. It is reasonable to expect that speech therapists and all others who work with pupils within shared school programs should work cooperatively, should have integrated lines of command and adequate communication with each other, and should understand the basics of each other's work and problems. Chapman,[1] Ainsworth,[2] and other leaders in speech correction and education have tried to clarify and to remind us of our roles, our dangerous trends to become "separatists" rather than "participants," and of our need to reconcile the serious disagreements concerning our appropriate responsibilities in public schools. If we are to prevent "separatism" from developing in our teamwork within school programs, we must be careful that we do not indoctrinate separatism into our professionals from the beginning, when they are in training. Institutions which train teachers and speech therapists are finding that their students mutually benefit from certain courses and experiences. Perhaps when there is better voluntary cooperation between "specialists" and the "rank-and-file" of educators, we shall see a revision of certain inappropriate legislation which has been erected in the past to enforce this educational cooperation.

Who, then, belongs on a speech therapy team working in a public school setting? Ideally considered, the team includes the speech therapist as "captain" and all others who are in positions to have therapeutic influence upon the client —the client's teacher, his parents, and his classmates. For some problems, the team may require the cooperation of the remedial reading teacher, the school psychologist or diagnostician, the school nurse or the family doctor, the visiting teacher, the school's social worker, the counselor, bus drivers, custodians, and the principal, who has over-all responsibility for the client's school. In addition, in some cases involving organic, emotional disturbances, economic, and other special problems, the speech therapist may enlist aid from child guidance centers, speech and hearing clinics, service clubs, welfare agencies, and other organizations. It is important, therefore, for speech therapists and others to know about these local, state, and federal agencies and how to procure their aid.

The Teacher's Responsibility and Acceptance

Speech therapists and teachers who recognize their rightful positions on the therapy team will willingly cooperate, since both realize that they are working toward the same goal—the welfare of the child. Yet at times there are forces which reduce their dedication to serve the child. These frank expressions of classroom teachers and speech therapists concerning their cooperation in speech correction do not represent the views of the majority, but they do reveal some insidious trends of varying degree which may spread and hamper services for children. The following remark was made in a teachers' lounge by a fourth-grade teacher concerning her sense of responsibility and involvement in public school speech correction:

> Why should I have to work to correct speech problems? Our school district hires speech therapists to come around to work with children with speech problems. That's their job; that's all they have to do. I'm swamped with more than enough duties as it is. Besides, people in special education are paid at a higher scale than we are. On top of it all, their work is easier and less confining.

The following teacher, although not antagonistic toward speech therapists, held a view which had the same effect—to relieve her of the responsibility for working with speech problems:

> Before our school had the services of speech therapists and remedial reading teachers, I felt and assumed a greater responsibility for my pupils when they had speech and language problems. I'll admit that at times I wasn't sure how to help them, but there was no one else around to do it, so I felt that I had to do what I could. I'm afraid that most of what I did was just plain common sense, since I've had no speech correction course in my teacher training. But now that our school has a speech therapist, I feel that she is handling our speech problems and is doing it in a professional way, better than I can. In fact, I might do things that would conflict with what she does. So, I leave well enough alone and let her handle the speech correction end of it.

The next teacher indicates another unfavorable relationship between the speech therapist and herself:

> Personally, I don't think that our speech therapist really wants or expects any help from us classroom teachers. She hasn't come right out and said so, but her attitude surely makes me feel that way. She doesn't ask for any information concerning the pupils I refer to her. She doesn't give me any reports on her work, or on their progress in therapy, unless I really corner her. She hardly notices me and probably doesn't even care to know my name. But it bothers me to think that our poor relationship may be keeping me from helping with my pupils' speech problems, especially since I'm confronted with their speech problems every day in my classroom.

The bitter resentment expressed by the next teacher indicates that the cooperation between this teacher and this therapist would be difficult, unsatisfactory, and short-lived:

Frankly, I just can't stand that guy and his airs of superiority! From the beginning, he's been waging a campaign to make us call him a "speech therapist" instead of just a lowly "speech teacher." He tries to impress us by flinging around high-powered psychological terms, and even I can tell that he misuses some of them. But he really revealed himself the other day in the teachers' lounge, where he spends more time than any of the rest of us. Someone asked him why speech therapists were started at a higher base salary than regular teachers are. He gave two dumb reasons. First, he stated that general "ed" students don't have to put in so many hours as speech therapists in their college case practice. Second, he reminded us that speech therapists are specialists, whom he defined as someone "trained to work with individuals, not just with a whole class." Imagine that! Doesn't he think that we must teach individuals within our classes? I'd like to see him prepare my lesson plans and take over my class for even one day.

A high school chemistry teacher compares the degrees of tactful understanding shown by different speech therapists when he says:

Scheduling high school students for speech correction has always created problems, and always will. Students realize it; their teachers realize it. But not all therapists seem to understand that a student must often make up the work he misses when his regular class schedule is interrupted by therapy. Some of these make-ups are difficult, requiring extra time and work for both the student and his teacher. Grades may suffer. Speech therapy often becomes unpopular and even may be refused by high school students and their parents if these complications are not handled compromisingly.

But when a therapist understands the over-all situation and shows consideration for everyone involved, better solutions are usually found. Therapists generally schedule therapy during a student's study hours. If for understandable reasons a study period cannot be used, a therapist sometimes arranges therapy at another period when problems of make-up can be reduced. Students, and their parents, are less likely to resist therapy when they realize that we teachers are solidly behind the speech therapy program. I've seen teachers stay after school to help speech cases with make-up work so they can get badly needed therapy. Sometimes a therapist will work with a case after school hours or during a part of the lunch hour.

The Teacher's Opportunities
and Capacity for Helping

The following discussions assume that the teacher has available the services of a speech therapist. The therapeutic work of a teacher and of other team members occurs in two related areas: diagnosis and treatment. A perceptive therapist describes help she receives from teachers:

Two of the most obvious ways by which a teacher helps me in speech correction involve her referral of speech cases and our exchange of the information I need in scheduling and treatment. But a teacher helps me and our pupils in many other ways. She helps to sell therapy to pupils and their parents. She conveys information to parents and relays information from them to me, relative to speech problems and therapy. A teacher can often serve as my co-therapist, working under my direction. In this way, I can extend into her classroom many of the therapeutic practices which otherwise would be limited to my therapy situations with the pupil. In therapy our biggest task is to strengthen the pupil's newly learned skills and attitudes, so they will carry over into his daily life. Since classroom experiences comprise the major part of a pupil's daily life, his classroom teacher certainly controls important opportunities for habituating these skills and confidences.

In my diagnosis and therapy planning, too, I gain important help from a classroom teacher, who is in a better position than I am to know pupils fully—their home backgrounds, their social behavior on the playground, their assets and liabilities in other areas, and their speech in a wider range of situations. A teacher's position is well equipped with materials, practices, and openings which can be directly or indirectly applied to speech therapy. Many of the teacher's regular activities have therapeutic effects upon speech, even though she may have other goals in mind, such as reading, spelling, conducting recitations, modeling speech through her usage, etc. I should feel frustrated and my speech program would fail in isolation if I didn't have the cooperation of teachers, and I let them know I need and appreciate their help. Too often in our educational jobs we do not sense the credit we deserve.

At times it may appear that we ask teachers to assume responsibilities which only speech therapists should be expected or qualified to do. What we should require of a teacher will depend upon many factors: her ability and dedication as a teacher; her understanding of speech and language problems and their correction; her burdens in the teaching situation; and, to a great degree, the ability of the therapist and other team members to work with her in the speech correction program.

The Role of the Speech Therapist

We sometimes hear speech therapists complain that their roles are misunderstood. When they are introduced to parents, and even to other school personnel, they are frequently met with the remark, "Oh, you're a speech therapist? Now, I'll have to watch my *ain'ts* around you!" Remarks like this may reveal the two misconceptions which Johnson[3] points out: that correct speech is often measured too narrowly, either in terms of language alone or with regard to the separate control of articulation, voice, breathing, fluency, or other factors. It may be wiser, as Johnson suggests, for parents and the general public to be more language-conscious than speech-conscious, at least until specific speech problems arise to justify focus upon faulty details of speech. The public school therapist who does not unduly separate speech from language and who identifies his or her role more closely with teaching and teachers will not resent being called a "speech teacher" in school. Although the speech therapist is a "very special sort of teacher," as Van Riper[4] indicates, he or she has more in common with classroom teachers than with most of the special education employees.

A public school director of special services compares the role of speech therapists with that of other professionals in school:

> Speech therapists lead charmed professional lives, somewhat as junior practitioners of specialized psychiatry. Accordingly, they enjoy that profession's immunity to definite responsibility—unlike classroom teachers, whose work must meet the stern requirements of state achievement standards; unlike the school nurses, who must diagnose the incipient scarlet fever or face an epidemic; and unlike the athletic directors, who must produce winning teams "or else"! Speech therapists deal with vague and elusive individual problems which may challenge their complete funds of knowledge and still fail of solution with justifiably little damage to their professional standing. Enough is known about the nature of speech defects to assure that the honest speech therapists will not assume full credit for "cures," will not feel abashed at failures, and will not sink to the alibis of incomprehensible pseudo-professional jargon.

Because this book is designed mainly for teachers and their roles in speech correction, we shall not include many of the ways by which speech therapists work with speech and language problems. References have been included within each chapter to give additional information on the special therapeutic equipment and methods used in the speech therapist's profession. These references list further sources of information such as textbooks and articles. Although written principally for speech therapy students, these sources are valuable supplements. A comprehensive orientation of the work of speech therapists may be gained from texts by Van Riper,[4] Johnson,[3] Berry and Eisenson,[5] and other authors. Specialized information on therapy directed toward individual problem areas in speech correction may be gained from such books as the *Foundations of Speech Pathology Series*, edited by Van Riper.[6]

Many teachers have added to their general knowledge of speech correction by taking extension courses, field service courses, and workshops conducted by departments of speech pathology and audiology. Education departments have recognized this need for interdisciplinary understanding and have granted credit for such courses taken to fulfill requirements for teaching certificates. Another effective way for teachers to learn about speech therapy has been through conferences and observations of therapists at work. Although not all teachers can arrange to observe therapy sessions and not all therapists will invite direct observations of their therapy sessions, some therapists who have offered these demonstrations, either openly or through one-way mirrors and intercoms, strongly support this method to give teachers and parents insight into therapy procedures for their pupils.

The American Speech and Hearing Association[7] has repeatedly attempted to clarify the role of speech therapists in public schools and to differentiate between the functions of therapists and the functions of the "curriculum-oriented instructional personnel" such as classroom teachers, special teachers of the deaf or mentally retarded, and teachers who work for general speech effectiveness. When a speech therapist is employed in hospital settings, in rehabilitation centers, in speech and hearing clinics, his role is more clearly defined. But in elementary and secondary schools the work of the therapist may become confused when it must overlap and harmonize with the surrounding educational goals of other instructional personnel.

Speech therapy must be adaptable within the general goals of the setting —in a medical orientation when therapists work in hospital settings and in correlation with education when they work in school settings. Consequently, this correlation calls for a delineation of the speech and language problems and the responsibilities which distinguish the teacher's role from that of the school's speech therapist. Similarly, when speech therapy is conducted in medically oriented programs, such as Medicare's, its direction or supervision may require further classification and adjustment. The term *speech therapist* may be conflicting in programs where therapies, except speech therapy, are under medical jurisdiction. Therefore, the term *speech clinician* has been proposed by the American Speech and Hearing Association as a more appropriate title for Americans who practice speech correction, since we are not trained in medicine, as speech therapists are in some countries of Europe.

We shall define and separate problems of speech and language into two broad categories: problems which fall within "normal limits" requiring "speech improvement" and the more significantly handicapping speech and language disorders which require "speech therapy." Under the category "speech improvement," we usually have in mind the general problems and goals which apply to *all* children, such as the improvement of pronunciation, vocabulary, grammar, verbal output, fluency, vocal control, speech poise and adjustment, and the ability to "think on one's feet." "Speech improvement," therefore, is identified with the total instructional programs under the primary responsibility of classroom teachers, with subordinate responsibility assigned to the speech therapist for consultation and planning with the classroom teachers.

Although there is no sharp distinction between problems which call for "speech therapy" rather than for "speech improvement," therapists should feel primary responsibility for the relatively small group of speakers who are handicapped in their language communication and speech adjustment. "Therapy" is generally directed toward cases whose speech and language problems are not expected to improve solely through normal maturation and educational means. Here, too, it is difficult for us to predict whether "speech therapy" or "speech improvement" will be needed to remedy a first-grader, for instance, who misarticulates several of his speech sounds. However, one of the speech therapist's functions is to identify the ordinary problems from the extraordinary ones which demand diagnosis and special treatment—which tends to be individualized, intensive, and coordinated with other services. But, as we have emphasized earlier in this chapter, the responsibilities and functions of teachers and other instructional personnel cannot be overlooked in speech therapy.

Speech therapists are sometimes inclined to think that their roles are removed from the "speech arts" curriculum, which gives instruction and practice in the general development of oral language skills and uses. Although the therapist is not primarily responsible for the teaching of reading, public speaking, debate, effective discussion, creative dramatics, oral interpretation, etc., we believe that he cannot afford to neglect the opportunities which this curriculum provides. Therapists who are acquainted with the "language arts" and the "speech arts" areas will be in a better position to lend their consultive services within these practical areas. In the following statement, a speech therapist expresses his appreciation for this cooperation with the "speech arts" teachers of his school:

> Experience has taught me that I'm not such an educational specialist as I had thought. When I started public school therapy, I felt that I was in a rather self-contained and self-sufficient field. I even resented the predominantly educational atmosphere in school. For a while I resisted the forces which reminded me that I had a part to play in other school programs. But I soon learned that speech therapy demanded close cooperation with teachers and other activities. In fact, I observed in various school programs that teachers were doing things that were directly or indirectly therapeutic for speech and language. In the kindergarten and first-grade programs I learned that teachers do much to improve and build speech and language. I found that young children, on my waiting list for speech therapy to correct their articulation, were corrected as readily under the influences of good teachers as they were when my therapy was added to their program. Some of these "cures" could be chalked up to maturation, but I had to admit that classroom teachers do many things which coincide with my work in therapy. Speech therapy can be complemented by teachers at every grade level and in all subjects.
>
> I find that many teachers are as interested in the speech welfare of their pupils as I am. They are glad to cooperate with me. Our speech teacher, who directs plays, teaches public speaking, conducts projects in oral interpretation and creative dramatics, does more to provide my speech cases with supportive experiences than I could possibly arrange for them. Previously, I had to rely upon assignments for pupils to do outside the school and trust that they would carry them out and profit. Or, if I put pupils in speech situations under my device and direction, the situations were often too artificial or limited to have much value. The teachers who work with me in our therapy assignments easily provide realistic experiences to facilitate therapy.

The Remedial Reading Therapist

We single out the remedial reading teacher from the other instructional staff members of the school to illustrate that speech therapists and teachers of reading have more in common than they may realize. Classroom teachers variously express our common aims and practices in their teaching of reading, spelling, and speech. Teachers realize that "phonics" helps children to listen more carefully to the spoken parts of words, to perceive the similarities and differences of phonemes, and to associate speech sounds with their corresponding written symbols and meanings. These goals are usually needed in therapy for misarticulation. The teaching of reading includes projects on the learning and use of plurals, suffixes, and prefixes—areas which are sometimes at fault in misarticulation. What speech therapists call "auditory training" is variously referred to by reading teachers as "word analysis"; "word-attack skills"; "recognition of rhyming"; "the ability to listen for and to recognize specific sounds and to enunciate them correctly"; "the ability to 'work out' the recognition, pronunciation and meaning of new words"; "word-form analysis"; "structural analysis"; "sounding out words", and so on. Teachers of reading, remedial reading specialists, and speech therapists do more in common than they may realize. At times the main difference lies in the professional terminology which labels the activity.

The Parents' Role in Speech Correction

No role in speech correction is more important and yet more often bypassed than is the responsibility of parents. Whether we work with children in school, in speech clinics, in Head Start programs,[8] or in hospital settings, a weak and neglected area in speech therapy is often found in our failure to enlist the cooperation of parents. Whether our clients are of preschool age or older, whether they have problems of misarticulation, language deficiency, non-fluency, or speech maladjustment, there are likely to be many opportunities for parental help. One speech therapist has declared:

> If we are to work upon the environmental factors which cause and cure speech and language problems, we cannot exclude parents and their roles in these matters. We prove in our diagnoses and prognoses that we recognize the importance of parental influences upon speech problems, and, although we may be ready to recognize and to blame parents for their inadequate influences and teachings, we are not always so ready to help parents to teach their children. Our large caseloads and crowded schedules offer excuses for our inaction in this dilemma. We may

sincerely feel the need for "outside" help with problems; but we may lack the time, facilities, personal security, or professional assistance to implement the added parental cooperation in our therapy programs. Then, too, we may lack faith in parental ability to learn and help in our professional work.

Speech therapists, family physicians, teachers, and others are inclined to warn parents that speech correction is a specialty, a job only for trained and qualified professionals. Under these convictions, we may induce parents to ignore a real speech and language problem, perhaps giving them a false trust that the problem will be "outgrown" by school age. We may feel that parents will handicap our therapy if we admit them into our therapy team. We may rationalize that parents will not understand, may get wrong impressions of us and our therapy, and may do wrong things beyond our supervision. Nevertheless, many parents have proved to us that they can gain interest, understanding, and skills in speech therapy, especially if we help them adapt therapy to fit the parental roles in the home situation. Some parents learn to be better therapists for their children than we are—when we give them a chance to join with us in therapy. As a personal bonus, we therapists find that our own therapy is upgraded by the extra incentives, information, ideas, inspirations, and better preparations which come from our face-to-face dealings with our clients' parents.

We learn, however, that not all parents make good speech therapists or teachers of reading and other school subjects. Therefore, before we assign any parent to help with a speech or a language problem, we should determine and insure, if possible, the parent's ability to help. But we find also that parents who are most in need of our counseling and instruction are often the ones who mostly will determine the success or failure of our work with children. We cannot afford to be neglectful or to lose faith in our efforts to help parents who at first may appear hopelessly apathetic, ignorant, or even harmful in the face of children's problems.

Classmates

Every able teacher knows that the art of teaching includes the ability to make use of that effective source of learning which comes from peers—through peer teaching. Our speech clients' classmates can be important members of our therapeutic team. The perceptive teacher knows that classmates are continually setting all kinds of examples, good and bad. She will be alert to the behavioral patterns which should be portrayed and reinforced by classmates. She will know the social lines of influence within the group—the social "peck order," the leaders, followers, the sociograms of her class. For speech and language problems, which often require social adjustment and modeling, the teacher can pattern class participation in ways which constructively harness group dynamics.

School Psychologist, Nurse, and Others

For ordinary problems of speech and language, the members of the therapy team include only the therapist, teacher, parents, and classmates. In cases where causal factors and remedies involve organic, medical, and the serious psychological problems, other professionals and agencies are needed in the team effort. The speech therapist generally makes the initial referral for this extra help, while subsequent referrals may come from examinations given by these added team members. For example, a third-grade girl was scheduled for therapy to correct several misarticulations in speech. Her therapist, observing that the client had a chronic nasal congestion and a tendency to mouth-breathe, verified the fact through the teacher's observations and referred the child to the school nurse. The nurse contacted the girl's parents, who acted on the recommendation that the condition be checked by their family doctor. The physician diagnosed the problem, a chronic middle-ear infection caused by an allergy. He corrected the infection but suggested that an allergist be consulted to determine and to eliminate the cause of the allergy, found to be feathers in her pillow. Thus, in securing cooperative medical services to solve a problem which was aggravating this girl's speech difficulty, her speech therapy team had temporarily utilized three added members.

There are times when speech therapy teams require the special services of school psychologists, physical and occupational therapists, visiting and home-bound teachers, audiologists, psychiatrists, and various agencies. In speech therapy programs for the blind, deaf, mentally retarded, or crippled children, we usually find the need for extensive as well as intensive cooperation. A report[9] which analyzes the problems and successes of a young speechless child, blind from retrolental fibroplasia and crippled from cerebral palsy, credits success to the integrated way in which his parents and all staff members at his hospital school teamed to help him achieve normal speech. In this case, the team members, under the guidance of a medical staff comprising a pediatrician, two orthopedists, and a director of special education, included the child, his parents, two speech therapists, a classroom teacher, his classmates, two occupational therapists, two physical therapists, school attendants, the school's manager —and even his huge, lovable boxer dog. Later, this child continued his education at a state school for the blind where his continued successes came from further cooperative work by new teams. In the analysis of the teamwork which solved this case's complex speech problems, *understanding* and *communication* were the essentials which made the teamwork effective. An effective working relationship in diagnostic and remedial teaching depends upon communication between services, the avoidance of red tape and disintegrated authority, and the efficient use of space, time, and equipment.

Education and speech correction have been reluctant to adopt the team-teaching approach in their professional work. Lately, we see a rising need for team-teaching and the creation of new supportive personnel because of teacher and therapist shortages, the realization that our fields have many facets requiring specialists, and the inadequacy of present specialists to handle some of the new roles which are being indicated in our programs. Pope and Crump[10] have shown the values which have been gained in education from the use of special assistant teachers, while Irwin[11] and Ptacek[12] have clarified the needs and implications surrounding the issue of bringing certain new professional aides into speech correction and audiology.

References

1. M. E. Chapman, "The Speech Clinician and the Classroom Teacher Co-operate in a Speech Correction Program," *Journal of Speech Disorders*, VII (March 1942), 57–61.

2. Stanley Ainsworth, "The Speech Clinician in Public Schools: 'Participant' or 'Separatist'?", *ASHA*, 12, (1965), 495–503.

3. W. Johnson, S. F. Brown, J. F. Curtis, C. W. Edney, and J. Keaster, *Speech Handicapped School Children*. New York: Harper & Row, Inc., 1967.

4. C. Van Riper, *Speech Correction: Principles and Methods*. Englewood Cliffs, N.J.: Prentice-Hall, Inc., 1963.

5. M. F. Berry and J. Eisenson, *Speech Disorders*. New York: Appleton-Century-Crofts, 1956.

6. *Foundations of Speech Pathology Series*. Edited by C. Van Riper. Englewood Cliffs, N.J.: Prentice-Hall, Inc., 1965.

7. "Services and Functions of Speech and Hearing Specialists in Public Schools" by Executive Council of American Speech and Hearing Association. *ASHA*, 4 (1962), pp. 99–100.

8. G. O. Egland, "Parents in Head Start Programs," *Young Children*, XXI, No. 5 (May 1966), 293–96.

9. G. O. Egland, "An Analysis of an Exceptional Case of Retarded Speech," *Journal of Speech and Hearing Disorders*, 19, No. 2 (June 1954), 239–43.

10. L. Pope and R. Crump, "School Dropouts as Assistant Teachers," *Young Children*, 21, No. 1 (October 1965), 13–23.

11. John V. Irwin, "Supportive Personnel in Speech Pathology and Audiology," *ASHA*, 9, No. 9 (September 1967), 348–54.

12. Paul H. Ptacek, "Supportive Personnel as an Extension of the Professional Worker's Nervous System," *ASHA*, 9, No. 10 (October 1967), 403–5.

Questions

1. Discuss the professional status of speech therapists.

2. Is it just to consider speech therapists as "the elite," separate from regular classroom teachers?

3. Who should belong on the team working on speech therapy in the public schools?

4. Discuss the types of negative attitudes of speech therapists which will hinder cooperation with classroom teachers.

5. Discuss the concrete help which the classroom teacher may give the speech therapist.

6. Define the difference between the functions of public school therapists and those of "curriculum-oriented instructional personnel."

7. Compare the methods of remedial reading teachers with the methods of the speech therapists.

8. How important is the parents' role in speech correction?

9. What is the value of peer teaching in speech therapy?

10. Describe a speech client in need of aid from (1) the school nurse; (2) the family doctor; (3) the school psychologist.

Suggested Subjects for Term Papers

1. A survey of state requirements for certification of speech therapists.
2. Why I Chose Speech Therapy.
3. The reasons for and against allowing direct observations by teachers and parents of therapy sessions.
4. How to deal with parents who:
   a. dominate therapy
   b. say: "Oh, he'll outgrow it. Leave him alone!"
   c. show jealousy of the child's emotional loyalty to you
5. Ways of preventing professional isolationism.

four

Problems of Speech
and Language

It is not surprising that problems in speech and language occur, when we consider the requisites for speech, its standards and variations, and the intricacies in its development. As suggested in Chapters 1 and 2, a study of normal speech and language behavior gives insights into the causes and effects which are associated with various speech and language problems, and keeps abnormality and normality in proper relationship to each other, for better orientation of corrective procedures.

Our corrective work as speech therapists and teachers will remain diffuse and indiscriminate and even potentially harmful if our procedures do not correspond closely with the client's problem. We have emphasized that careful diagnosis and correct evaluations provide the bases for our efforts to correct speech. If we have only a vague understanding of deviation problems, our procedures in speech therapy, remedial reading, language rehabilitation, etc., will miss the crucial aspects of the situations and may even create new problems in the process. We shall continue to stress the importance of getting a clear definition and analysis of a client's problem, because observation, testing, and diagnosis should be neither separate from, nor incompatible with, teaching and therapy. One experienced speech therapist expressed the following views on problem-detection, problem-analysis, and problem-solving:

> I learned from our state psychological consultant in special education that a broad base of information is needed in diagnosis. This capable diagnostician cooperated with us in the public schools and children's hospital centers of our state, giving tests, evaluations, and guidance in cases involving exceptional problems of learning and school adjustment. She knew and was certified to give every test in the book, and at times she found a need to give each of them. But she gave a particular test only when it was indicated, and her indications usually came from her extensive observations of the child and from information gathered from his everyday setting of learning and adjustment. She often devoted from three to five full days, studying a client within his daily environment, observing him at work in classes, on the playground, in speech therapy class, and visiting his home.
> Her observations were supplemented and verified from information gained from

teachers, pupils, parents, therapists, and others. Moreover, her own psychological tests followed, rather than preceded, this collection of field information. As she admitted, her formal follow-up tests often did not disclose any new leads; they served mainly to verify and measure more objectively that which she and we already thought. Nevertheless, her services were very helpful. When her study of a client was completed, she met with all of us—teachers, therapists, parents, and others—to help plan for problem-solving. But in all of this observation, testing, and counseling, this outstanding psychologist did not ever lose sight of her client's problem area.

Defining a Speech Problem

The ideal first step in treating a speech problem is to identify the problem according to a clear concept of what designates a speech problem to be a handicap deserving our aid. Speech and language problems are not easy to define and measure. Van Riper[1] and Johnson[2] have provided commonly accepted criteria for identifying a speech problem and for measuring its handicap value. Van Riper suggests that speech becomes handicapped when it interferes with communication, causes its possessor to be maladjusted, and calls attention to itself. Johnson adopts similar criteria by his representation of a speech problem as a three-dimensional cube, composed of the speech characteristics, the listener reactions, and the speaker reactions. Both of these definitions emphasize that a speech problem must be judged not only in terms of the muscle movements and distorted sound waves, but also on the basis of the speech fault's effects on communication and other aspects of the speaker's and the audience's reactions. Each of the following statements indicates how one or more of these dimensions of a speech problem has been noted:

"We can understand him all right, but some of his third grade classmates are starting to tease him because he 'talks like a baby' on some words."

"If it weren't for his gestures, we couldn't understand half of what he says in kindergarten. But so far, he talks merrily on, as if nothing were wrong."

"I feel so sorry for him when he recites and stutters. He gets completely stuck on certain words, struggles so hard, and sometimes cannot finish what he has started to say. But the other first-graders don't seem to mind it yet. They're curious but patient."

"Our girl is tongue-tied. She can't say some of her words right."

"Mary will hardly ever talk in school. When she does, she talks so softly that none can hear her."

"I have two Mexican children in first grade. They rattle off Spanish between themselves, but they speak very little English. It leads to some frustration for them and others. Of course, it is handicapping their school work."

"In my junior high classes I have had boys whose voices were changing. Their voice-breaks often sound comical. They create giggles. Usually the adolescent takes it good-naturedly, but sometimes he gets sensitive and won't recite while this change is going on."

"A sixth-grader brought a beautiful accent up from South Carolina when her family moved here. Everyone accepts her and her Southern speech, although at times we must do a little translating when she says her 'r' words as true Southerners do. But the speech therapist and I have decided that her speech difference presently is not a problem for special therapy."

"Phil talks so fast and mumbles his words together. We often miss some of the important words in his sentences. I've told him to slow up and try to speak more distinctly, but he doesn't seem to be able to change or to feel that it's a problem. Perhaps only a few people in his life have regarded it as a problem."

"That's not a 'wabbit'; that's a wabbit!" retorted an indignant three-year-old, hearing her mother intentionally imitate her misarticulation of *rabbit*.

"What's the matter with your lip? Why do you talk funny?" (Questions asked by first-graders of a classmate whose scarred lip and cleft palate caused her to speak with nasal emission and misarticulation).

Each of the foregoing statements describes one or more of the aspects of the speech problem which it describes. These statements indicate that we can learn from what laymen and even young children have to say about speech problems. Their observations are often expressed with simplicity, conciseness, and frank objectivity. We see factual and illuminating information on a speech problem being discussed by the following teacher and her third-grade pupil:

"Miss Brown, why does Ralph talk funny? He talks like Porky Pig. When he says my name, he says, 'W-W-W-W-Wilbur'."

"Wilbur, you shouldn't say that! Ralph stutters but we shouldn't say that he talks *funny*."

"Well, some kids think it's funny; they laugh at him and kid him when he talks. Porky is funny. People laugh at him."

"Yes, but Porky the Pig is supposed to be laughed at. His feelings can't be hurt."

"But Ralph doesn't care if we kid him. He just smiles. He kids us about things too. We're friends."

Effects of Speech Handicaps upon Behavior

The three dimensions of Johnson's concept of speech problems do not correlate uniformly in quality or in degree. It is evident, also, that only one or two of these dimensions may operate. One speaker may be maladjusted because of his concern over a speech problem which no longer exists, while a younger person may not be alerted to an existing problem—although others may be concerned about it. The relationships which exist between the person, his speech defect, and his society tend to be kaleidoscopic.

The Factors and Dynamics of Handicapped Behavior

The diagram below portrays how a speech problem may become a behavioral handicap, entangled with interrelated forces which determine either success or failure in the handicapped person's goal-directed activity. The diagram emphasizes the need for consideration of a person's problem "as a whole" —the physical and psychological aspects, the social involvements, and the

EFFECTS OF SPEECH HANDICAPS UPON BEHAVIOR

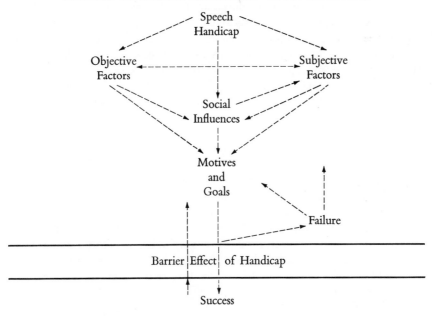

dynamic system in which all these factors contribute toward the person's ambitions and activity leading to success or failure. At times we must deal with certain meshes of this network, but we should not forget that the rest of the network exists. This diagram indicates how speech problems fit into this dynamic scheme.

SPEECH HANDICAPS

The earlier part of this chapter defined a speech problem and proposed criteria for measuring the extent of its handicap in personal and social behavior.

Speech handicaps are variously revealed: some are obvious to audiences; some are subtle and hard to detect. Moreover, no two persons, having what may seem to be the same outward handicap, are affected in exactly the same way or to the same degree. We must be cautious in judging the severity of a handicap from its outward symptoms. Some handicaps are greater below the surface. A high school senior, for example, continued to be handicapped in school recitations because of his extreme shyness, caused by being teased during his freshman year when he suffered from a temporary problem of uncontrolled pitch breaks in his voice. Although the physical and social causes and symptoms of this problem had been overcome, the personal insecurities remained to haunt his classroom speaking.

OBJECTIVE FACTORS

The objective factors of handicaps are the physical or intrinsic limitations of the disorder. They are generally overt, measurable, and may be identified in body structure and function. For example, in cleft palate cases, the objective limitations may include the abnormality of the speech structures, the excessive nasality of voice, greater susceptibility to ear infections and hearing complications, the abnormality of facial appearance, etc. These objective limitations would exist even though the person might be in complete mental harmony with them.

SUBJECTIVE FACTORS

These represent the limitations which come from the speaker's unfavorable interpretations and evaluations which he builds around his speech disorder. Subjective factors are the personal fears, prejudices, frustrations, anxieties, and other negative attitudes which tend to operate, often apart from the objective limitations, to hamper the person's aspiration, happiness, and achievements. It should be remembered, however, that body and mind are not separable, and that physical changes, like ulcers, may result from emotional maladjustments generated by a speech handicap, such as stuttering. A person with cleft palate may become further handicapped if he harbors such subjective problems as: feeling that his appearance is repulsive; fearing that his speech will be misunderstood or be comical; believing that his defect will be inheritable; and sensing that his cleft palate symptoms cause audience embarrassment. Some of these subjective views are based on fact; others are fanciful. But even when these subjective attitudes rest upon assumption instead of reality, they may lead to handicaps which are as real and potent as physical ones. Because a maladjusted person is not always aware of the piecemeal concepts which make up the disturbing aura of subjectivity surrounding his handicap, a main goal in speech therapy is to help him probe and review experiences, to give him insight into cause-effect relationships, and to help him reconcile the imbalance between subjectivity and objectivity.

SOCIAL INFLUENCES

A person's speech handicap may be adversely or favorably affected by other persons in numerous ways. These social influences may be verbal or nonverbal, intentional or not. A listener's facial expressions, for example, may tell a stutterer that his speech is being received with pity, embarrassment, uneasiness, humor, understanding, acceptance, or rejection. Through language there are endless ways to encourage, discourage, help, or hinder the handicapped speaker.

An important reciprocal interaction operates between social influences and the handicapped person's subjective attitudes. Two types of responses, empathic and sympathetic, exist in this relationship. The attitudes and reactions expressed by the handicapped person tend to determine similar attitudes in his audiences, acting back on the handicapped speaker, who tends to gauge his handicap as the others interpret it. A teacher may say, "I feel so sorry for pupils who struggle and get embarrassed when they stutter in recitation." A pupil tells how he is affected by this teacher's reactions when he replies, "I have a hard time reciting before my teacher because she feels so sorry that she almost bleeds for me. Then I try to keep from stuttering and becoming an object of pity. That really makes me stutter."

There are times when social influences are predetermined—in latent or perennial prejudices which are associated with certain speech handicaps, ready to be expressed when those handicaps appear. A teacher revealed this prejudicial misconception and faulty basis for handling a stutterer when she stated: "I've never had a pupil who stuttered, but if I should get one, I'd certainly not call on him to read or recite because the embarrassment would add to the emotionality which goes with stuttering."

Social influences upon a handicap sometimes spring from an audience's reactions to a specific external symptom which is judged apart from its true context with the handicap. A social influence of this type is seen in the following parent's statement: "When Fred stutters, his tongue gets stuck up in the roof of his mouth. I've told him time and again to practice some exercises to make it more limber, but he just gets irritated with me."

MOTIVATION AND GOALS

These are considered jointly because voluntary action toward goals implies incentives, even though the goals may be vague. The handicapped person's incentives and goals impinge from three sources: the objective features of the handicap; the subjective make-up of the speaker; and the social influences which affect his goal behavior. These three types of influence which shape the activity of a speech-handicapped person are illustrated in the following discussion of an eight-year-old boy with cerebral palsy:

We are in a dilemma with Phil. He wants to answer our phone at home; in fact, he has been urged by his speech therapist to use the phone as much as possible.

But his father relies upon our phone for business call-ins, and since Phil's speech is so difficult to understand at times, we don't want to lose important business because of this practice. Yet we don't want to discourage Phil from using the phone, because he needs all the speech practice he can get. Besides, he seems to apply his speech controls better over it. What would you suggest we do?

The foregoing case illustrates how a handicapped speaker and his desire to use the phone are affected not only by the physical realities of cerebral palsy but also by the several social factors which blend with his personal needs and attitudes to mold his ambitions and courses of action. Social influences, which often are dominant in determining a handicapped person's motives and goals, may help or hinder. Indiscriminate advice, unsound encouragement, discouragement, overprotectiveness, and domination from his associates can not only blight his individuality but can also confuse and misdirect his undeclared motives and goals. We find solicitous parents who, by their constant anticipation of and provision for their speech-handicapped child's needs and desires, reduce his motivation, confidence, and opportunity for developing speech. In their conscientious desire to ease the burdens of the handicapped speaker, struggling under obvious difficulty, they too often do too much *for* him but *without* him.

BARRIER EFFECT

Earlier in this chapter, the consideration of the criteria of speech problems indicated how speech handicaps may act as barriers. In Diagram 1, the negative value of the barrier indicates that a speech handicap may thwart success in a temporary, partial, or complete sense. Often, only time and experience will tell whether a barrier will be temporary or permanent. Much depends upon the changeable array of objective and social factors which constitute the barrier against the forces which lead to success. For instance, in the case of a severely maladjusted stutterer giving his first oral book report, the actual blocks which slow up his speaking may represent an objective problem if he is speaking in a situation where a time-limit is imposed upon his talking. His reluctance to let the class know that he is a stutterer may be a subjective aspect of the barrier. An impatient teacher who interrupts him with attempts to help on blocked words may become an added social barrier in making his recitation difficult or impossible.

SUCCESS

The attainment of a goal has the effect of reducing the negative significance of the handicap's limitations with feelings of confidence, self-reliance, optimism, hope, faith, security, courage, promise, adjustment, etc. The beneficent circle of success encourages greater interest, effort, and learning along lines leading to repetitions of that success.

When failure occurs after effort has met too great resistance and falls short of its goal, the effects are referred to by such popular terms as frustration, inferiority, bitterness, let-down, defeat, hopelessness, disappointment, insecurity, giving up, and so on. For the handicapped person, barriers contributing to failure assume greater negative force.

Reactions to failures may take other more devious forms; some are misinterpreted and their link with failure is overlooked. Illustrations of some of the more common reactions are listed below:

Withdrawal. "We have noticed that our nine-year-old boy, who stutters, has begun to retreat from the social scene when guests come to our home. He told us that he has too much trouble answering the 'dumb' personal questions that they often fire at him, and that they don't give him a chance to answer when he tries to."

Substitution. "When we look back on the extracurricular activities in Mary's high school life, we see several instances when she failed because of her cleft palate problems and then substituted something else, usually a second choice. In the band, before she settled for the kettle drums, she tried out several wind instruments and became convinced that her nasal emission ruled them out. She also tried out for the debate team, but the coach, who wanted winning teams, suggested that she would find more success in journalism, working on the school paper and annual—which she did."

Projection. "John has developed a strong dislike for substitute teachers. At first we thought it was the fault of poor substitutes; then we learned that his aversion to them came from the fact that he stuttered more around new teachers. Instead of blaming himself, he saw *them* as the source of the evil."

Self-blame. "Chet's stuttering has been a problem in his school life, all right, but not to the degree of handicap that he attributes to his speech defect. At times, I think that he unduly blames his poor speech for his failures. It disturbs me to see how he's becoming more ready to blame things upon his speech defect."

"Laziness". This term is placed within quotation marks to acknowledge that many perceptive teachers and therapists consider it to be taboo, worthless, and dangerous to use, because it is used often in a degrading sense without disclosing the valid and specific reasons for the indolent person's failure to work as hard or as fast as others expect him to work. Two examples of reported "laziness" follow:

"Before Susan was found to have a severe hearing loss, was fitted with a hearing aid, and given a front seat in her classroom, her teacher thought that she was 'uninterested and lazy.' Well, until she could hear and understand what was said around her in the classroom, she was uninterested, of course. But she wasn't *lazy*, in the usual sense of the word. Since she has gained the means to participate in class, she has become one of the most alert and hard-working members."

"In my conference with Roland's speech therapist she complained that he was 'apathetic and lazy' in speech class. I pointed out that Roland worked on his faulty *r* for seven years, under three speech therapists, and he's still stuck with that fault. He has complained to me that many of the exercises and drills have been repeated over and over, that he has lost hope of correcting his speech and considers therapy a bore and a waste of his time."

Alibis and Rationalizations. "Ruth would like to have plastic surgery to remove the faint scar that remains on her lip, stating that her lack of close friends in school may be due to that scar. She emphasized that if it weren't what others thought about her scar, she wouldn't give it a second thought. But she's more sensitive about the scar than she lets on."

Compensations. "Mike has always had a tiny, high-pitched, effeminate voice. Now since he has grown to be such a big boy, he sounds ridiculous. In his insecurity over his little voice, he tries to bolster his masculine image in various ways; some of his tactics are not so good. He has gone in for football and really plays a rough, bruising game. In fact, he has become a bully off the field too. He tries to assert his manliness in dress, haircut, and even by salting his informal speech with four-letter words. Actually, some of his adopted manners add to the incongruity of his voice, rather than counteracting it."

Rebellious or Negativistic Behavior. "John's speech problem is getting under his skin. Lately he has developed a dislike for school, complaining that the kids tease him about his cleft lip and faulty speech. He carries a chip on his shoulder, has been in several fights resulting from teasing, and he resents being called on to recite."

The frustrations and failures caused by speech handicaps may take other more obscure and puzzling forms. Often the behavioral reactions to speech problems are misjudged and the roots of the problems are overlooked. Many children who are thwarted in communication are tagged with terms which refer to secondary symptoms of their problems rather than to primary causes. When children are thus mislabeled, the resulting treatment may go astray and compound their basic problems.

Types of Speech Problems

The various classifications of speech and language problems may be indistinct and divided broadly on the basis of their origins in organic or in functional causes. Organic and functional factors are often intertwined. Examples of organic problems which lead to speech problems are: faulty anatomical structures in cleft palate cases; the loss of the larynx or tongue from cancer operations; the loss of neuromuscular control from cerebral palsy or strokes; and vocal effects from ulcers and nodules on the vocal cords. Other organic abnormalities, like loss of teeth, malocclusion, "tongue-tie," and abnormal size of tongue may or may not cause defective speech. However, these various organic elements usually become linked with functional factors which also determine a speaker's ability to adjust and to compensate for these organic deviations.

Speech problems of a functional nature refer to the emotional factors and the elements of learning and habituation which enter into the speech act. Most cases of misarticulation can be explained on the basis of functional or environmental conditions, such as poor teaching methods, insufficient motivation, inadequate experience, faulty models for learning, the lack of practice, and emotional states which interfere with learning. Stuttering, for instance, is usually regarded as an emotionally based problem, growing from conflicts which overburden speech during its formative stages in early childhood. A child's speech output may be inhibited by emotional maladjustment, which may induce a substituted form of language based upon gestures and other devised symbols for communication.

The classification of disorders becomes more discriminative and practical when we group these disorders on a more analytical basis, in terms of their affected elements or processes, rather than solely on their broad organic or functional origins. There is limited value in concluding that a person has "brain-injured" speech. That statement indicates only where the primary source of the fault may be, but nothing else. It does not guarantee classification of what aspects of speech or language are affected. A more informative and useful statement of the problem would be to say that the person has the history and the symptoms of being "brain-injured," that he has retained his comprehension of words and spoken sentences but has lost the ability to express word concepts and to arrange them in correct grammatical order unless he can immediately imitate them verbatim after someone else. In this more detailed description, there is an attempt to analyze the total problem and to assign the difficulties to specific areas and processes within speech and language. The last statements suggest better guidelines for therapy.

Thus, another classification of speech problems refers to the behavioral elements of its language aspects, the oral articulation of these linguistic units, the voicing of linguistic patterns, and the rhythm or time patterns of speech. The following classification of speech disorders indicates how each of these areas may become disordered.

LANGUAGE PROBLEMS

Chapter VII will disclose how language may be lacking or faulty and how various deficits are labeled. *Aphasia* and *dysphasia* refer to language problems associated with brain injury or diseases which interfere with neurological control. *Delayed speech* or *retarded speech* are broad terms which usually refer to slowness in the development of spoken vocabulary and grammar. Delayed speech or language may have many causes, extending into the categories of articulation, emotion, language, and others. An impairment of the central nervous system may cause disorders in language forms other than speech. *Alexia* applies to reading ·disorders based upon neurological cause; *agraphia* relates to disorders in writing. However, one should avoid using these terms loosely in referring to miscellaneous problems which are not brain-centered. Concluding prematurely that the problems arise from "brain-injury" may deny the cases their needed treatment.

MISARTICULATION

In this category, too, descriptive terms may be vague, overlapping, and misapplied. A speaker may be described by a speech therapist as having *misarticulation* but by a teacher as using poor *pronunciation* or *enunciation*. Although a dictionary shows that these terms are synonymous, a speech therapist is inclined to think of misarticulation as being faulty production of the sound alphabet which composes language, while a teacher tends to notice articulatory errors when they mar language at the wider word and sentence levels of speech. There is justification for keeping both points of view in mind if we are to judge and treat speech as spoken language rather than as mere sound production of a repertoire of phonemes. Furthermore, the spoken sounds in language units may be faulty in several ways: through *substitution, omission, distortion,* and *addition.* For example, when a child says, "I tsaw dat appol fa down," he is distorting the *s* in *saw*, substituting a *d* for the *th* in *that*, adding an *o* within the *pl* blend in *apple*, and omitting the *l* in *fall*. Chapter 6 will consider these types of articulatory errors and will indicate how their severity and treatment may depend upon their type of error.

VOICE PROBLEMS

In *aphonia*, the failure to voice the articulation will cause speech to be whispered or merely mouthed—as it is when voices are lost from laryngitis or when vocal cords are removed by operation for cancer. But speaking voices may deviate in other ways, with problems of *pitch, intensity,* and *quality.* When the pitch level of speech is not in harmony with the person's sex and age, the effect may create personal and social handicaps, according to the criteria discussed earlier in this chapter. When a person does not use the customary inflectional patterns required for the numerous shades of meaning in his language, his listeners realize how much communication depends upon the vocal· "key" and the meaningful "tunes" of each language. They sense this importance of voice patterns when they have difficulty in understanding the monotonous speech of the congenitally deaf person who has never had the chance to learn these tonal patterns in speech. The importance of pitch is revealed when an audience tries to understand a foreign speaker who reads their language in a word-by-word fashion, using foreign inflectional patterns which do not fit the language. From the standpoint of intensity, the speaking voice may be too loud or not loud enough. The child must learn to monitor his voice and to vary the loudness of his speech according to the demands of situations. Teachers complain about the "shy" voice of the insecure child who cannot be heard in noisy, large classrooms; however, parents may have repeatedly reprimanded that same child at home for speaking too loudly. Chapter 10 will continue the analysis of some factors which enter into our judgments and treatment of inadequate intensity of speech.

No area of speech is more variable and difficult to describe or to standardize than is that of speech-voice *quality*. Speakers' voices, from the very birth cry, are as individualistic as fingerprints, with wide variations in voice quality causing problems when the vocal characteristics are odd and distracting. Deviations of resonance or nasality may characterize a voice as *husky, hoarse, harsh, breathy,* and *strident.*

RHYTHM OR FLUENCY

Chapter 1 indicated that normal speech is an integrated sequence of movements in which the timing and the patterns of rate are physiologically imposed upon the speaker, with their fortunate conveyance of linguistic meaning. A voice scientist, when asked about the problems in inventing a machine which would simulate normal human speech, replied:

> One of the most difficult speech features to program and to produce mechanically would be the variable changes in rate which mark the flow of oral language. We do not grind out sounds, syllables, words, and phrases at an even and steady pace, you know. Even if we could make a machine which would articulate correctly each of the correct speech sounds in proper order, its speech would be strange and meaningless if it spaced sound units equally. Speech like this would be as obliterated as a tune would be from a music box from which every note of a tune was cranked out as an evenly spaced full note.

Stuttering and *cluttering* are two disorders of fluency described in Chapter 8. There are many degrees of nonfluency which differentiate speakers, and the standards for judging normality are not clear. The rapid rate of the facile auctioneer may make his speech unintelligible to some listeners, but to others in his audience his speech may seem normal and easily understandable. The slow and hesitant speech of other speakers may lack communicative impact if it distracts listeners. Chapter 8 will point out that some problems in speech fluency are neglected in the confusions over recognizing the vague bounds which separate normality from abnormality in speech rate and fluency.

Diagnosing Speech Problems

Although timely and accurate diagnosis must precede the treatment of speech disorders, it also continues with the treatment and should never become separate from it. Johnson, Darley, and Spriestersbach[3] discuss in detail the diagnostic methods in speech pathology: the necessity for gathering information on the developmental history of a problem; its present status, its causal and maintaining factors; a tentative formulation of treatment; and an attempt at prognosis.

A school teacher has an important role in diagnosing speech and language problems. Often she is the first school professional to notice the problem and, if necessary, to refer it to speech therapists, physicians, and others for help in the problem's diagnosis and solution. Speech therapists depend upon classroom teachers to supply information for defining the problems and for charting the course of therapeutic action. A teacher's role fits into four phases of the diagnostic process: recognizing and defining the problem; judging its importance; studying the cause-effect relationships which surround the problem; and conducting diagnostic trial therapy.

RECOGNIZING AND DEFINING THE PROBLEM

The first steps in correcting any problem should recognize that a problem exists and should clarify and pinpoint its nature and location. The initial awareness and concept of a problem are often vague, but systematic observation, testing, and verification clarify the picture and judgment of symptoms. A capable first-grade teacher, who had worked extensively with speech therapists, gave the following views concerning her recognition and appraisal of speech problems:

> At first, my pupils' speech problems were rather hazy to me. I had feelings that something was not right, but when I tried to describe the problem in words, I realized that my descriptions were not specific enough. After I took a course in speech correction and had worked around speech therapists for a while, I became acquainted with the parts and mechanics of speech, the symptoms of various problems, and standards—and the vocabulary for describing this information.

In each of the chapters of this book, we shall study the symptoms which identify each speech disorder. When a problem is well described and well defined, it is often half-solved. Problems must be pointed and freed of irrelevancies, not left in an umbrella-like form of safe generalities. One diagnostician has made the following appeal for more careful preparation of the problem area before launching forth into therapy:

> Therapy, like an artillery attack, would be more effective if we'd bracket, triangulate, and then zero in on the problem, rather than to bombard the target area with a standard battery of rounds fired indiscriminately, without correction from observed misses.

Having noted and defined the child's speech or language problem, the teacher, often with aid from the therapist, then must judge its importance, its severity, its handicap value, and whether or not corrective measures are indicated, then or later. One kindergarten teacher has stressed the need for cooperation in making referrals for speech therapy:

> Our school has a general policy that no kindergartners will receive speech therapy unless their speech problems are severe. Well, this division point is not always clear to me or to the speech therapist, either, when I refer doubtful cases to her. We must decide not only how far a problem exceeds the norms, but also whether or not the problem in question will respond to treatment which she, I, or both of us can give—or whether others should be called upon to help. Of course, the answers to some of these questions are often delayed until the therapist and I have done further investigation and trial therapy with the case. Whenever I'm in doubt, I confer with our speech therapist.

Another important requirement in the diagnosis of speech and language problems rests upon our knowledge of the causal factors which underlie each speech disorder. It is important to know the processes by which the problem grows and becomes complicated, and the signs which indicate these favorable or unfavorable trends in the problem's development. There are many unanswered questions in these important areas of speech pathology, despite the thousands of research projects that have been aimed at them. Yet in speech pathology, as in all sciences, a mounting fund of information from research is steadily establishing our guidelines for a better understanding of the life settings of speech and language problems, the factors which create problems, and the dynamics by which problems develop for better or for worse. The director of a noted training center for speech and hearing therapists emphasized the need for understanding cause-effect relationships when he said:

> Too much of our past emphasis in speech correction courses has been devoted to What? ... What? ... What? ... classification ... pigeon-holing of isolated "facts" ... the faithful itemizing of symptoms placed under properly assigned tabs. A share of this stuff is worth teaching and learning, but we must do a lot more. We must follow up with sincere, tough-minded attempts to answer such questions as: Why-so? ... What-if? ... So, what? ... Why? ... If this is true, what then? ... How can I tell if this is so? ... Is this a true cause-and-effect relationship? We cannot be content to be glib name-callers; we must try to explain, too.

In speech correction we should proceed as we do in any problem-solving process, especially since speech and language problems are relatively complex and difficult to understand and solve. After we have spotted and defined the problem, and have gathered and analyzed sufficient information pertinent to it and its treatment, our next phase in speech or language therapy becomes more creative. Often as we work at a speech problem, either in preparation for therapy or in the course of trial therapy, we change our concept of the problem; consequently, we change our goals and procedures in therapy. As Osborn[4] explains, preparation and analysis go hand in hand, while our progress toward the solution of a speech problem will be determined by the extent to which we pile up hypotheses. Our speech therapy must often be based on our most creative and educated hypotheses; while the results from this trial therapy will indicate the efficacy and direction of these chosen hypotheses. An experienced speech therapist has explained trial therapy in this way:

> Much of my understanding of a case and his problem comes after I start therapy with him. After I spend a reasonable amount of time and effort upon diagnosis, I begin therapy. Therapy itself, however, is often diagnostic, providing the answers which verify whether or not my diagnostic hunches were right, whether I should follow this or that approach. Problem-solving in our field must be a step-by-step process based upon information, ideas, and moves correlated around the client—not a prepackaged set of formulas. //

Prevention of Speech and Language Problems

A state consultant, addressing a convention of speech therapists, once made this challenge:

> If we directed our efforts more to the prevention of some of our obstinate speech and language problems, instead of waiting until the problems develop and become chronic and then trying to cure them, we'd accomplish much more than we do. Or if we started therapeutic action earlier, during the incipient stages of some of the disorders, like stuttering, we'd have a higher percentage of "cures." Better yet, many of these speech problems would never exist.
>
> Why do we work on correction more than on prevention? Does our training as speech pathologists create too much of an attraction in us for the pathological end of the human behavioral spectrum? Can we derive as much satisfaction from working to prevent problems through cooperative work with other persons? Can we feel as professionally important by nipping problems in their early stages before they become spectacular and crying needs? Perhaps we are not as well trained to prevent problems and to give "first aid" measures.
>
> Regardless, the hope for greatest results from our service lies in the prevention

of certain disorders. To accomplish this, we may be required to limit our present efforts to correct the relatively fixed terminal cases which attract our help. As in the case of polio, if preventive research and treatment had not occurred, we should still be swamped with efforts to correct the ravaging effects of the terminal disease. As with preventive medicine, there is more credit and glamour in preventing speech or language problems than in alleviating developed ones.

References

1. C. Van Riper, *Speech Correction: Principles and Methods.* Englewood Cliffs, N.J.: Prentice-Hall, Inc., 1963.

2. W. Johnson, S. F. Brown, J. F. Curtis, C. W. Edney, and J. Keaster, *Speech Handicapped School Children.* New York: Harper & Row, Inc., 1967.

3. W. Johnson, F. L. Darley, and D. C. Spriestersbach, *Diagnostic Methods in Speech Pathology.* New York: Harper & Row, Inc., 1963.

4. A. F. Osborn, *Applied Imagination: Principles and Procedures of Creative Thinking.* New York: Charles Scribner's Sons, 1953.

Questions

1. How do Van Riper and Johnson define a speech problem?

2. Have you known cases of speech problems which fitted these definitions?

3. Can laymen, even young children, make accurate observations of speech problems?

4. Is there a consistent correlation between the outward symptoms of a speech handicap and its severity?

5. Describe the objective factors of a speech handicap other than cleft palate.

6. What are the subjective factors which may inhibit the handicapped speaker?

7. Is it possible for adverse social influences to initiate and crystallize a speech handicap?

8. What organic defects may cause speech defects?

9. How many functional causes affect speech?

10. Define: aphasia; alexia; agraphia.

11. What are the causes of misarticulation?

12. What opportunities exist to correct voice problems of pitch, intensity, and quality?

13. Rhythm patterns have been compared to thumbprints. Why?

14. Why is the classroom teacher an important factor in diagnosing speech problems?

15. How may a teacher develop better awareness and concept of a speech problem?

16. In schools without speech therapists, how may a teacher find help in diagnosing speech problems?

17. In searching for a successful method of therapy, may the teacher dare to try more than one or two?

18. Which appeals to you more: an apparently fixed terminal case crying for help or an early case with a vaguely defined problem?

19. What is the effect of a person's dialect or foreign language on his speech production and reception?

20. What is the effect on a speaker of a wide variation from the norm—such as a high-pitched voice in a boy or a guttural monotone in a girl?

21. In what way does a faint voice create a speech problem?

22. The normal "Me, too!" enthusiasm of babyhood may continue in timid children as a withdrawn fixation centered on self. How would you interest him in the *you's*, and the *they's* around him?

23. How would you aid a child handicapped by a disagreeable tone of voice?

24. Discuss the value of setting up a recognizable goal for the handicapped child.

25. What may be the effect of hand and body gestures on speech?

26. When do most parents begin to worry about speech handicaps of their children?

27. Questioning aroused by curiosity is a useful aid to speech for the average child. What are the devices which speech-handicapped children must use to acquire information?

28. Children from seriously substandard environments are often ignorant and bewildered enough in new situations to become lethargic or antagonistic. What is the best preliminary treatment for such behavior?

Suggested Subjects for Term Papers

1. Describe some concrete social influences which may thwart the handicapped speaker in reaching his goals.
2. Prepare a questionnaire to investigate public attitudes on the seriousness of speech problems. Compile your findings from fellow students, landladies, librarians, store clerks, and others.

3. Make a survey of a dozen cities regarding their school policies of deciding at what stage speech problems should receive attention.
4. Make a survey of twenty-five parents on their views concerning the causes and correction of various speech problems.
5. Make a survey of twelve classroom teachers on their views concerning the causes and correction of various speech problems.

five

Problems of Speech
Output in the Classroom

In this chapter the problems related to pupils' speech output or talkativeness in school will be described and evaluated. Causal factors will be analyzed and case histories presented, suggesting a few procedures by which teachers have helped children with problems involving speech output.

Types of Problems

It is difficult to define and measure problems which come under the category of "speech output." A speaker's production of talking must be judged against a background of many considerations, depending upon subjective and objective factors. Talkativeness may be measured in terms of talking duration, the number of words or sentences spoken, the length of the verbal response, the number of different persons with whom the speaker talked. We often differ in our interpretations of these patterns of speech output. For example, a sensitive pupil who has been snickered at during recitation for having substituted a *w* for an *r* may become less talkative in class, reciting reluctantly in a telegrammic manner in order to minimize the likelihood of disclosing his errors. However, if a teacher observes that this pupil is highly verbal on the playground, she may view his classroom reticence to mean that he does not know his subject matter or that he has a poor command of language. The conditions which cause variations in speech output are often overlooked or misread.

Various problems of speech output are illustrated in the following cases described by teachers, parents, and pupils.

THE "CHATTERBOX"

There are children, like adults, who talk too much, who "don't know when to stop," who "talk out of turn," who irritate by being noisy "magpies," etc. There are conversationalists, young and old, who make excessive use of

82

the language which we popularly refer to as small talk, chitchat, idle talk, gossip, chatter, babble, prattle, tête-à-tête, chewing-the-rag, etc. At times these conversational skills fulfill worthwhile purposes, but when they predominate and interfere with listening and other skills in the art of conversation, they become personal and social handicaps.

A teacher describes overtalkativeness in pupils in this way:

> Having taught in all elementary grades, I have made some interesting observations of children who talk too much. Usually, in every classroom there are one or more children who are too talkative. Unless I can curb their verbal flow and teach them to regulate when and how much to talk, problems arise. Children who monopolize recitations and who talk more than their share tend to upstage other children and create in them feelings of inferiority, subservience, hopelessness, and so on. It's frightening to see how quickly pupils in my class establish their "peck order" of who is to have the first and last word, and who is expected to have the most important "say." Even we teachers soon learn who the "eager-beaver" speakers are, and unless their verbosity interferes with our poise and philosophy in teaching, we may give in to their speech domination and even cater to them at the expense of the more quiet pupils.

The father of five young children makes the following complaint about how his eldest son and daughter talk more than they should during the family's meal conversations:

> Our family's meal situation is often noisy and hectic. It's about the only time the seven of us are together to share news of interest, to give and get information, etc. But, usually I find myself acting as a sergeant-at-arms, trying to check the endless flow of dialogue between Phil and Sue, who keep the rest of us from entering their verbal duel. Although we have allotted Joan, our five-year-old, the dubious honor of saying grace, she barely gets the "Amen" out before either Phil or Sue takes over. The three youngest children don't have much leeway to get in their two cents of conversation, even on subjects which rightfully belong to them. I don't like to get tough and crack down on their enthusiastic jabber, but I'll have to do it. The rest of us have things to say, too, and there's tension building all around the family circle.

THE "SHY SPEAKER"

When pupils fail to talk as much or as often as the average, they appear to be shy. Just as shyness, introversion, insecurity, and fear are conditions which ordinarily tend to inhibit speech output, so outgoing, aggressive, well-adjusted, and sociable traits encourage speech. However, teachers, parents, and others may have different standards for judging a lack of verbal output in children. There are parents who believe that children should be seen but not heard in conversation between adults. They would not rate a shy talker, brought into adult conversations, the same as would parents who feel that children should be heard from as well as seen in adult situations. Teachers who value the personal freedoms of thought and speech in their pupils tend to be more concerned about the shy talker, while teachers who favor an orderly, quiet, and receptive atmosphere in their classroom may be less inclined to expect and to desire more speech from the shy speaker. This is the comment of a teacher to the parents of a pupil who she felt did not speak enough in class:

> Joan is a capable and cooperative pupil. She is interested in all subjects and really could contribute more than most pupils do in class discussions. But so far she has not found herself in recitation. She speaks when she is asked questions, but she hesitates to volunteer or to give her opinions in class discussions. I'm working to encourage her to do more of this, though. Lately she has shown more confidence; she doesn't cut her recitations as short as she did at first.

The following remark was made in a teachers' lounge in reference to pupils who do not talk enough:

> Well, it may be that some of our pupils don't talk enough in class, but give me a roomful of pupils who speak only when I want them to talk. I'm cramped enough to get the chance to say what I want to say in class, without having to ration and regulate what comes from thirty other mouths. Children get enough chance to talk outside the classroom. After all, pupils come to school to learn from teachers and books, don't they? If we let our pupils talk as much as they'd like, we wouldn't have much chance to talk, and our rooms would be in more of a hubbub than they are.

THE SPEECHLESS PUPIL

A child's failure to speak may be due to an inability or an unwillingness to speak. It may be limited to the classroom or school situation, or it may apply to his entire life area. Obviously, teachers are quick to notice a speechless pupil, especially in the elementary grades, and to feel strong concern over the many problems which may arise from his failure to communicate. As one teacher has stated:

> It's not surprising each year to find several emotionally immature children who refuse to speak for a while upon entering kindergarten. Usually a child's silence lasts only several hours, days, or weeks. But sometimes he continues to be a non-talker for months and even years. Then it really becomes a major problem which may tax our wits and patience, especially if it's a child who indicates to us that he can talk but won't, that he does talk freely on the playground or at home but won't speak in our classroom.

ABBREVIATED SPEECH

This term refers to the use of incomplete language units. Pupils who speak in a skeletal style may have an insufficient command of language or a speech problem which makes the act of speech difficult or embarrassing for them. They may have forms of emotional maladjustments which inhibit and induce speakers to adopt telegrammic styles of utterance or to learn a pattern of language which is required for communication under certain limiting environmental conditions. However, the use of shortened speech does not necessarily mean that the speaker is shy, has failed to learn complete language structures, or has an underlying speech problem. Abbreviated speech sometimes represents a style of communication which the speaker's environment has forced him to adopt. A teacher who has taught in a ghetto neighborhood of a large city describes a speech-handicapped second grader in this way:

> Julian is sociable and talkative, but his speech is full of grammatical gaps. He tries to make single words serve to convey the meanings which are usually carried by sentences. Even some of his words are clipped short, like a verbal shorthand. Moreover, he assumes that we understand his verbal shorthand and gets impatient when we can't catch what he says.
>
> But when the speech therapist visited Julian's home in the tenement district and observed his speech environment, she saw that Julian's mother and two pre-school-aged brothers were talking similarly. They lived in a noisy and crowded flat where talking had to be conveyed by shouted word signals rather than by normally spoken sentences. The interruptions and hubbub of activities made listening a hit-and-miss and momentary matter. Speech had to be "catch as catch can" in order to be heard or attended to. The therapist reported that the younger children and their mother communicated much better with each other than they did with the therapist in that home situation, when she tried to speak with them in full sentences.

"FABRICATED" SPEECH

This term refers more to the nature of what is said than it does to the amount of speech output. However, it should be included with the afore-mentioned problems of speech output because when a child or an adult stretches the truth, spins tall tales, or lies, he may also be looked upon as a person who talks more than he should. "Lying" is relatively common in childhood, when the division between fantasy and reality is unclear. As one kindergarten teacher says:

> In my show-tell periods, I have learned to expect and tolerate a mixture of truth and untruth in what young children say; some do not speak much else than fantasy, in which there may be more excitement and satisfaction than in their more drab realities. But I'd much rather have a verbal "story teller" than a silent daydreamer who does not share his thoughts with us. Most children eventually learn to separate fact from fiction. In the process they exercise language and are given a chance to reveal and fulfill some of their personal and social needs.

Causal Factors and
Correction

Unless the cause or causes of a particular problem involving speech output are known, treatment of it may be ineffective and may even worsen the problem. The pupil who incessantly chatters in the classroom may not do so for the same reasons that prompt other speakers to talk too little, to lie, or to refuse to speak at all. Suppose, for example, that a child had been encouraged by her parents and teacher to recite freely and excessively during her three years of kindergarten, first, and second grades, and that her effervescent verbal nature had been fostered primarily by her conscientious desire to gain and to cultivate the approval of her teacher. Suppose further that this girl suffered a reversal when she met her third-grade teacher, who sharply disapproved of talkative pupils and who traumatically punished her by changing her seat to a neglected far corner of the classroom, a move to keep her shamefully reminded that her verbal output was offensive to the teacher. Under this change of influences within the classroom, this former "chatterbox" may become a "shy" speaker in the judgment of succeeding teachers with their differing standards concerning pupils and their speech output. And later there may be failure to recognize that in this girl's background had been both a "chatterbox" and a "shy" speaker and that both patterns of her speech output were fed from the same primary source, her conscientious desire to please the teacher and to maintain her approved standing as a pupil. As one professional states: "Suspected causes are at best just educated guesses. Therapy proceeds on the best known evidence, but diagnosis is continuous. A therapist must be flexible enough to evaluate new evidence and make needed changes in therapy."

Since patterns of talkativeness are often established during the child's preschool years, his parents and home conditions are important areas to explore. At times, home factors continue to influence a child's speech output during his school years. The next case, described by a speech therapist, illustrates how the home may condition a child to become nearly speechless at school:

> Stephanie was referred to me by her kindergarten teacher, who reported that the girl had not spoken a word in school. No one had observed her speaking in any school situation, not even on the playground, riding on the bus, or at lunch period. When Stephanie's problem was referred to me, two months after she had begun school, I started by observing her in various situations, being careful not to let her know that I was around specifically to observe her. She was attentive and interested, but silently cooperative in classroom activities. On the playground she was sociable and appeared to enjoy games and children. Other children seemed to accept her, and there were no signs that she was being penalized for not speaking. I heard her laugh several times during play, but there were none of the shouted interjections that young children spontaneously utter during play. Having observed Stephanie in these various situations at school, I decided to visit her home and interview her parents while she was in school. Her one-year-

old brother, who was at home, appeared normal. But her home gave me some hints of possible causes of her silence at school, even though her parents were not yet aware that Stephanie was not speaking there. Her mother reported that Stephanie enjoyed school and readily answered questions her parents asked about her school experience. I observed that the home was neat and orderly, showing strong religious overtones in the form of framed mottoes, plaques, and statuettes. It was interesting to learn that Stephanie attended Sunday school, in a class taught by her mother, who took pride in the fact that Stephanie knew her weekly lessons better than the other children did. In the Sunday school program, she participated in singing and speaking, although she spoke only when asked questions.

But, despite the mother's intelligent concern and sincere desire to help with her daughter's school problem, I ended that home visit without much reliable evidence to explain the child's refusal to speak. We agreed that it would not be advisable to mention to Stephanie the purpose of my visit, nor to disclose to her that her parents had learned of her refusal to talk at school.

Stephanie's teacher and I held a conference, pooled our information and ideas, and drew up a plan of attack which emphasized two goals: to strengthen Stephanie's security at school in every way and to build a warm and solid relationship between Stephanie and her teacher. We decided that presently I would not schedule the child for any direct therapy with me.

Well, within three months we had Stephanie talking, thanks mainly to her teacher's wise implementation of our planned program. The teacher accomplished this rapport by discovering Stephanie's interests and points of success and sharing her feelings of pride and gladness over her various achievements. Within the classroom, the teacher created informal social situations in which the pupils, singly or in pairs, could help the teacher with certain enjoyable "chores" before and after school, between bus schedules, etc. Later, after Stephanie had begun to talk in these chore projects with the teacher, some of the activities were moved into the regular class periods. For example, Stephanie and one of her favorite classmates were given the chance at noonhour to help arrange educational posters and displays around the classroom. They also helped to erase blackboards. During classtime, she shared with other pupils the appreciated chance to distribute art paper. She enjoyed her turn to operate the projector in a phonic lesson which was designed around strip films. While waiting for the bus, she was given the satisfying opportunity to help the teacher paste and mount pictures to be used later in classroom phonic practice. In all of these helpful activities, the teacher did not intentionally press Stephanie for speech; she worked only to create an atmosphere in which a child could normally feel like speaking in a spontaneous, "natural" way. Later, when the girl began to talk, the teacher was careful not to make any special ado over it.

Stephanie was soon talking as much as her classmates. It was interesting that her classmates offered no special comments or questions concerning Stephanie's change from silence to speaking. At home, too, the parents gladly learned of their daughter's victory without making any fuss over it.

Not all "speechless" pupils are handled as successfully as the foregoing case. Ted and Cheryl, who were classmates in the same grades and were taught by the same teachers, are examples where the problem continued and grew.

Cheryl's refusal to speak lasted until the third grade, when it was partially corrected; while Ted's problem became so chronic and complicated that his asocial and introverted behavior was finally diagnosed as autism, a case in need of intensive psychiatric help which was not available. The following summary of their long-standing speech problems was made by the speech therapist when she initiated a speech correction program in the school during their third-grade year.

When I began screening for speech problems, it was obvious that everyone in school knew about Cheryl and Ted and the notorious campaigns which had been tried for three years to get them to talk in school. Active interest in Ted's problem had subsided because he had not talked for three years in any school situation; Cheryl's problem had become increasingly exasperating because teachers had observed her talking on the playground and on the bus, and yet she refused to talk in their classrooms. Many persons had tried to crack Ted's and Cheryl's silence: their three teachers, two principals, their parents, a bus driver, the janitor, other children, a family physician, the school nurse, a county diagnostician, and a child guidance clinic. Reportedly, all had failed. But all these attempts and failures had left an aura of mystery and challenge. As the principal commented, "The reputations and honor of different professionals have been at stake; glory lies ahead for anyone who finds the combination to unlock their mouths."

So, when I came upon the scene, I met all kinds of theories on what should be done or what should not have been done. I was told that the kindergarten teacher had followed an inconsistent policy, starting with an assumed gentle disregard of the children's refusal to speak, then shifting to a period of several weeks while activities were structured so that speech would bring rewards while failure to speak would be penalized. Finally, after the teacher had failed to get results from a personal talk with each of the children, openly appealing to their reasons for talking, she resorted to a policy of trying to put pressure on them by deliberately ignoring them for the remainder of the school year.

The first-grade teacher had followed from the sidelines the futile strategy in Ted's and Cheryl's first year of management. She maintained that a child was sent to school to learn, that his teachers knew best what he should do in school, and that his education demanded from him self-discipline and social conformity. Cheryl and Ted were expected to participate in speech activities and were told to do like the rest of the class. Their refusal to speak was met by reactions which were designed by the teacher to make them feel "left out" and variously penalized for not speaking. At first, these reactions were expressed only by the teacher; later, she induced her pupils to assume added responsibility for showing rejection, disrespect, and intolerance toward Cheryl and Ted for not speaking in classroom activities. I am convinced, however, that this teacher meant well in all of this. Perhaps, in addition to her concern for the children's welfare, she felt that their failure to speak was a reflection on her teaching ability, although both children showed that they were learning to write, spell, and read silently. Except for speaking, both children were cooperative. Cheryl, who spoke only outside the school building, switched to playing mostly with kindergarten children. Ted remained completely nontalkative at school and began to show increasing signs of asocial and dreamy tendencies. His tight silence at school had attracted the interest of other school personnel. The janitor and bus driver had tried to stimulate him to speak through friendly attempts at conversation. When that approach failed, the janitor turned to bribery, offering Ted "five dollars to buy anything you want" if he would talk. The principal arranged with his teacher to send Ted and Cheryl on errands to his office, hoping that he could influence them to add verbally to the written information they carried to him. It should be noted, however, that the school had not yet approached the children's parents for help with their speech problem.

Cheryl's and Ted's second-grade term was marked with a series of referrals and examinations. During this year the teacher ignored their speechlessness, hoping that solutions would come from the work of specialists and agencies to whom the problem had been referred. The school nurse arranged a conference with the parents of each child. She pointed out the seriousness of their speech problem and recommended physical examinations by their family physicians. Their doctors found no physical abnormalities and diagnosed both cases as being psychologically caused, since both children reportedly were talking at home. Next, the county's school diagnostician was asked to give each child a series of psychometric tests. Because they would not speak to this school psychologist, only nonverbal performance tests could be given. The tests confirmed that both children were within the range of normal intelligence. Observations of them in the test situations and information gathered from parents, teachers, and others, led the psychologist to diagnose the problem as being emotionally based and to recommend that the parents contact the county's child guidance center. Ted's parents refused to apply for help at the child guidance center; Cheryl's parents waited seven weeks for the first of the three appointments which they and Cheryl attended before the close of that school year. The following conclusion and recommendations were sent to Cheryl's school by the center's child psychiatrist:

"We believe that this child's refusal to speak at school is a symptom of emotional conflicts, originating from traumatic preschool experience and reinforced by broadening influences and experiences which have fixed her concepts and reactions as a nonspeaking pupil. However, except for her failure to reconcile herself as a speaker in the classroom, we do not regard this child to be emotionally maladjusted in a broad sense. But, unless this speech conflict is removed, her maladjustments are likely to grow and create new problems.

"We have given Cheryl's parents counseling on matters which should improve her security at home and at school. Her parents have aired their concerns, and they may have gained insights into their daughter's situation and how they can help her to feel more adequate at home and in school. Efforts in counseling were focused upon reducing the parents' perfectionistic views and high standards, their puritanical ideas about living, and their intolerance of errors and failure. We attempted to show them how these factors may relate to a child's failure to speak at school, before teachers, etc. The parental conferences ended after three sessions, reportedly because of the parents' difficulty in arranging transportation and time off from work.

"Our most hopeful recommendations for solving Cheryl's problem are directed toward her daily school situations. As you indicated in your school's reports to us, many different approaches have been tried, and it is apparent that failures to help her may have resulted not because certain goals and methods were mistaken but because of the difficulties which prevented your working sufficiently and consistently toward these goals. Nevertheless, we believe that Cheryl will start talking in school only when she develops a true self-desire and confidence to talk there."

"Although we are not in touch with your everyday school situations in which therapeutic influences may be channeled and adapted for Cheryl, we shall be glad to arrange conferences with you to discuss methods for helping her there."

At present, halfway through their third-grade year of school, Ted remains speechless; Cheryl's tongue is showing signs of loosening. Since fall, when I initiated the school's speech therapy program, I have scheduled both children for individual therapy. My goals for Ted have been mainly to earn his respect and affection. By sharing his interest in stamp collecting, by bringing books on stamps, and through exchanges of our stamps, I have at least won from him a few thin smiles, headshakes, and nods in our dealings. Reportedly, he told his parents that he likes me and our work with stamps. I'm hoping he will learn that people and speaking can add enjoyment for him at school.

As for Cheryl, the situation looks brighter. Fortunately, the kindergarten teacher and I picked up a valuable clue last fall when Cheryl's brother started in kindergarten and it was noticed that she had a close and affectionate interest in him. Moreover, she freely talked with her brother during recesses, before school, on the playground, and even in his classroom, where she was inclined to visit. Cheryl's teacher, her brother's kindergarten teacher, and I held a conference to decide how we could use this favorable brother-sister relationship as an opening wedge to crack her speech problem. We decided to let Cheryl visit her brother's kindergarten room during one of her daily recess periods, giving her some acceptable duties as a teacher's helper in an activity which invited speaking with her brother and later with the class as a whole. Cheryl welcomes this chance to visit her brother's classroom.

For several weeks she was given non-speaking chores, such as distributing and collecting art materials and holding up attractive composite pictures of action scenes, around which the teacher guided interesting class conversation. During some of these chores, Cheryl spoke comments and directions to the kindergartners and to the teacher as well. Then the teacher conducted a series of story-reading sessions in which Cheryl and the class listened while the teacher read stories from second- and third-grade books, readers which Cheryl had learned in her class. The next move was to invite Cheryl to read a story to her brother while they stayed in his room when his classmates were out for recess. She willingly took the opportunity, showing no inhibition in the presence of the teacher, who busied herself with other tasks about the room. Next, the kindergarten teacher arranged a dual story-reading period in which she divided the class into two groups, one consisting of Cheryl's brother and three of his classmates, who were seated around a table with Cheryl. The other members of the class were seated on the floor around the teacher at the other end of the room. The teacher announced that she and Cheryl would read the same selected story to their groups. Cheryl read with enthusiasm, and both audiences openly expressed appreciation for the stories when the teacher pointedly made a bid for their response, done for Cheryl's benefit.

At this point, the kindergarten and third-grade teachers and I held another conference to decide how Cheryl could make a transition to speaking in her own room. Her teacher suggested that the kindergarten children be brought by their teacher into her room during the regular third-grade reading time, to share seats individually with each of her pupils and to hear the story of the day. Cheryl's brother would be assigned to Cheryl, of course. Several of these visitation periods were carried out with success. Cheryl welcomed this reading assignment and continued to accept invitations to read within her room without the direct kindergarten support. We feel that Cheryl is finding more and more that it pays for her to speak.

Several principles have been illustrated by Ted's and Cheryl's speech problems. Their repressed output of speech appears to have been developmental, caused and maintained by factors from home and school. The disorder spread or became fixed, especially in Ted's case. Except for the coordinated plan to help Cheryl in the third grade, efforts to correct the problem were ineffective. The reasons for failure were those which commonly obstruct progress in speech therapy. Treatments varied according to variations in the diagnoses of cause and the case's needs. Since some of the diagnoses were conflicting, the resulting treatments were in disagreement, perhaps causing more harm than good. Because of the complexities of a classroom teacher's role, it is often difficult for her to give these special problems the attention they deserve. The need for team action was indicated, not only in diagnosing the problems but in the day-by-day implementation of the goals. Although the final breakthrough in Cheryl's speechlessness during her third year was largely accomplished by the two classroom teachers, the background help from other professionals should not be overlooked. It is likely, too, that Ted's and Cheryl's problems could have been prevented if the children's early preparation for school had been different. It is also conceivable that their problems could have been solved earlier in school and by more than one procedure. There are as many factors determining the cause of such disorders as there are in the correction.

The problem of the "shy" speaker, the inhibited pupil who does not recite as much or as often as he otherwise would, is often caused by the same conditions and is corrected along the same lines as those which were discussed for the speechless child, the difference being matters of degree. A teacher with experience at elementary, secondary, and college levels, has stated:

I believe that one of the most insidious evils which occur in education comes from the curbing effects which schools often produce upon pupils' speech and the resulting denial of an important vehicle for their free thought, creativity, and establishment of a strong self-image. In kindergarten we usually encourage more of this self-expression from pupils; but it becomes increasingly difficult at following grade levels for teachers to provide for speech development when they feel obliged to cover the prescribed subject matter and teach the skills which cram their curricula. Consequently, speech from pupils tends to be rationed, governed, and censored. Some teachers regard speech by pupils as an extracurricular exercise; some teachers obviously use it merely as a basis for grading, at times in an onerous way. It's no wonder that for some of our pupils it's safer in school not to speak much, or in some cases not to speak at all. Later we may blame these shy speakers when they enter college and show "stage fright" or when they are passive and nonresponsive in seminars which call for verbal participation.

Many problems of "shy" speakers in our classrooms would be prevented or corrected if more teachers regarded teaching as an integrated process calling for classroom talk between teacher and pupils. Pupils at all grade levels would develop greater confidence and skills in oral communication if their teachers would follow the previously mentioned principles advocated by Amidon and Hunter[1] in their book on how to improve teaching through a teacher's analysis and better use of verbal interaction in her classroom. The authors explain how classroom verbal interaction should correlate with the seven teaching activities: motivating, planning from the course of teaching, informing, moderating, discussing, disciplining, counseling, and evaluating.

Teachers share many good ideas on how to free the shy pupil who does not talk sufficiently in the classroom. One kindergarten teacher provided pictures of interesting topics, such as a circus, a farm, an aquarium, and stimulated class discussions around them. She also invited shy speakers along with other pupils to draw on the blackboard easily made snowmen, or fish, or rockets, to be used in free class discussions. She employed class-wide guessing games of charades, in which shy children had the chance to act out meaningful things without using speech. It is commonly observed that shy children are more relaxed around relaxed teachers whose voices and faces are pleasant, who genuinely enjoy children and teaching, and who have a good sense of humor.

Another teacher found that speech shyness could be thawed through creative dramatics, the silent or verbal dramatization of stories or skits. In one of her variations, the teacher told the story while her pupils acted it out. She found that masks and other stage props often gave the needed security to timid speakers, enabling them to fall into the spirit of the occasion and to lose their shyness. Choral speaking in games or play will give shy children support in speaking. Shy speakers may be caught in a vicious circle; they fail to speak because they are shy, and they shrink from speaking because they have not heard their own voices sufficiently to identify themselves as speakers. Tape recorders are valuable aids in providing the shy child an opportunity to hear and to regard himself as a speaker within situations which had become tabooed. Teachers have used projectors and silent strip films to stimulate and support verbal commentary from shy pupils. Live creatures, brought for "Show and Tell," may be more stimulating than inanimate things, and some children will respond better if they are allowed to sit or to walk around and personally show and demonstrate what they are talking about. Teachers learn to avoid limiting pupils to static solo performances so that shy pupils may seek and gain support from other pupils. Even in later grades, during high school and in college, pupils often need this support from peers. Besides, there are important special skills which come through panel discussions and from book reports that are shared by more than one pupil. An elderly teacher, auditing an adult extension course in speech correction, made this comment to her instructor:

> I am rather ashamed to say, but glad to say also, that this is the first class since I started school fifty-three years ago in which I have recited without being stiffened from insecurity and bothered by cold sweat and a dry mouth. As I see it, my courage to talk in this class comes from the good class atmosphere, with its demo-cratic, informal, and acceptable participation by class members. Second, I already had a vested interest in the topic for that panel presentation in which two other second-grade teachers and I were assigned to bring our familiar teaching materials and to talk informally about how our reading programs correlate with speech correction. Third, in that panel discussion, where we were seated around a table and equipped with our displays of materials and bolstered by each other, I gained that secure "we" feeling for the first time in recitation. Finally, I'm surprised to know how much relief came from the fact that I was auditing this course and was not being graded. It makes me appreciate how pupils feel under continual pressure to maintain good grades.

In each class there usually is at least one pupil who talks excessively or too often, creating problems for the teacher and fellow pupils, who must compete for the limited shares of talking time. One teacher made this comment on "chatterboxes":

> In my many years of teaching, first in one-room schools and later in classrooms at each grade level, I have noticed some interesting trends with children who talk too much in school. In the early grades I've found a higher percentage of "talkers." Later, as children establish a "peck-order" among themselves and as other curbing influences are applied, many of these talkative pupils pull in their necks, leaving perhaps one or two children to compete as chief spokesman. There are all sorts of pressures brought to bear upon pupils who talk too much. During adolescence, when children tend to think more about their social images than they do about their future needs for education, or even of their grades, some of the more talkative pupils become inhibited when they find that their talkativeness in class threatens their popularity with other pupils. We teachers, too, have different views about the preferred amount of talking by pupils at this or that age, in this or that class, in this or that subject. Moreover, it takes artful handling by the teacher if she is to encourage and regulate talking by thirty pupils and yet leave time for every-thing else that goes into class time.

Teachers sometimes must encourage some children to talk more, while teaching the overtalkative to share the talking, to become better listeners, or to gain security and attention in other ways than through excessive talk. With a philosophy of education and teaching which allows for the verbal interaction proposed by Amidon and Hunter,[1] teachers will find that the problems and correction of shy talkers and of chatterboxes have much in common.

There are cases where the problem of speech output relates more to the truth of than to the amount of what is said. Kindergartners and first-graders may have difficulty in distinguishing between reality and wishful thinking. But when older pupils spin yarns, bluff, and lie, then their problems will become serious, as a third-grade teacher explains:

> Usually, when pupils reach the third grade, they have learned generally to be dependable in what they say around us. Before that, when we hear them mix fancy with fact, we are more tolerant of this tendency, especially in kindergarten while they are being socialized and given free rein in exercises of self-expression. But for several reasons a child may continue to indulge in fantasy—if he is an insecure child and finds more satisfaction from telling falsehoods than to deny himself verbal exercises in the wonderful world of make-believe. If his life of reality is deficient, he cannot be severely blamed for trying to make up for it through wishful thinking, done aloud. I believe that it is much better for a forlorn child to express some of these longings openly than to bottle them up and create a lonely dream world for himself. A teacher or parent has a better chance to help the child who doesn't keep such problems to himself. But I've known teachers who absolutely won't tolerate any "tall tales" in the classroom. Yet these same teachers may be equally intolerant of the bitter truth as in telling "white lies," keeping some of the unpalatable truths from pupils, and failing to reward children for telling the truth, even though that truth is hard to take.

Haim G. Ginott's popular book, *Between Parent and Child*,[2] applies wisdom to school situations and teachers' roles. If teachers, like parents, punish a child for telling the truth, they create the feeling that it does not pay to be honest. They must realize, too, that lies hold diagnostic value, to reveal a child's fears and hopes for what he would like to do or to be. In their teaching roles and in the presence of a roomful of other children for whom they feel responsible, teachers may not only reject the unpalatable truth when it comes from pupils but may even provoke them to lie. A first-grade teacher expresses this dilemma in handling pupils who spoke falsehood as well as unadulterated truths in her classroom:

> Each year I seem to have at least one first-grader who gives me a bad time, either with his habit of lying or with the tendency to tell raw truths that shouldn't be told in school. Unless I control such tendencies in a child, he may have a contagious effect upon other children, with each trying to outstrip others in what they say. This year I had such a problem with a little fatherless boy from a poor home on relief. He would repeatedly relate class topics to fantastic experiences which he claimed he had had with his father. I knew he was stringing us along, but the children accepted everything in good faith, until finally his claims became so sensational that even his classmates began to doubt his word. At Christmas, for

instance, he claimed that his father had come home with a new jet airplane and was teaching him to fly it. Later, when he proceeded to tell about the flying adventures with his father, two other imaginative boys were so taken in by the tales that they began to hatch up some flying exploits of their own. At this point I contacted the school's psychologist and asked for advice on how to handle the situation.

So far, I had merely listened in a neutral way to the boy's fantasies, showing neither a denial nor an acceptance of their validity. The psychologist suggested that I take a more dynamic or active stand toward the falsifications, letting the boy and his classmates know that I knew that he was expressing *wishful* thinking, helping him to feel that there is some room for wishes in our thoughts and speech, and teaching him to employ his expressions of fantasy as outlets, rather than as substitutes for reality. So, when he made his next statements about his airplane up in the wild blue yonder, I followed with such remarks as: "You wish you had an airplane, eh, Chester; I sometimes wish I had a helicopter and could land right on my front yard. Maybe then I could pretend that I was Santa Claus and land on my roof." In two or three of these exercises in wishful thinking, I invited some wishes from others in the class. Before long, Chester accepted the fact that wishes and fact were on separate levels, that they could and should be employed separately and yet be satisfying. Soon he began to use the word *wish* in his own diminishing statements of fantasy.

But another problem can crop up in the face of naked truth, when a pupil relates something which is evidently true but which should not be openly told in school. One worried little girl from a home of marital conflicts had a compulsive need to tell us about her parents' drunken brawls, how she hated her father and wished he were dead. This created a delicate class situation too. My first impulse was to try to wipe these dishonorable thoughts from her mind, mainly to protect the class from hearing such things about home and parents. At times, we get back-lashes from parents when pupils carry home bad gossip which they pick up at school, and if it comes from the classroom, we teachers are sometimes held responsible.

Here again I consulted the school psychologist and the kindergarten teacher who had had this girl in class. We decided that she should not be scolded or given guilt feelings for harboring or saying such things about her folks, especially since her reports appeared factual. It was suggested that I react to her lamentable gossip in such ways as to make her feel that I understood, that I sympathized not only with her but with her parents, who have their problems too and who perhaps were sorry for the ways they handled some of their problems at home. It was also recommended that I provide her with some chances to talk out her personal problems—preferably in privacy with me, apart from class time. Of course, it was also decided that we would do everything possible to give this girl greater successes and personal security at school, so that her domestic reverses would not be such a threat to her total existence. I followed through with these goals and noticed that her outlook on life brightened. She dwelt less upon troubles at home and talked more about school interests. Little children can adopt wholesome philosophies about major problems in their lives if they are allowed to gain truthful understanding. We often underestimate the ability of young children to face stark facts in their lives.

Degrees of Seriousness

It would be difficult to establish standards for judging the seriousness of problems of speech output in the classroom. There are many considerations which must enter into the evaluations of whether or not a pupil's speech output is excessive, normal, or deficient. Judgments may depend upon whether the viewpoint is psychologically or sociologically oriented, or individual-centered or class-centered. It is possible to judge talkativeness on the basis of what is good for the child rather than on how he is affecting the class or the teaching program. At times, personal prejudices tend to rate others according to traits possessed or lacked by the observer. A professional cautioned against this tendency when she advised: "A teacher must examine her own attitudes and recognize her own blind spots. She should ask herself such questions as: 'Do I dislike aggressiveness? Do I mistake shyness for stupidity?' " Views concerning a pupil's verbal output may depend upon the teacher's philosophy for child-training, education, and the processes which underlie teaching and learning. Each speaker must be evaluated in his own right and within the speech situation at hand. In judging this problem area of speech, it is helpful to apply the three criteria which were suggested in Chapter 4 for determining the importance of speech and language problems generally: whether or not the trait interferes with communication, produces unhappiness and maladjustment in the child, and causes social problems.

References

1. Edmund Amidon and Elizabeth Hunter, *Improved Teaching, The Analysis of Classroom Verbal Interaction*. New York: Holt, Rinehart and Winston, Inc., 1966.

2. Haim G. Ginott, *Between Parent and Child*. New York: The Macmillan Company, 1965.

Questions

1. What are the terms of measurement of talkativeness?

2. Describe conditions which cause variations of talkativeness in the same pupil.

3. Who has the more critical speech problem: the "chatterbox" or the "shy speaker"?

4. What may be the causes of speechlessness?

5. Describe abbreviated speech.

6. Why is it preferable for a child to be a verbal "story teller" than a silent daydreamer?

7. What are the three criteria for judging the general importance of speech and language problems?

8. Describe a situation which causes a "chatterbox" to become a "shy speaker."

9. How would therapy differ for the "chatterbox" and the "shy speaker"?

10. What may be the effects of parents' perfectionistic ideals on the child's speech?

11. In the break from kindergarten to primary grades, how may changing discipline affect speech?

12. Discuss the principles which Amidon and Hunter advocate for correlating speech with teaching activities.

13. What are some concrete aids for thawing shyness?

14. How does "peck order" exert influence on speech development?

15. To what degree would you insist on truthfulness in speech from young children?

16. Describe the conflicts faced by a child from a home of substandard ethics, morality, and social mores.

17. How would you manage a school situation in which others laugh at a child with a speech defect?

18. How would you help a child with a speech problem which attracts negative reactions from the public?

19. Most children tell family "secrets." How would you deal with one who talks excessively of "secrets"?

20. In applying the principles of learning to a speech-handicapped child, is he best treated as an individual or as a type?

21. How would you treat a problem child who refuses to speak for fear of criticism and punishment?

Suggested Products

1. Summarize the findings reported by professional investigators, with your own observations, on the comparative effects of TV and radio on listeners' speech habits.

2. By personal visits, compare the speech and language patterns and the classroom climate for speech in schools attended by middle-class children with those in "culturally deprived" neighborhoods.

3. Write three skits aimed at giving the needed security to timid early primary grades speakers.

4. Observe your classmates with normal speech. Do the majority cling to current standardized speech and idiom? What percentage dares to be individual? Keep a tabulation for a month.

six

Helping the Child
who Misarticulates

A public school speech therapist once made this typical appraisal of misarticulation:

Most of my work in speech correction has been with the problem of misarticulation. In my caseload, required by state law to serve seventy-five to one hundred pupils, I usually find that 75 per cent or more of the problems are with the faulty articulation of speech sounds. Many of the problems are not serious, but some of them are. If I didn't provide help for the milder cases, more of them, too, would turn into serious handicaps to hinder educational achievement and personal adjustment. I find a relatively high percentage of misarticulation in young children at kindergarten, first, and second grades. I could quickly fill my quota of cases from our school population if I started at kindergarten and scheduled everyone with misarticulation from that level on up. We and our potentially handicapped children would be aided greatly if a valid predictive test of articulation could be devised to determine whether or not a kindergartner, first, or second grader will "outgrow" his misarticulation from the helpful influences which regularly come from home and school, without extra speech correction. But we have learned from experience that beyond the third-grade level a child with misarticulation is less likely to outgrow his faulty speech sounds. For this reason, I give priority in my selection and scheduling of cases to older children, proceeding downward to the younger grade levels. In this way, I'm more likely to schedule a higher percentage of children who need the extra help with their speech problems and who won't outgrow them. Of course, if a kindergartner has an unusual type and amount of misarticulation which handicaps him, makes him unintelligible, and threatens his educational achievement, then I give him priority too. This policy in selecting cases makes for a heavier case load of more difficult cases, and I show a slower or lower rate of dismissal. Nevertheless, I believe that since it is usually impossible for us to schedule and handle all cases with speech problems, we should direct our efforts where they are most needed. After all, I believe that we have the professional responsibility to help those children who most need our help—not to make professional work easier and outwardly successful.

An experienced kindergarten teacher states:

I have learned to expect that about one-third of my five-year-olds have one or more faulty speech sounds. But most of my kindergartners show definite improvement in articulation during their first year at school. Later, in follow-up checks with the speech therapist and the first- and second-grade teachers, I find that about half of the pupils who enter first grade with faulty articulation are partly or entirely corrected by the end of the first grade. Moreover, this early progress during the kindergarten and first grade seems to take place whether or not the child gets added speech correction. But when I follow the speech progress of children who are still misarticulating when they enter second grade, I find that correction of their problem becomes increasingly difficult, less likely to be outgrown without special help. From this point on, our speech therapists assume greater responsibility for helping these children who misarticulate.

Nature of Errors

Misarticulation, introduced in Chapter 4 with other types of speech disorders, may occur in the form of substitution, omission, distortion, or addition of sounds. The speech sounds which are usually most difficult for children to learn are those of *r, l, s, z, th, g, k, sh, ch,* and the blends of consonants.

SUBSTITUTIONS

The substituted sounds are often used instead of the above-mentioned difficult sounds; they may be sounds already learned and easier for the speaker to say. For examples, a child may settle for such substitutions as "wun" for *run,* "wet" or "yet" for *let,* "thee", "she" or "tee" for *see,* "dump" for *jump,* "fumb" or "tumb" for *thumb,* "det" for *get,* "tat" for *cat,* "tut" or "thut" for *shut,* "tair" for *chair,* "whiso" for *whistle,* "twuck" for *truck.* Children also have frequent difficulty in making the different sounds of "r" when it must be used in the sense of a vowel in connection with consonants. Thus, they may adopt the "Southern" vowel-like form of "r" when it is used in such words as "buhd" spoken for *bird,* "uhly" for *early,* or "huh" for *her.* These substitutions, common in young children during their preschool, kindergarten and first-grade years, normally diminish by the third grade. Early substitutions tend to be inconsistent, as when a child who says the "w" sound for "r" in most of his words may correctly say the "r" in certain combinations of sounds, especially in words which have been more recently learned. But as the child grows older and if environmental influences and learnings have not corrected or improved his misarticulations, his errors often become more consistent and widespread in his speech.

Children may also react to difficult sounds by simply omitting them. A child may say "ca" for *car*, "pot" for *part*, or "un" for *run*. He may say "ba" for *ball*, "tephone" for *telephone*, "hore" for *horse*, "i" for *is*, "at" or "a" for *that*, "bo" for *both*, "et" for *get*, "wa" for *walk*, "wa" for *wash*, "tu" for *touch*, "in" or "kin" for *skin*, "mik" for *milk*. Omissions are found more frequently on final than on initial or medial sounds of words, perhaps because these final sounds are often in unstressed parts of words or in frameworks of sounds where they are perceptually less distinct or are linguistically less important. For example, when a child says "Tha boy too my lello ba an balloon" instead of "That boy took my yellow ball and balloon," he may be revealing that he has perceived the "l" phoneme more correctly within certain frameworks than in others. However, when a child says the above sentence, it is likely that he considers and says the utterance in a connected, unitary fashion instead of as a series of eight words, each consisting of a "head," "middle," and "tail" sounds. But in the flow of connected sounds which constitute the language framework of this sentence, the child may perceive and articulate a phoneme, such as the "l," more easily within certain word positions and phonemic frameworks than in others. This principle may not only explain the inconsistency of a child's omissions of speech sounds but may also suggest where and how to correct his omissions of phonemes in these more obscure and difficult contexts of sounds. When a speaker omits sounds which constitute the key morphological units of language, he tends to be more difficult to understand than when he provides at least partial clues of the missing sounds. Omissions, therefore, tend to be classed at a lower developmental level of articulatory learning. But although they may cause greater unintelligibility in speech, they are not necessarily more difficult to correct. Perhaps a child who omits sounds and is less easily understood loses some reinforcement through reduced speech acceptance by his audiences. Another child with substitutions or distortions of patterns which are more generally interpreted and accepted is not offered remedial instruction by audiences.

A misarticulatory distortion is a speech sound which does not meet the acceptable standard of correctness established for the phoneme for which that sound is meant. Misarticulations classed as distortions are generally regarded to be of a higher order of mistake than are omissions and substitutions, because distortions usually are more easily identified with the speech phonemes which they represent and approximate. Older children and adults who misarticulate are more likely to distort than to omit phonemes or to substitute other phonemes for faulty ones. Distortions are often consistent and difficult to correct. If distortions do not significantly interfere with the intelligibility of speech, they may generally receive audience acceptance and thereby become habituated in the speaker through his self-acceptance and unaltered usage.

Although any of the phonemes of a language may be distorted, the most common distortions in English involve the *s*, *z*, *sh*, *ch*, and *l*. However, other phonemes may be just as phonetically distorted as are these sibilants, fricatives, and glide sounds. But audiences tend to overlook a distorted phoneme if it can be easily interpreted as that phoneme, especially if that phoneme is one which allows for a wider spread of variance. We are less inclined to be critical of misarticulation if they do not interfere with the intelligibility of speech or if they do not create distraction by their novelty. As one teacher said:

> I find that I have become more tolerant and less aware of speech sounds which are not made just right. When I began teaching in a large metropolitan school where various dialects, accents, and shades of pronunciations were spoken, I felt that I was teaching in a foreign land. Having previously lived only in an isolated and stable linguistic area of the Midwest, I had difficulty in understanding some of the pupils' "mistakes." I was especially critical of how children from the South and East spoke their vowels and *r*'s. But when I got accustomed to their usages, I became less discriminatory. Now, when I go back to my home locality for a visit, I notice differences in the speech of the hometown "natives" and can understand why some of my associates at school have identified me by the way I "shade" certain of my Midwestern vowels.

Troublesome Sounds

In the preceding discussion of sounds which are substituted, omitted, or distorted in speech, it is apparent that trouble may occur on any of the phonemes of a language, most commonly on *r*, *s*, *l*, *th*, *ch*, *sh*, *j*, and the blends of these and other consonants. Other consonants and vowels may be at fault, especially in young children who have not yet developed the perceptual distinctions and skills to produce them. There are fine differentiations between some of the phonemes and their related allophones. In severe cases of misarticulation, most of the phonemes may be faulty. One speech therapist has stated:

> We normally expect faulty sounds in the "baby-talk" of preschool children. Usually we are satisfied if we can understand preschool children. We're less critical of their variations, which are usually not fixed or of a very standardized nature at that time. But when these same sounds come from the older mouths of school children or adults, we become critical, especially when their vowels and "easier" consonants are at fault. At times it is difficult for us to agree on whether or not certain misarticulations are "normal," whether it pays for us to work on them now or later. Diagnosis is difficult; it must take many things into consideration.

Studies of speech and language have given us developmental scales which show the ages at which the average child should be expected to master the various sounds of his language. Other scales and tests have attempted to measure the severity of the articulatory problem and whether special therapy will be needed in addition to the help which accrues from ordinary maturation and learning. These studies reveal not only that some phonemes of a language are more difficult than others but also that children vary widely in the rate and sequence of learning phonemes. Some three-year-olds have mastered all the phonemes of their language, while many six, seven, or even eight-year-old children misarticulate one or more of their phonemes and yet are judged to be normal in their articulatory development. For this reason, some of the developmental scales of articulation give the norms in terms of age *ranges*. Other developmental scales express articulatory attainment in terms of the percentages of children who master certain phonemes at each of the age levels. In all speech therapy it is wise to guard against the tendency to generalize and to treat individuals and difficulties on the basis of statistical averages. A speech therapist points out the dangers of too close reliance upon statistical averages:

> At times in our well meant zeal to soothe parental concern over a child's mis-articulations, we cite statistical figures on age and error to try to convince parents that their child's articulation is as normal as can be expected. In doing this, we may be promoting mediocrity and denying this child the chance to prove his potentialities and to show that these statistics are not true limits for him. Scales have value for general reference, but too often they are based upon limited sampling of children whose individual differences have been statistically leveled. We must not let statistics rule our judgments of the individual—like the physician who told an oldster who had submitted to a check on rheumatism, "You're in exceptionally fine physical condition for a man of ninety-two years. In fact, according to the experience tables, you should be dead."

Misarticulation versus Mispronunciation

The term *misarticulation* may not be understood by laymen. Its concept is sometimes associated with *mispronunciation* or with the use of poor grammar, as in saying "ain't" instead of "isn't." Professionals, too, may have difficulty in differentiating these terms and assigning responsibility for correcting their errors. Pupils, ranging from the early elementary grades to college, are some-times referred for speech therapy to correct deficient grammar or careless usages, such as "Me ain't done dat 'fore." These deficiencies in grammar and pro-nunciation are worthy of correction, but they are not the primary responsibility of speech therapists. Classroom teachers generally work to improve these sub-standard usages. In upper grades, there are remedial courses for the student who says, for instance, "He done it dat way cuz he di'n't know no better." Such a student needs a correction of language and diction rather than speech therapy. His substitutions and omissions of sounds and language units represent a cultural discrepancy in grammar and pronunciation instead of an inability to articulate the complete set of English phonemes. Another type of English mispronunciation occurs when speakers are unduly influenced by the spelling of words, as in their voicing of the *l* in *calm* or the *w* in *toward* and in their putting three "k" sounds in *Connecticut*. However, when a foreigner has difficulty in learning English as a second language, he may misarticulate some of the English phonemes which are unlearned because they are foreign to his native language. A speech therapist who worked in school districts where children of Mexican parents were confronted with the problems of learning English as a second language with their Spanish explains how pronunciation and articulation are intertwined in bilingualism:

> In my caseload of eighty children, I have two therapy groups of first and second grade children whose parents are migrant workers of Mexican origin. Spanish is their family language, although their parents can speak some broken English. However, I find that these Mexican children misarticulate English as well as mispronounce it. They may substitute either Spanish or English phonemes for certain English phonemes which are not found in their native Spanish language. For example, they tend to substitute the "s" or "t" sounds for the voiceless "th," and they may substitute the "d" for the voiced "th" and the "sh" or "s" for the "ch" sound. Sometimes these substitutions seriously interfere with the communicability of their speech. "See seenks day washed her wen see chumped ober da wooedpile and urt er sheen" might be spoken for "She thinks they watched her when she jumped over the woodpile and hurt her chin."
> Other articulatory inabilities of this Spanish-speaking child may be classified as distortions—for example, trilling the "r" sound in *girl*. For the English "h" and "b," he may substitute somewhat similar sounds of Spanish, sounds which we may perceive as distortions but which he may feel are similar enough. He may add the "g" sound after the *ng* phoneme in the word *sing*, because in his Spanish the *ng* is used in the more limited context of being inserted between the *n* followed by *k* or *g*.
> However, for the correction of this mixture of misarticulation and mispronunciation which I observe in the English of my Mexican pupils, I find that speech therapy is very similar to that required for pupils who have phonemic problems in only one spoken language. Because there are some special learnings that apply to misarticulation therapy for the bilingual children, I believe that the best arrangement has been to schedule them separately as well as jointly with the American children who misarticulate. By so doing, the bilingual children are helped by the American children in ways which I cannot conduct alone. Of course, in the classroom, too, these Mexican children gain a lot from the speech and language teaching by their teachers and English-speaking classmates. Lately, our schools have found it necessary to employ Spanish-speaking teachers' aides to be good communicative links for the Mexican pupils in several of the classrooms where the pupils have not yet made a sufficient transition to the levels of English demanded of them.

The standard for our judgment of pronunciation, and even of misarticulation, should be actual cultivated usage, the outgrowth of the cultural and regional factors which determine this standard. There are times when colloquial, informal, conversational, or easy English forms of speech are in order. But in other situations, we expect and require pronunciation to be more formal, dignified, "cultivated," careful, precise, and clearly understood. *Clothes* has been pronounced without the "th," as *close*, so frequently that for centuries lexicographers have differed over whether the latter colloquial form is acceptable or faulty. If *Worcester* or *Leicester* are spoken with three syllables instead of two, residents of those cities rightly judge them to be mispronunciations by uninformed speakers. When pupils with a Southern heritage drop the "r" in saying "ca" for *car*, "pot" for *part*, they should be judged incorrect only with respect to the standards of regions where these "r's" are suitably sounded. Likewise, there are speakers who pronounce *creek* as *crick*—or vice versa, depending upon the region and common usage which they represent. Therefore, before we as speech therapists and teachers judge the correctness or incorrectness of speech variations in pupils, it would be well to consider cultural and regional backgrounds and to determine whether or not the differences actually are mispronunciations or misarticulations.

Reasons for Misarticulations

Since we do not yet understand the processes by which speech is normally learned, we cannot know the mechanisms by which it is disordered. Chapter 1 discussed the conditions which appear to be essential for normal speech development. Chapter 2 outlined the sequence stages and variations in its development, including the learning and habituation of articulatory skills. The complexity of the speech act and its development have been emphasized. Speech is a language act having many psychological and social functions. It is dependent for its acquisition and uses upon many physical, psychological, and social factors, operating in wonderful ways through maturation, learning, and habituation. It is also evident that articulatory skill, underlying the particular sounds of a language, represents only one of the many integrated facets of maturations and learnings which are needed for normal speech. Whether articulation is correct or incorrect may depend upon one or more of the following conditions.

NEURO–MUSCULAR IMPAIRMENT

The term "neuro-muscular" refers to the physical or organic structures of speech: the brain and its nerve tracts; the organs of hearing and vision, the tongue, lips, jaw, teeth, palate, breathing mechanism, vocal cords, etc.

Two types of misarticulation, *dysarthria* and *dyspraxia*, have been attributed to impairment of the central nervous system, causing a deficiency in the control of a part or all of the speech muscles. Dysarthria, often seen in cerebral palsy, may be characterized by a lack of muscle tone and control of the tongue and jaw, thereby affecting speech articulation and perhaps other fine voluntary and involuntary movements of these organs. Dyspraxia is a neuro-muscular deficiency which is not characterized by a lack of muscle tone or by general incoordination of the speech articulators, but instead shows lack of tongue-jaw control when speech actions are willful, volitional, or done on command. Thus, a dyspraxic speaker may find all degrees of difficulty when he consciously tries to coordinate speech organs in the willful process of talking. However, in the involuntary or automatic functions of these speech organs, this clumsiness associated with volitional speech may not occur—perhaps not even in articulation when he speaks spontaneously without deliberation. It is generally believed that dysarthria and dyspraxia cause only a relatively small percentage of misarticulation cases. Their diagnosis, often difficult to determine, should avoid hasty conclusions and should be based upon careful speech and neurological examinations, verified and tested by trial therapy and follow-up.

ANATOMICAL DEFECTS

It is obvious that anatomical defects cause some cases of misarticulation. Cleft palate produces an excessive nasal escape of air and thereby distorts speech sounds. In addition to its physiological handicap, the cleft may also lead the speaker to adopt poor compensatory habits which further interfere with his optimal control over articulation, thus adding functional cause to the organic insufficiency. Defects such as loss of teeth or malocclusion, "tongue-tie," irregularities in the shape and size of the palate, and partial excision of the tongue also hamper speech articulation. However, the encouraging fact that speakers with these handicaps of moderate severity can achieve normal speech should caution us against discounting a speaker's ability to make good use of what he has, defective though his physical structures may be. First- and second-grade teachers observe, for instance, how quickly most pupils learn to make satisfactory articulatory compensations during the temporary periods when their lost baby teeth leave gaps.

PERCEPTUAL DEFICIENCIES

Speech articulation is a learned skill, acquired through the perception and imitation of prescribed language patterns. The acquisition and maintenance of articulation depend upon combined cues from external and internal perceptions, utilizing auditory, visual, and kinesthetic senses. If these senses are impaired or if the speaker does not make adequate use of them in the learning and maintenance of speech, misarticulation may result. The child with a severe loss of hearing learns to articulate according to what he hears and sees in the speech of others, supplemented by his inner auditory and kinesthetic cues. Of these perceptual senses, hearing appears to be the most important one we use in learning to speak. The blind person relies more heavily upon the external cues from sound and touch, combined with his internal monitoring from self-hearing and muscle-feel. But even the child with normal organs of perception may fail to make sufficient use of them to learn the characteristics and discriminations which articulation requires. Milisen[1] thus explains his concept of the inverse process by which speech sounds are learned and self-regulated. In evaluating the adequacy of his own articulation, the speaker initially may depend more upon his audience than upon self-perception of his speech. Restrictions and reinforcements of the child's articulation are environmentally imposed upon the child from the communicative situation. They are perceived by him and eventually become the basis of his self-regulatory system which may then operate with less dependency upon external patterns. The poor articulation of some autistic children may be partly explained by their lack of observational feedback from audience reception and reaction to their speech patterns.

LOW INTELLIGENCE

Children who are mentally retarded are often lacking in their speech and language development. But the factor of low intelligence is sometimes unduly blamed for being the main or sole determinant of misarticulation. Many children of subnormal intelligence acquire normal articulation of their language through extra measures to cultivate their motivation and to facilitate their perception, imitation, and establishment of correct articulatory patterns. One speech therapist expressed the following observations of mentally retarded children:

> I have known a number of children with IQ's around 50 or 60 who have attained normal articulation and yet have not acquired the vocabulary and grammar of the average three- or four-year-old child. These children are usually in homes where their parents have worked patiently and persistently with them, instilling in them the pleasant desire to imitate and clearly exemplifying for them the correct speech patterns, scaled to their comprehension and frequent daily usage. Some of the children's speech patterns, which were especially well articulated, were in the form of polite "social talk," trained into them along with nice social manners. At times a mentally retarded child is trained to utter some verbal expressions more clearly than he understands them; but even so, this speech training can bring him more social acceptance than he would get without this verbal front.

INSUFFICIENT OR FAULTY LEARNING

Most cases of misarticulation appear principally to have functional causes, the result of faulty or insufficient learning. Obviously, when neurological, organic, perceptual, or intellectual impairments occur, the burdens upon learning become multiplied and the functional processes in acquiring articulation become more complex. But the majority of children who misarticulate appear to have normal equipment for speech and language. Their problems often center around such functional factors as the failure of their speech and language environment to provide them with the incentives for learning speech or the models, instruction, and unhampered opportunity to practice and habituate the skills of articulation to suit their environment. Chapter 2, which discusses the course of normal speech and language development, offers information on what must be learned in normal speech, the approximate timetable in acquiring the skills and their stages of development, and some conjectures on how speech learning takes place. Later, the present chapter will consider the measures by which teachers, therapists, and parents correct misarticulation and will suggest in more detail the functional causes. It should be emphasized that the learning of articulation is only one facet of the total language act, dependent upon an interplay of physical, emotional, intellectual and social factors. As one therapist remarked, "It is far more complex to teach a pupil to shape a faulty phoneme in his repertoire of speech sounds that to teach him how to sharpen a pencil."

How Misarticulations May Handicap a Child

Misarticulation can be one of the most insidious of the speech disorders. A child's misarticulation may go unnoticed for years, then suddenly become a serious issue to threaten and handicap him. A college sophomore, majoring in education, made this comment about her lisp upon being enrolled in a university speech clinic:

> I feel bitter about my shpeech, shpeech correction and my whole outlook on life. Now, in my sophomore year, I finally find out that my lisp is a serious problem. Occasionally I have been told that I didn't make shome of my *s*'s just right, but nobody ever made any fush about it until thish year. Now the education department tells me that I must correct my lisp or I cannot expect to graduate in education. During my grade shchool years, I attended a little shchool which didn't have a shpeech therapist. Several teachers have made a few brief attempts to correct my *s*, but even they didn't act like it was a sherious problem. Then, when I moved to a consolidated high school, I was given a shpeech test and told that I had a lisp that should be removed. But the shpeech therapist said she was overloaded with other cases in the grades and couldn't find time to shchedule work at the high shchool. So, here I am, referred here to the Shpeech Clinic, hoping now to remove this lisp or else I'll have to shwitch my major and lose most of the credits I've earned sho far. Besides, I want to teach—at the elementary level. That's the level they shay this lisp would be most harmful to children. I shee their point.

There are many borderline misarticulation problems like that of the lisping education student, with relatively common defects which are ignored during the years when their correction would be more convenient and effective and which later becoming chronic and critical. Many similarly handicapped pupils do not get the later chance to receive speech therapy. The following high school graduate tells how misarticulation has handicapped his life:

"My hife ha' be' a' met up—an' a' atount of my peet. In too' I taut to nobody, but my fen' undetoo' me. Da teea, day eft me a'one. I wa' dood in aitmatit, do, an' I ten wite an' wead toay, but da' wan't 'nuf ta eveh det me any de'ent dob. Aw I ten eveh det i' manu wabo."

Translated, the preceding misarticulated paragraph reads:

"My life has been all messed up—and all account of my speech. In school I talked to nobody, but my friends understood me. The teachers, they left me alone. I was good in arithmetic, though, and I can write and read okay, but that wasn't enough to ever get me any decent jobs. All I can ever get is manual labor."

The foregoing complaint of an articulatory handicap is not as unique as one may think. Misarticulation affects the intelligibility of speech in all degrees of severity. Speakers with unintelligible misarticulation may go unnoticed by the general public because of their being forced into relatively silent and obscured niches of life. It should be remembered, however, that the degree to which a speaker's misarticulation detracts from the intelligibility of his speech sounds is not always a good measure of his handicap. In school we find "mild" appearing cases of misarticulation which are burdened by heavy costs. A high school counselor cites the following example of a student who illustrates how an inconsistent error on one sound can become a widespread handicap:

I'll never forget Sam—"Tham," as some of the children at school called him. I personally got acquainted with him when he reached high school, but I learned about his grade school life from the speech therapist who had worked off and on with him since the first grade. His speech defect had always been limited to one sound, an interdental lisp—substitution of the "th" sound for the "s," the appearance of which made the fault more conspicuous than just its sound. But of most importance was the fact that the children had learned to expect eventual lisps from Sam, since he bore that nagging name of "Tham" from earlier years. Unfortunately, he had developed a gnawing sensitivity toward this teasing and his speech in general. He avoided recitation and refused to take part in plays, debating, and other school activities where his fault would be displayed.

In high school, Sam's expanding problem came to my attention when his grades began to decline in courses where speaking was required. His intelligence and aptitude tests and his performances in other subjects had placed him in the upper quartile of his class. Oddly enough, after years of acceptance of his defect, his parents wanted him prepared for college and hoped that he would become a lawyer like his father. But Sam had no faith and interest in being a lawyer or anything else which required good speech. Rather than take all courses needed for college entrance, he planned either to enlist in the armed services or go to a business college and take accounting, where his speech problem would be less of a problem. He became aggressive and rebellious, seemingly because of his speech insecurity. His social life and reputation deteriorated from his association with a gang of boys who accepted his lisp. However, in all of Sam's academic, social, and counseling problems, it would have been easy to overlook the fact that his lisp was at the bottom of it. It operated in subtle ways to spread its personal and social handicaps.

Generally, articulatory problems are often corrected with cooperative help from teachers, parents, and speech therapists before a pupil reaches the second or third grade. Teachers and speech therapists not only expect to find a relatively high incidence of articulatory faults in children at kindergarten and first-grade levels but also recognize that these unlearned skills in oral language lead to various handicaps if they are not corrected. One kindergarten teacher summarized her views on the importance of speech improvement as follows:

> I believe that speech is the most important learned skill which a five-year-old brings to school. If it's defective, and it often is at this age, the pupil faces handicaps in communication, preparation for reading, and social adjustment. His effectiveness in speech often helps to determine whether or not he likes school. If his speech is unintelligible, it bars him from some school activities, leads to frustration, threatens his school progress. In such cases, a kindergarten teacher should seek help from the speech therapist. Parents, too, may need to help.
>
> We kindergarten teachers generally learn to appreciate the importance of language and speech skills in our pupils. Throughout our curriculum we must rely upon speech and work to improve it. Our speech therapist, too, emphasizes the importance of helping children with their speech problems at this time, even though she cannot spend as much time in direct work with kindergarten cases as she spends with her required caseloads of older children who are less likely to improve their speech under the ordinary corrective influences from kindergarten and home. Our speech therapist, however, closely cooperates with me by suggesting and even demonstrating in my classroom some ways I can integrate more and better speech teaching into my total kindergarten program. I find that her efforts not only improve the articulatory skills of children but also correlate with my efforts to teach them the correct sounds of letters for reading and writing. Pupils learn to recognize and accept errors in speech as a respected part of school work. Social problems are prevented too. Teasing is not likely to occur, and problems are outgrown without complications.

How the Teacher Can Help

Classroom teachers correct misarticulation in many direct and indirect ways. Teachers' corrective roles are prominent, whether or not speech therapists are available to share responsibility in this work. Teachers at kindergarten and first-grade levels, where immaturities and errors in speech are common, are especially aware of the need to incorporate speech correction with general teaching. As one kindergarten teacher said:

> I expect to find about half of my entering pupils with faults on one or more of the speech sounds. Most of their errors are of the types frequently associated with

young children. But in each class there may be two or three pupils whose mis-articulation exceeds ordinary limits, causing their speech to be unintelligible and handicapped. Hopefully, I can get help with these exceptional cases from the speech therapist, but this is not always possible to do. Even if a speech therapist is available to give special help with the several worse cases of misarticulation, I find that there is still plenty of help I can give them, because the therapist relies upon me for many aids which cannot be conducted within only his area of work. In the first place, he appreciates my help in locating these cases and in referring them to him. He seeks my supplementary observations and evaluations of the problems, even though he conducts his own survey by coming into my classroom during the first several weeks of school to screen the class for speech problems. We realize that kindergartners with mild and moderate speech problems must rely mainly upon my help. Besides, the therapist usually has an overflowing schedule with other children having critical problems or with older children who have failed to improve from the regular influences and practices in the classrooms.

A speech therapist has made the following general statements about classroom teachers and their roles in correcting misarticulation:

Classroom teachers help with speech problems in more ways than they realize. I may also add that many speech therapists do not realize how much classroom teachers improve and correct speech problems. If one becomes specialized and too removed from the classroom scene, he may fail to realize that in the teaching of subject matter, like the three R's, there are many ways to teach better speech and language. Although attention to speech may be divided and secondary when a teacher is focusing upon reading readiness, reading, and spelling, gains in her pupils' speech usually accrue too. When a speech therapist sees a teacher modeling and teaching pupils the specific sounds and the letters which represent them in reading, he may fail to recognize and appreciate that this teacher may be doing essentially what he does in his therapy for misarticulation. While pupils learn and practice phonics as a tool in determining words, their articulation tends to improve. Therefore, it is no wonder that many problems of misarticulation are corrected during the kindergarten, first, and second years when so much interest and activity center around speech, spoken words, and speech sounds.

Chapter 3 considered the responsibilities, opportunities, and capacity of the teacher as a member of the team working with speech and language prob-lems, including misarticulation. Chapter 4, which suggested further important functions of classroom teachers, discussed the effects of speech handicaps upon behavior, the recognition and diagnosis of problems, and their referral and prevention. The following section of this chapter will limit consideration to the ways by which a teacher can specifically help in the correction of this disorder.

RECOGNIZING MISARTICULATION

A first step in therapy is to detect that the fault exists and to define and locate it within the pupil's speech patterns. A full recognition of misarticulation in a pupil requires that observation and analysis be made of an adequate sample of the pupil's speech. A classroom teacher has many good opportunities to get this sampling of the pupil's articulation from the various speech situations which she stimulates and observes in his school life. It is possible for an observant and speech-minded teacher to make helpful surveys of articulatory errors without setting up special situations to stimulate and test speech. After screening, however, she or the therapist will find it often helpful to give the child a formal and systematic test of articulation to elicit complete samples of speech revealing his ability or inability to articulate all the phonemes of his language. It is important to determine how the sounds are spoken in various positions of words, within the different phonemic contexts, and in the language framework of informal conversation and in reading. Testing by the therapist will grade the child's ability to duplicate the phonemes—spoken in isolation, in words, and in sentences—after being given the chance to hear and see the correct patterns spoken by the examiner. Picture tests of articulation have been prepared for this purpose, such as the standardized one devised by Templin and Darley.[2] However, a teacher may easily devise her own test of articulation by using pictures, objects, or written words and sentences which contain the speech sounds to be elicited for testing. Or she may stimulate pupils to give speech samples through conversation or by asking the child questions. A child's misarticulation may be quickly revealed when he is asked to count from one to twenty, name the days of the week, recite "Humpty Dumpty," tell the story of "The Three Pigs," etc. The following first-grade teacher used a positive method of detecting misarticulation in her classroom:

> During the first two weeks of each school year, I make a special effort to "tune in" on my pupils' speech and to locate speech problems they may have. I find that misarticulations are the most common errors, usually on the sounds of s, l, r, ch, j, and the consonantal blends. These errors are picked up in all sorts of speech situations: during pupils' recitations, in reading, and in conversation with me and with classmates. I find that many of our sets of picture cards used in teaching phonics of letters and words are excellent for testing articulation. The pictures and strip-films used in kindergarten for reading-readiness are also easily adaptable for this testing. In fact, any pictures of collections of objects will provide the chance for me to zero in on a child's faulty articulation.
>
> When I hear a child misarticulate one or more sounds, I aim to elicit and record at least ten different words in which each error occurred, underlining the faulty part of each word and noting whether the mistake was a substitution of another sound, an omission, or a distortion of the sound. I also note whether the error was made while reading, conversing, or while the word was repeated after me. Our speech therapist has suggested that I note and record inconsistencies of the error— words in which the child correctly articulated the troublesome sound. We have found that these occasional successes in his saying the difficult sounds can be useful footholds, instances to serve as models to expand success within his speech. A child may not realize that he can already say the difficult sound correctly in some words. When he learns this fact, his confidence often rises.

The testing policy followed by the above teacher is a recommended one, helpful not only to the teacher but also to the speech therapist who made the following comments about her policy:

> The detection of speech problems in our speech correction program depends partly upon teachers and their yearly referrals. Although I do my own annual screening of children in kindergarten and odd-numbered grades, thereby screening each child at least every two years, I find that most of the teachers and I have about 90 per cent agreement in recognizing speech problems. Teachers help me not only in first locating problems but also in keeping me posted on follow-up evaluations of children whom I have dismissed from my therapy program or who have not been scheduled because of their lack of severity at the time or for other reasons.
>
> I depend upon teachers' referrals not only at the beginning of the school year but also throughout the year—especially near the close of the year, after each teacher has had an ample chance to know the child and to appraise his problem. These speech evaluations became valuable additions to the pupil's records which are given to his next year's teacher. But when I started speech correction at this school, some of the teachers were not trained to recognize and make informative referrals of speech problems. The teachers were given some mimeographed information and guidelines on the characteristics of speech problems; we held some staff conferences; and now I find that some of the teachers are better at screening than I am. Teachers who observe children speaking in a much wider variety of speech situations than I do often get a broader perspective of the problem itself and the particular conditions surrounding it.

EVALUATING ERRORS

Having recognized that an articulatory problem exists, and after sufficient samples of speech have been elicited and recorded to show the errors and their variations or exceptions, it is important for the therapist to make an evaluation of the problem's severity, to estimate its prognosis and to search for clues which indicate appropriate therapeutic goals. The severity of misarticulation may be judged on two bases: the probable difficulty in correcting it and the extent of its handicap, judged according to the three criteria credited to Van Riper[3] earlier in this text. In this chapter we shall consider severity as it relates to the difficulty in correcting a problem, since the appraisal of handicapping effects has already been discussed. Studies have suggested that the cases of misarticulation most stubborn to correct tend to be the ones with the most consistent errors or cases having the greatest number of different phonemic flaws, especially if the vowels are faulty. But at times it is more difficult to remove a single established error in one speaker than to correct several errors in another speaker. A speaker who misarticulates a phoneme in all positions of his words is likely to have a more stubborn problem to correct than one who has trouble with the sound in only one position—the final position, perhaps. Consistent errors of articulation, showing little or no variability, are usually more resistant to therapy. When a troublesome phoneme is spoken correctly in some words, a favorable prognosis is indicated and constructive therapeutic opportunities for teaching and learning are provided by these "key words."

A *Stimulability Test*, devised and tested by Milisen and his associates,[4] indicates that faulty sounds of a speaker are more readily correctable if they show improvement when they are repeated in imitation of an examiner who provides vivid and correct modeling and positive motivation for the speaker. For this reason, before completing a test of a child's misarticulation, it is advisable for the therapist to note the change which occurs in each faulty phoneme when the child repeats it either in isolation or in words directly after clear and correct pronunciation by the examiner.

McDonald[5] explains how "deep testing" of misarticulation adds to therapy by going beyond the mere recognition and labeling of errors. His approach has indicated the need for testing the sound-errors in a sufficiently wide variety of phonetic contexts of the speaker's language. It gauges the pupil's ability to make the troublesome sound in various contexts where it is adjacent to or blended with other speech sounds. This testing often reveals that a speaker can make the sound more easily and correctly when it is associated with some sounds than with others. Because deep testing is respectful of linguistic principles which operate in spoken language and affect articulation, the method does more than classify errors and note whether the faulty sounds occur in the initial, medial, or final positions of words. It follows the belief that speech is a sequential flow of connected articulated sounds made as overlapping ballistic movements and that articulation, therefore, should be tested in its normal sequential contexts of language units. A therapist who includes "deep testing" in his evaluations of pupils' misarticulation has remarked:

> For years I tested articulation merely by using a list of words or objects to elicit singly spoken words from my clients. Then I learned that a client often articulated sounds in single words differently than when he joined them in words, phrases, or in sentences. So, by testing the articulatory errors in a series of sentences, I gained better guidelines for therapy because therapy is usually easier when one starts work upon errors within phonemic contexts which have been partially learned.

An evaluation of misarticulation should include not only an analysis of the sounds in error but also an appraisal of the speaker's attitudes and other attributes which relate to the problem and its correction. It is important to note whether or not the person is aware of his faulty phonemes and whether or not he can consider his defect objectively and constructively and is willing to work on its improvement. A speech therapist with many years of effective service in the public schools has said:

> During my first two or three years of professional work with articulation, I treated the defective sounds but did not consider the person who made them.

One might say that I centered my attention and efforts on the pupil's articulatory region—extending from his neck to his nose. I was like a piano tuner who had little interest in the piano except for its poor notes and their mechanical adjustment. I soon learned, however, that the pupil who misarticulates had to be considered more fully. The client's intelligence and his attitudes toward himself and his speech are important angles to allow for in therapy. In testing and prognosticating, it's necessary to test and evaluate the psychological and social factors of the pupil. I don't mean that one must delay speech therapy with a pupil until complete data on the client's intelligence, personality and social life can be gathered. Many of these valuable appraisals come from the pupil's behavioral reactions during speech examinations, therapy, and from information provided by classroom teachers and parents through conferences. Diagnosis and therapy go hand in hand, because the person and his problem hopefully change as therapy progresses. A therapist must keep up with these changes and allow for them.

Helping the Pupil to Correct His Misarticulation

It may be more appropriate to think of *helping* a person to correct speech errors than of *teaching* him to do so. The concept of *helping* places greater reliance upon the person who has the problem and who must perform the actual correction to it. While teaching is basically necessary and important, it often must function in supplementary or subordinate ways—as a resource of aids, influence and support for the person who must perform the correction. If a therapist or teacher loses sight of the fact that the person and not his defect must be the point of reference, speech therapy becomes an administration of indiscriminate lessons, drills, and teaching devices. A teacher expresses this viewpoint in the following thoughtful statement:

In speech correction, I've found that the element of teaching follows the same principles that hold in teaching a child to read, write, or do arithmetic. In teaching reading, for example, we follow manuals and workbooks which specify certain goals and outline procedures for all the children. It becomes obvious, however, that children differ in their needs. When problems develop, the teacher must recognize that solutions depend upon these individual differences. If a pupil is subjected to teaching measures which do not apply to him, his reading problem may even be intensified. In one's zeal to correct and to teach a pupil, it is easy to forget that *he* is the one who must eventually achieve the mental processes and physical skills which must be combined into the act of genuine reading. It is not enough to lead him across page after page of print, faithfully pronouncing word after word for him. Much more is needed before he can enter the act and become an independent reader.

So it is with children who cannot say some of their speech sounds. It is obvious that there is as much of a teaching-learning process in speech correction as in remedial reading. My association with speech therapists has convinced me that their success depends upon educational principles that are similar to ours in the teaching of reading and other subjects. In the first place, the child must be inspired to talk better. As with reading, he must know what's wrong and what should be done and, if necessary, given some guidance and practice in acquiring those goals.

When the role of the speech therapist or teacher is considered from the point of view of the pupil who has the problem to correct, five areas in teaching are suggested. Stated in the form of questions which the pupil might ask if he could realize his needs in correcting misarticulation, they are:

Why should I articulate better?
What's wrong with my present articulation? What should I say?
How can I say it correctly?
How can I get to say it easily and habitually?

In correcting misarticulation, the needs suggested by the above questions are not necessarily met in their stated order. Goals in the correction of speech problems are usually interrelated; they are not met and fulfilled one by one and then dismissed. For example, the strongest incentive for correcting misarticulation may arise in a pupil only after he has been taught to correct a faulty sound and when he begins to experience the new rewards from improved speech. It should be remembered that instructional goals must fit each person's stage of developmental learning. The same goals and their relative weight and sequence do not apply equally to all cases of misarticulation.

WHY SHOULD I ARTICULATE BETTER?

Perhaps no goal is more important and yet so neglected as this one. Unless a pupil is sufficiently convinced that his present articulation is faulty and inadequate, efforts to change his articulation will be futile. It is easy for therapists and teachers to project concerns for a client and to assume that he shares their desire to remove the faults which they have been trained to recognize in him. But unless a pupil's misarticulation has become a definite concern or handicap in his life, he may show apathy and even resistance to the efforts by therapists and teachers to force him to make unwanted speech readjustments. However, a pupil who has not yet recognized the handicap of misarticulation may become motivated to work upon it mainly to please his therapist, teacher, or other persons. There are many ways by which therapists, teachers, parents, pupils, and others have motivated pupils to correct their misarticulation. Some of the more common influences which have prompted pupils to work upon their faults are found in the following excerpts gathered from therapists, teachers, and parents.

A speech therapist describes his method of stimulating five- and six-year-olds to correct their relatively commonplace misarticulations:

I've found that a majority of children in kindergarten lack sufficient desire to correct their faulty sounds. Sound-errors are not novel in these young children.

Unless a child has been teased or penalized in some way for his misarticulation, he may not care. He may become uncooperative and even resistant to our efforts to change it. Again, if he has suffered too much because of his problem, he may be oversensitive and also defensive and unwilling to work upon it. In either case, we therapists have a selling job to do. The child must like me, respect me, and want to please me by doing what I ask of him. This approach requires that I clarify for him the rightness and wrongness of his articulations. When I put my stamp of approval on the right and sufficient disapproval on the wrong, he will often move in the direction I want him to go. Praise and all types of rewards are used to encourage his efforts and to reinforce his progressive steps.

Another therapist evaluates other positive ways to entice a pupil to work on his misarticulation:

Usually there are more effective ways to get a child to work upon his speech than merely to tell him "That's good!" or stick stars after his name or tie his efforts and successes in speech work to the winning of various competitive games. I try to find some special interests in which each child already has developed a vocabulary and a desire to communicate the interests. I look for words related to the important topics and containing his wrong sounds. We work upon these words in conversation where they are communicatively important. When work is carried on within this area of interest, I find that the child will attend to words more closely and will take a greater personal responsibility for their improvement. For instance, if a lisper had a strong interest in camping, we would collect many words containing *s* and associated with camping activities. I've worked with groups of boys on Cub Scout and 4-H projects in which speech work was made an integral part of the achievements.

The following therapist explains how he motivates children by creating new interests for them and then rewarding them in tangible ways for their efforts and successes in speech work:

For the past several years I have devised a system of motivation which not only provides children of various ages with an incentive to work on speech errors but also leaves them with newly developed interests and hobbies which provide values beyond those of speech correction. One approach centers around seashells. My wife and I collect lots of miscellaneous seashells during our summers spent in Florida. I keep a supply of the shells at school and develop the children's interest and knowledge about seashells and seashore life. We work on the articulation of words and sentences about shells and seashore. I reward the pupils for their efforts and successes by giving them seashells. Incidentally, when I dismiss a case from therapy, I give him a little mounted display of shells as a "graduation" gift. To the ones who have severe problems and are slow to "graduate," I periodically give shells for their steps of achievement along the way.

A therapist and classroom teacher who cooperated closely in stimulating unmotivated children described their use of peer influences:

We have cooperatively worked out a rather unique way to spur children to work upon their speech. Formerly, we strictly followed the usual policy of grouping misarticulation cases of the same age or grade. Now we find that problems and personalities are more effectively handled in groups of mixed ages, such as putting a fifth-grader, a fourth-grader, and a third-grader with two second-graders. But we should group similar problems. By focusing therapeutic efforts on one or two of the older children, who are picked for having model attitudes and good work habits, we encourage the selected leaders to act as prime movers for the others. The younger children tend to emulate their leaders' actions; the older ones get satisfaction from being helpers of the young. One can also take advantage of the built-in motivating force which comes from the older children's wanting to work so as to get rid of the speech characteristics which classify and hold them with the young. In the process, they act as bellwethers to make the younger children work and move along to overcome their unlearned sounds.

Although praise and various positive rewards are usually recommended to get children to work on their misarticulation, penalties and other negative forces sometimes act effectively. A speech therapist experienced in public school work explained his philosophy and policy:

During my first few years of professional work, I went overboard to make speech therapy sweet and pleasurable for the children. I tried to keep them from feeling any stigma over their unlearned speech sounds. We played speech games which were fun. I strove to make them eager to come for speech therapy. In fact, I saw signs that the rewarding fun from therapy made some pupils want to continue in my program year after year rather than to correct their problems and stop coming. Pupils were given a fair chance to work and earn worthy rewards from their work—including the right to be dismissed. For instance, some of the teachers were dubious about the occasional scheduling of a pupil's speech work on two of his five recess periods each week. But teachers accepted the idea when they realized that in certain cases it placed therapy on a more businesslike basis and brought better results. Besides, teachers saw that these therapy sessions may also serve as "breaks" from classroom routines and confinement, giving the children satisfying individual outlets for expression.

Teachers and therapists soon learn that a speech client's feelings about his speech problem are influenced by various outside sources which therefore must be considered in therapy. A therapist's sincere desire to correct a child's misarticulation may not be a sufficient reason for the child to feel the need and make the change. Sometimes parents, classroom teachers, and others are in better positions to influence the child to work and to change his speech patterns. For this reason, therapists often work cooperatively with parents and teachers to stimulate them to show greater interest and appreciation for the child's work and progress in speech by providing them with evidences of the child's work and suggesting ways they can encourage the child and reinforce his gains.

There are other ways to motivate a person to correct his misarticulation.

Teasing a child for faults which he can correct may not necessarily be harmful. Teasing can be helpful if it is not excessive, if it brings necessary awareness of his deficiency—provided the child has access to sufficient support to help him overcome the teasing and meet the acceptable articulatory standard of his social group. In the belief that "he will outgrow it," teachers and parents may be too ready to accept a child's misarticulation and successfully learn to understand his speech. But they impose a false show of confidence on his inward uncertainty and frustration. A first-grade teacher voices her philosophy on this point as follows:

> I believe in being direct, honest, and factual with my pupils when they have articulatory mistakes which deserve my help. I treat speech mistakes with the same objectivity that I give mistakes in reading, arithmetic, or other factual matters. I point out mistakes as mistakes. I treat them as matters to be taught and learned. I try to understand what a child is saying even though his speech intelligibility is low, but I do not try to guess if I don't understand. I let him feel some responsibility for not being understood. If a child is not aware of his mistakes and if I feel that he should be made aware of them, I help him to realize his deficiencies. Hearing himself on a tape recorder may also aid him to realize that something is wrong in his speech and give him a desire to correct the mistakes.
>
> If other pupils inquire about mistakes in a child's speech, I try to give them open, informative, and satisfying answers. Under these policies, I find that there is little teasing of misarticulation or of other speech problems. Problems are respectfully regarded as matters to be given mutual help.

WHAT'S WRONG WITH MY PRESENT ARTICULATION? WHAT SHOULD I SAY?

The dual question "what is wrong?" and "what is right?" is considered jointly because it must be resolved through joint action in therapy. As previously stated, the corrective process cannot be neatly divided into distinct steps which follow a definite sequence. The client must gain a clear perception of what is right along with what is wrong. This important differentiation is not easy to teach or learn. Teachers and therapists observe that a child can usually detect and judge an articulatory error in others' speech more readily than he can in his own.

The perceptual training of what is wrong and what is right in one's articulation appears to be a comparative process involving the learning of contrasts through interdependent circuits—external and internal. In learning to speak a language correctly, a child must learn the characteristics of the many phonemic patterns from information which he hears and sees in the speech of others. From this flow of externally perceived information, and guided by the regulatory internal circuits of his self-hearing and self-feeling of his speech, the child learns to produce, match, and fix similar phonemic patterns in his own speech. If there are gaps or insufficient data within these interdependent perceptual circuits, the speaker may fail to meet acceptable standards of articulation.

In this intricate process, he must learn not only *what* to do but also what *not* to do. While articulatory patterns are being learned in his early formative stages, a child appears to regulate himself through self-perceptions which are shaped primarily from information on the hearing and seeing of articulation in other speakers. Later his articulation, correct or incorrect, tends to become automated. The automation is seemingly regulated by the feel and sound of himself, with diminished reliance upon his perceptions of external speech models.

Whenever teaching and learning depend heavily upon perceptions, as they do in correcting a pupil's misarticulations, it is important first to determine whether or not the child has normal acuity of hearing and vision. If this information is not obtainable from school records of the auditory and visual tests which every public school child should have, attempts should be made to provide these tests in the school.

Teachers and speech therapists should not only consider the child's test results but should also insure that sufficient use is made of his perceptual capacities. He may need training in the fuller use of his ears, eyes, touch, and feel of muscle movement. His perceptual skills need development not only for mastering articulation but also for learning reading, writing, and many other achievements. Harris,[6] for example, explains how a pupil's reading ability depends upon his perceptual training in the auditory and visual characteristics of sounds and the discriminations between them.

Speech correction profits from the knowledge and procedures which have been developed for phonic instruction in the field of reading. The speech therapist who is acquainted with the perceptual requirements for reading is less likely to violate the linguistic principles which underlie spoken language generally. Teachers of reading, for instance, have found that phonic training is easier and faster when words are left whole and are not divided into sound segments of less than the syllable unit. The perception of parts depends upon configurational aspects. When we dismember a unit of speech, we may be obscuring or distorting the perceptual distinctions which identify the profile of that unit. In reading, the pupil is trained to listen for the sound in *known* words where he may be aided in his perception by having the sound lettered, underlined, dramatized, or highlighted in other ways. In speech correction too, perceptual training is likely to be more effective when an analytic rather than a synthetic approach is followed, when learning proceeds from *wholes* to their *parts* and from the *known* to the *unknown*.

Unless perceptual experiences in speech correction, as in reading instruction, carry sufficient impact upon the pupil, they will not make lasting imprints. Perceptual training in the sound, sight, and feel of speech events should not leave the pupil with the thought, "So what?" Perceptual experiences should have conceptual significance; they should be personalized and enriched with emotion and clinched with judgment. The following therapist emphasizes how she teaches pupils the characteristics of speech sounds by working analytically, starting from meaningful and larger wholes and then delving into the characteristics of their parts:

> Although I still do a limited amount of perceptual training on isolated speech sounds, most of my work is upon sounds fitted within their natural language settings—within the framework of words and sentences. Previously, I drilled systematically on speech sounds in isolation where they not only meant little to the pupil but also did not give training on the true sounds of that phoneme as it occurred in various language settings where the pupil eventually had to learn and use it. Oh, I dressed the sound up in fancy letterings, identified it with associations with sounds made by tea kettles, fire engines, snakes, tigers, geese, Indians, etc., but these efforts often became dead ends—too far removed from the child's need to regard and use these sounds in his everyday language. I had meant to simplify the task for him, but really I was teaching him perceptual and articulatory patterns which were often unimportant, irrelevant, and even foreign to the ones he needed for speech. In fact, in some cases I found that a pupil had more difficulty in distinguishing isolated sounds than when realistic variations of those sounds were made in larger units of speech.
>
> I recall a third-grade boy, for instance, who had the error of substituting the "th" sound for the "s". I did not insist that he must learn first the characteristics of these phonemes in isolation and to practice the "snake" sound by itself. Instead, I selected words and short sentences in which the substitution of "th" for the "s" sound produced meaningful linguistic differences for him. I found pairs of words like *thumb* and *some*, *bath* and *bass*, *think* and *sink*, *mouth* and *mouse*, etc. He learned not only to perceive the phonetic and visual characteristics and contrasts between "th" and "s" in these spoken words but also learned to associate these sounds with their written symbols and their differences semantically. I trained him to perceive differences and to indicate his judgments of correctness when these sounds were interchanged in various ways to create right, wrong, and even humorous effects upon language and meanings. For instance, I might ask the child to nod or shake his head in judging my usages of "th" and "s" in such choices as:
>
> "Look, am I opening my mou*th*?" in comparison with "Look, am I opening my mou*s*e?"
> "I caught a ba*th*," with "I caught a ba*ss*."
> "I *s*ink it will *th*ink" and "I *th*ink it will *s*ink."
> "Please pa*th* me *s*ome," "Please pa*ss* me *th*umb," and "Please pa*ss* me *s*ome."
>
> After the client proved that he could clearly distinguish the phonemic differences in my spoken words and sentences, I trained him to perceive and adopt these usages in his speech while I served as judge and gave timely instructions in this developmental process. Later he and I searched our vocabularies for numerous *s* and *th* words, saying them rightly or wrongly, in words and in sentences, trying to trick each other into overlooking mistakes. I have found that even kindergartners are keenly impressed by hearing and saying words which create amusing, novel, or preposterous meanings from being misused in words and sentences which they know. This approach makes a child motivated and perceptually

attentive, and it bridges that difficult gap which occurs when one is taught new sounds which are too separate from his adopted speech usage.

According to the next therapist perceptual training to correct a phonemic distortion may be more difficult when alerting a pupil against substituting one correct phoneme for another:

A child may find difficulty in perceiving a distortion of his *s* phoneme, for example. When he distorts a phoneme, he must learn to identify that phoneme and to bring it within the boundaries of normality for that phoneme. It is not easy for him to determine the standards of correctness for his *s*. But until he does make this perceptual reorientation, he will be unable to revise his articulation of it. The therapist, teacher, or parent must help the child establish these new standards. Suppose a child distorts the *s* by lateralizing it in a fashion which allows the air to escape broadly over both sides of his tongue instead of directing it through a groove to his middle front teeth. The resulting sound may be a strange combination of an "l" sound with an "sh." I would imitate the child's distortion as closely as possible, not only to show him how his faulty phoneme looks and sounds but so that I can learn what he does wrong in the production of it. Here too, I usually find that the distorted sound can be more effectively worked at within words and sentences. However, after the child perceives that his *s* is perceptually incorrect I may then make incorrect and correct isolated models of it in order to pinpoint the faulty features of his production of it. But as a rule, I work upon the flaw within the contexts of words and sentences, because speech sounds make sense when they are judged in language where they ultimately belong. Another difficulty arises when a pupil cannot appreciate and accept our imposed standards of correctness for a phoneme. He may adequately perceive the gradations in our produced sound patterns but yet may not accept the level at which we want him to fix it. He may be induced to form a more definite conviction concerning a produced pattern if this pattern is associated with words which already carry important semantic values for him. For instance, suppose that a child is working to raise his acceptance level and satisfaction toward a revised *s*. On the negative side I would find words containing this phoneme and representing things which he did not like: perhaps *sour milk, spinach, sick*, etc. To offset these negatively imbued words, I would pair them with words like *sweet milk, celery*, and *squirrel*. By working to limit his substandard *s* within these few words associated with undesirability, I find I can more easily tip the scales in favor of his correct *s*. His new *s* is made more positive by this semantic reinforcement with words symbolizing preference.

The effects of semantics upon misarticulation may also be therapeutically employed when a child omits sounds from his words. Patient perceptual training is required in the correction of sound omissions, not only to make the client aware of his omissions but also to instill in him the conviction that it pays to include the missing sounds where they belong. The following kindergarten teacher explains how she helps her pupils recognize their omissions:

Most of my pupils who omit sounds in their speech are corrected by the work we do in learning the letters and sounds of the alphabet and in the related phonic work of sounding out words from their letters. In all of this teaching and learning, we rely upon careful listening, looking, and even upon the feel of how we make our speech sounds. Our speech therapist has given helpful pointers in this work. The children are taught from the beginning that they must rely upon their "speech helpers"—their ears and eyes—to tell them how to use their lips, teeth, tongue, voice box, etc. We learn to listen for wrong sounds as well as for right ones in words. I pass out small mirrors so that each member of my class can check on his mouth actions in making sounds which may be causing difficulty. This individual check on their actions, coupled with my silent demonstration of speech for lip-reading practice, helps to correct misarticulation, including sound omissions.

When pupils omit speech sounds, saying "boo" for *boot*, "pay" for *play*, "cool" for *school*, etc., I work at their problem from several angles. I exemplify these words in a clear and correct way whenever possible, sometimes exaggerating the sounds they omit. When children have learned to read, I point out the letters of the sounds they omit, reminding them that these sounds, too, are meant to be in the words. I may underline or encircle the letters of these neglected sounds, to remind pupils not to omit them in speech. I give them imitations of the mis-spoken words to help them recognize the nature of their errors. I show them that in some instances their sound omissions create entirely different words. For instance, I may ask them:

"Do you like to *pay* at recess? Or do you like to *play* at recess?"

"Is this a *cool* room? Or is this a *school* room?"

Children notice and feel more responsibility for their sound omissions when they are impressed by the differences their mistakes create in language.

The following teacher indicates how she uses word-rhyming exercises and a classroom game called "Don't lose the sounds when you pass them around," to help children who omit parts of words:

Some pupils leave out sounds and syllables from their words. For some children this seems to have resulted from a failure to hear and learn these omitted parts; in others, it seems that they have been careless in speaking. At the rate some children speak, it's no wonder they cut corners and miss the low spots of their racy utterances.

I believe that classroom teachers may help these pupils in several ways. First, we teachers must set adequate examples of correct speech in an atmosphere where pupils are interested, looking and listening. Of course, this requires that our class-rooms must be sufficiently quiet and free of distractions while we set these good examples. It also means that the pupils must feel respect and admiration for the teacher, or else they won't feel much desire to speak as she does. Recitation and oral reading should be conducted in an unhurried atmosphere, with patience and respect shown all speakers.

We can help pupils in formal ways too. I've found that rhyming exercises help to remind children of their word endings. We recite the published rhyming material which is available for teaching, and we also think up rhymes of our own. I may, for example, present them with the line, "I opened my book," inviting the class to come up with such a response as "And took another look" or "And read about the zook."

Another enjoyable classroom game, called "Don't lose the sounds when you pass them around," offers wide possibilities in teaching children to listen and imitate carefully. In this game the children stand up, elbow to elbow. I cup my hands to the ear of the first pupil in the line and speak either a syllable, a word, a sentence or a nonsense utterance. Each successive pupil receives and passes this vocal utterance along through cupped hands to the ear of the next recipient, the object being to keep the spoken sounds from being lost or altered in passage. I may step into the line at any point to check whether the sound has been changed or lost; if so, I restore it and send it on its way. Easy words, like *boy* and *moon*, are included with utterances of more challenging difficulty. In this game the pupils are stimulated to pay close attention to speech and to imitate well.

Speech therapists and teachers frequently use tape recorders to help pupils recognize personal errors in articulation. It is likely that the growing use in the home of small and inexpensive tape recorders is assisting children of all ages to hear and judge their speech. The following speech therapist comments on his use of tape recorders to solve misarticulation problems:

> I credit much of my success in correcting misarticulation to the use of tape recorders. First, they help in my analysis of the errors and in keeping accurate records of these errors for purposes of measuring progress. Second, the tape recorder gives the children a more accurate and easily acceptable picture of how they talk than I could show or describe for them. When children are given a chance to hear recorded samples of their speech, "before and after," they realize progress and are motivated to continue. I'm not saying that the use of a tape recorder has lessened the need for personal teaching skills, however. If anything, it calls for greater fidelity in teaching. For example, when I let a child hear himself on a tape recorder, I also try to show him my imitation of his error. I make recordings of these imitations too, and if my imitations are not close to his, this deficiency in my teaching is more clearly evident. Tape recorders may enable everyone to examine problems more objectively and to create constructive attitudes toward therapy.

> Teachers, too, have found greater uses for tape recorders in their classrooms. Our district supplied a recorder to every classroom from kindergarten to high school. These recorders not only serve academic purposes but also generate interest and inform everyone about speech. As one teacher said: "Our tape recorder has become one of our most popular tools for learning in the classroom. The children quickly learn to operate it under my supervision, and they have suggested some excellent uses for it. From the use of it, I have discovered some faults in my speech behavior, too. I tend to talk too much, too fast and to slur my words. We also use it to check on the volume and quality of our voices. Pupils who have speech problems can be made nicely aware of the fact. But I am careful to use it as an aid, not as a threat merely to expose weaknesses.

HOW CAN I SAY IT CORRECTLY?

"I can't say that."

"I don't know how."

"That's too hard to say."

"Show me."

These are statements which indicate that a pupil is trying to correct his misarticulation, that he knows he still is not speaking correctly, and that he seeks help in saying a sound correctly. It is evident that the solution to the problem of "How can I say it?" is closely related to the previously considered stages of the corrective process, pertaining to the issues of "What is wrong?" "What is right?" and "Am I saying it well enough now?" Perceptual training is needed not only to clarify for the pupil *what* the articulatory difference should be but also *how* he can achieve this difference. A therapist who emphasizes the importance of providing perceptual information declares:

> In teaching our clients to modify their articulatory productions, we may make the mistake of acting too much as trainers rather than as helpers and resourcers. In a therapist's or teacher's eagerness to bring corrected sounds from a client's mouth, it is easy for them to treat him in a manipulative fashion without recognizing that a speaker must regulate his own speech act ultimately and as soon as possible. Even though we may become skilled in our diagnosis of what a client is doing wrong in articulation, if we become too oriented around methods, techniques, exercises, and applied skills, we may deny that speaker the chance to employ his own senses and to correct himself. However, the therapist who acts more as a resourcer and helper in time of need is one who more completely diagnoses the case in terms of when, where, and how that speaker needs help. The relationship is client-centered, working to open channels of information, perceptions, and motivation for the client to use in correcting his problem. This type of therapist generally works in a more indirect manner, helping the client to have successful experiences and acquire self-responsibility as soon as possible. A client under this working relationship is more likely to succeed.

The next speech therapist has observed that a client who has been given basic perceptual stimulation often needs relatively little direct instruction on how to manipulate his tongue, lips, and other articulators in the correction of his faulty sounds:

> I used to move right in with tongue depressors, fingers, and a flood of wordy directions to get a child to move his tongue, lips, and jaw as I thought he should use them in order to make the speech sounds that I had in mind for him to say. I would work diligently to modify his defective sounds, but the alterations didn't last; they didn't appear to mean to the child what they meant to me. Then I noticed that some of my pupils were expert at imitating ricocheting bullets, screeching brakes, the clicks of hammers, and numerous other complex sounds which were easy for them to make but impossible for me until I went through the process of taking careful stock of these playful imitations, practicing them in a

joint manner with the children until I could match their patterns. The children certainly had proved that they did not have "lazy" or uncoordinated articulators in making these complex sound imitations. So I decided to give more attention to the preparing of children for making the new sounds of speech, by helping them to create genuine interests in the improved sounds and subjecting them to vivid impressions of the visual and auditory characteristics of the sounds. I learned that most clients with functional misarticulation can and will learn to maneuver their own tongues, jaws, and lips properly without much immediate manipulation from me, provided they are set up for this acquisition.

In the discussion of the following ways to teach a pupil how to articulate correctly, it will be apparent that the measures will relate to all stages of the child's learning process. Some of the teaching devices would appropriately fit under the previously discussed categories of motivation and perceptual training —a further reminder that the therapy process is not a route which is divided into distinct steps, each of which is traversed only once. Like a repeatedly traveled highway, the course requires maintenance, to patch holes and to reroute traffic when indicated. Occasionally the irregularities of old, hardened configurations must be scarified and rebuilt with freshened materials. The therapy route must be duly patrolled and regulated with directions from adequate information and signs to insure a correct course of action. For instance, in a comparison of six methods of aural stimulation, Webb and Siegenthaler[7] found that a child made more correct productions in work upon misarticulation when he was provided with evaluations of his responses and when opportune verbal instruction was given to point out his specific mistakes. The least effective methods of stimulation in their research experiment were obtained when the child was given only aural stimulation, or when stimulation plus hearing was provided, or when the child was given aural stimulation simultaneously with his utterance. This lack of immediate evaluation and on-the-spot instruction is one of the difficulties in the use of teaching machines and programed instruction to correct misarticulation.

Another requisite in therapy for misarticulation appears to be the client's need to escape from "old ruts," to loosen and alter his habituated faults in using the tongue, jaw, lips, etc. As previously mentioned, this process requires "unlearning" as well as learning. It depends upon a resensitizing of the speaker's senses which provide him with the information he needs to make the changes in articulation. When a speaker with functional misarticulation is sufficiently motivated and equipped with this information of *what* needs to be articulated, he will usually learn *how* to do it.

As donors of faith and patient reliance which the client deserves from us in the correction of his misarticulation, we can find many appropriate ways to help him. In the following excerpts, teachers, therapists, parents, and others have suggested some of the ways to facilitate learning and progress along the therapeutic path. The first quotation pertains to a speech therapist's use of tactile cues:

In my speech therapy with pupils who are learning to correct their faulty sounds and who have trouble in learning new placements of the tongue, I find that the common toothpick is one of my most useful tools. At first I used tongue depressors and orange sticks to point out where a pupil should or should not place his articulators. But toothpicks proved better and cheaper. In each of my therapy rooms around the schools I keep a box of them ready to use, for instance, when a child is slow to learn by himself where the tip of his tongue should go for the *l*, the *k*, *r*, *th*, *s*, *sh*, etc. With the toothpick's flat end I can safely chafe the part of the child's mouth where the tongue must make contact, leaving a tactile sensation which lasts for several minutes to direct him in making a particular sound. This method has the effect of drawing one's tongue to the sensitized spot—as the tongue tends to seek the gap from newly pulled teeth. I believe that these tactile sensations aid in the proprioceptive controls which we get from our muscle action—cues needed for the control which must take over in speech before articulation can become a smoothly integrated and automatic act. It is important for speakers to hear and to see articulation, but eventually they must regulate themselves on a more internal level, and the toothpicks, judiciously used, get right to the nerve endings of the muscles that need retraining.

Another therapist describes one of her methods to help a pupil locate the specific points in his mouth where articulatory changes are being established:

We sometimes use bits of tissue paper and mirrors to mark and sensitize the different contact points where we articulate the problem sounds of speech. I first demonstrate to the child where I place the little tab of tissue on my tongue, roof of the mouth, lips, etc., in order to make the desired sound. Then I give the child a tab of tissue and let him spot it correspondingly in his mouth, afterwards using a mirror to compare his position with mine. We continue to make the sound, using our tabs as focal points to remind and direct us in the right postures. The tissues remain stuck in place for a number of trials. If the tissue moves before we are through working with it, we replace it, thus refreshing our perceptions of where the sound is made. In this method, I believe that much of the value comes from the reliance placed upon the child to map and touch his own mouth contacts rather than from having someone else point the way, stroke the spot, and try to keep him reminded through verbal instruction. This method is usually much more effective than my trying to direct him only by telling him what to do and what not to do.

One therapist effectively used photos of the mouth in various articulatory positions:

With photographic help from a friend, I have developed an effective way of instructing pupils through close-up snapshots taken of my mouth in making speech sounds. This set of pictures, mounted separately under durable plastic, is used in various instructional games. Pupils verify the snapshot postures by viewing themselves in mirrors. We direct each other also through verbal descriptions of what we do right and wrong. The photos help to motivate children to use visual cues; they facilitate lip reading for persons who are in special need of that com-municative skill. I have also used models and sketches to show speech postures. But I prefer photography. It is more accurate and versatile in its uses. For instance, I have used photography to motivate a child to work and achieve correction by taking snapshots of his mouth in wrong and in right positions. I've used snaps in speech books being built for him to keep and display at home. Parents are usually favorably impressed with these photos too. Some of the teachers of kindergarten and first grade have asked for reprints of some of my photos to use in their teaching of letter-sounds and the phonics of word-beginnings. I am convinced that it pays to cooperate with classroom teachers in this area of phonic work.

Speech therapists and teachers have devised various other gadgets to help in the identification and production of correct sounds. Puppets, which are frequently used as motivational devices and as instructional go-betweens, are discussed by the following therapist:

I prefer to use homemade puppets for therapy rather than to buy them. When children make, decorate, name their own puppets, and know that they may eventually keep them, they show greater interest and responsibility in working with puppets. Our most popular and easily made puppet is made of sacks. We make even the sacks—hand-sized or finger-cot size. We usually draw and color a face on the sack-puppet and write on its back the letter which represents that puppet's sound. When a child has learned to say that sound in a "key word," the successfully spoken word is written on the back or side of the sack. As he learns to say correctly more words having that sound, these words are added to his puppet's list. The puppet becomes a concrete incentive for work, a record of the child's progress, and a growing reminder and supply of key words to show the child how to say the problem sound. Sensitive and shy children work more easily when they can share their problems with someone. To children, a puppet can become an important someone. Occasionally, I let the children take their puppets home to show their family. These puppets, with their guiding symbols and records of successful words, display and expand the children's achievements in speech work. Whenever possible, at parent conferences and in my talks before P.T.A.'s, I suggest that parents make good use of all types of schoolwork which their children bring home. When a child has earned the right to keep a puppet, learning to say its sound and to fulfill a certain quota of correctly spoken words, I may find that his mother has proudly pinned it to a kitchen curtain or bulletin board.
Finger puppets have an advantage over fist puppets by enabling a child to operate two or more puppets on his hands at once. For instance, a child's speech confidence may be boosted if he is given five finger puppets: four with easy sounds, such as "m," "p," "t," and "k," and one with a problem sound, which may be "s." By exercising his correct usage of the four easy sounds in various sound and word games played with the puppets, he realizes that his total articulation is more correct than faulty. Our finger puppets become actively engaged in teaching and evaluating each other.
We have made mask-faces on larger head-sized paper sacks, with holes for our eyes and mouths, worn over our heads as live puppets. When these masks with

large mouth openings are worn before a mirror, they help to focus upon the visual aspects of the mouth, to point out the right and wrong articulations of sounds. Here, too, I find that even sensitive children will face their problems and will work more intently with masks than they may act in the open.

Other techniques and gadgets have been invented to suggest either the nature of the sound to be taught or the manner in which it is produced. A therapist explains some of his techniques in teaching certain sounds:

When a child misarticulates a sound, I first try to determine a predominant feature which accounts for his faulty production. Then I try to find some way to vivify for him the perceptual and mechanical feature which determines rightness or wrongness for that sound. For example, a child may spoil an *r* and give it a *w* quality by uttering it through the round opening of his pursed lips. I may point out this faulty lip action in a combination of ways: telling him to "smile" while he says words beginning with the "r" sound, thus eliminating the pursing; stretching apart the corners of his mouth with my thumb and forefinger while he says words with *r*; reminding him by tape not to purse his lips, by taping an inch or two of plastic bandage or scotch tape from the corners of his mouth to his cheeks; and using the mirror to give further information of what he does. I have placed adhesive tape on the skin for other sounds too. A short strip of tape stuck at the midpoint of a speaker's upper lip will help to direct him to raise his tongue-tip for the sounds of *t*, *l*, and *n*; a patch of tape below the rear part of his chin will help to direct his tongue toward the *k* or *g* if he has the tendency to substitute them with *t* and *d*. For a cerebral palsied speaker, who may lack coordination and perceptual awareness of his muscle action, I have used adhesive tape in longer strips, placed over various parts of his face, to give him a better perceptual picture of what he is doing, so that he may learn to stabilize competing reflexive movements of his musculature.

We therapists have used all kinds of gimmicks to instruct lispers to sharpen or narrow the stream of air for the "s" sound. At times I have had success by stroking down the midline of the client's tongue or laying a length of string along its midline, telling him to press his tongue against the roof of his mouth while I pull the string outward between his middle front teeth. This leaves a sensation and a suggestion for him to narrow that escaping stream of air for the *s*.

There are other methods to point out that this narrowed, constricted passage of air is necessary for a good *s*. I may stroke the inside edges of his upper teeth and tell him that his tongue must touch along these gum borders—except in front, where he must leave a little opening for the air to come through nearly closed teeth. These directions are conveyed by showing, telling, touching, and even by dramatizing them. For example, I have made paper cones of the approximate size of ice-cream cones, with a tiny opening at the small end and a flattened opening at the large inch-wide end. When the little opening of the cone is held close to the client's teeth, which are positioned for the *s*, it helps to suggest and direct a narrowed emission of air. When the large opening is presented, the client is directed to relax the front of the tongue and let the air gush through the wider openings. I have identified the "s" sound with the sound that a tire makes when it is punctured and leaks air, but pointing out that some "flat tire" sounds are good and some are not the kind we should make. We find pictures of tires and punch holes of various sizes in them, ranging from a large pencil-sized hole for the substituted "sh" and the "th" sounds to the small pencil-point size for a good constricted *s*. Even children of preschool age will get the idea of these two types of sounds and their productions from these holes. They try hard to make flat tires with the small-puncture sound.

Another therapist explains why he keeps a little flashlight in each of his schools' therapy rooms:

> We frequently use a little flashlight of pen-light size to examine our mouth positions in articulation. It not only lets us see by lighting up the shaded interiors of our mouths but also helps to focus the attention of pupils upon the mouth areas being studied. We also find that the flashlight helps in our viewing before the mirror. It enables us to see the palatal areas in making sounds like "r" and "k," after we "freeze" the tongue positions required for these sounds.

The next therapist uses several homemade devices to intensify the auditory characteristics of sounds being taught:

> I make simple cardboard megaphones but use them in a reversed fashion as ear trumpets, to clarify and amplify the sound I direct into a child's ear. If one uses it as a megaphone, its mouthpiece should be large enough so that it doesn't restrict the speaker's lip or jaw action.
>
> We have also made some "self-telephones" from quart milk cartons to aid self-hearing of speech. By cutting a hole in each end of one side of the carton, a child can speak into one end and more clearly hear the sounds carried through the carton to the other hole before his ear.

Classroom teachers also give pointers in the production of speech sounds by teaching their pupils the sounds of speech and the symbols that represent spoken language in reading and writing. The following first-grade teacher tells of several phonic exercises which she and speech therapists have exchanged, adapted, and found useful for speech and language training:

> We have shared many valuable exercises which are as adaptable to the classroom as they are in the speech therapy room. One game is called "Follow the Leader." I tell the children to watch me, to do what I do and say what I say, while I follow a routine designed for each sound. For example, to demonstrate the sound of "f" I wet my finger, hold it horizontally along my lower lip, and cool it with a prolonged "f" sound. For the *k* I place my fingers on my throat, open my mouth, tuck my tongue down, and say "k-k-k".
>
> We play a game called "Hitching Posts for Consonant Sounds." I tell the pupils to make three "posts" (vertical lines placed in a row on their papers), to listen and decide the relative position of the *s*, for instance, in the word *mouse*. Games like

this help the children learn to improve speech sounds and also their letters and word spellings.

We have an "Echo" game for careful enunciation. I group the children who need help in their articulation or pronunciation. I say a word on which the group needs practice, and the children respond as echoes of what I say. They try hard to duplicate my sounds and actions in this game.

My pupils also enjoy a game called "Backward Phonics" in which they try to guess short words which I sound out as the words would be spoken in reverse. For example, I may ask what a reversal of "oh—t" or "oh—s" would say.

We have a listening game called "Busy Phonics" in which the pupils listen carefully while I stretch out and somewhat separate the sounds which make up a selected word in a sentence, such as: "Let's see if you can all sss—mmm—ile." In this exercise when some of the sounds of a word cannot be truly spoken in isolation, I say them in their syllabic setting; otherwise I am likely to sound out the word in a mispronounced way and give the pupils a faulty pattern to judge. Another favorite game with the children is called "Phonics up Front." In this exercise a child volunteers to come forward and stand to the left of me, another child on my right. I secretly give each of them a spoken sound and ask each to say his assigned sound loudly and clearly when I tap him on the shoulder—while I speak a chosen vowel between their utterances. For instance, I may tap the first child, who says his sound, "fff"; I say "i"; the second child says "sh." The class is to respond with "fish." In this game I mostly assign sounds which I know can be correctly articulated by each child, but occasionally I assign a sound which I know the child will misarticulate. But I do not let the children's errors slip by without some corrective attention. I may imitate the error as well as demonstrate its correct articulation. If the child who made the error is working on it in speech therapy, I respectfully point out this fact and explain that this is one of the reasons we play this speech game. When a child through careful effort has shown that he can correct a sound, I make it a policy to assign him this sound so as to give him more confidence and practice in using it.

The following teacher describes some of the games which she and the speech therapist have used to improve speech and language for pupils in kindergarten and elementary grades:

"Toss the Block" is a game played by one or several children with alphabet blocks around a blanket spread on the floor. The children take turns tossing the blocks on the blanket, noting which letters come up on top. They think of words beginning with the sounds of these letters and speak them clearly and as well as they can. We sometimes toss two blocks at once, one with consonant sounds and the other with vowels, and then think of words containing syllables formed by the pairs of sounds. There can be many variations to this game.

We play another game that focuses upon initial sounds. I may begin with the unfinished sentence, "Billy likes butter and . . .," and the children finish with words beginning with *b*, such as *beans, baloney, beer, biscuits, basketball*, etc. An easier variation of this exercise calls for any words, beginning with an assigned sound, that Billy can "pack in his big box." Or, to make a game with more personal interest, we pick a child in the room and find all sorts of words which begin with the first sound of that person's name and represent things that that person might like to do, such as, "Mary likes to make money" or "Mary likes muskmelons and monkeys." If words are mispronounced, I clearly correct them. We have a game that requires the children to listen and focus upon the middle sounds of words. They are asked such questions as: "Which one can fly, a board or a bird?" "Which one grows on trees, a loaf or a leaf?" "Which one can crawl, a beetle or a bottle?" "Which word means to cook, to fry or to fly?" It's obvious that these games teach more than speech sounds; they develop vocabulary and grammar too.

Interesting ways have been used to teach children about their "speech helpers," the organs of speech and how they function in speech. One teacher reports:

> In kindergarten we talk about our speech helpers. My pupils learn about their speech helpers—the tongue, jaw, lips, teeth, hard and soft palate, breathing, and their voice box. They locate these parts and identify their uses in speech. I may say to them: "You can feel your hard palate when you move your tongue back over the roof of the mouth, and you can feel the soft palate working when you make a gargling sound or when you say "ung-ga" or "ink."
>
> We do many exercises to teach pupils a better use of their speech helpers. I have collected numerous jingles and stories which are designed to stimulate and direct children in the physical mechanics of speech. Five good sources of teaching materials which have been recommended by our speech therapist are:
>
> Clara B. Stoddard, *Sounds for Little Folks: Speech Improvement* (Magnolia, Mass.: Expression Co., 1940).
>
> Empress Young Zedler, *Listening for Speech Sounds: Stories for the Speech Clinician and the Classroom Teacher* (Garden City, N.Y.; Doubleday & Co. Inc., 1955).
>
> Louise B. Scott, *Soundie's Magnetic Learning Board* (Atlanta, Ga.: Webster Division, McGraw-Hill Book Co., 1964).
>
> Charles Van Riper and Katherine Butler, *Speech in the Elementary Classroom* (New York: Harper & Row, Inc., 1955).
>
> Stanley Ainsworth, *Galloping Sounds?* (Magnolia, Mass.: Expression Co., 1962).

Because children adopt the speech patterns which are most regularly heard and seen in their speech environment, their total daily experience strongly affects their standards of articulatory achievement. Yet many children correct their commonplace misarticulations without receiving any special or consciously given instructions at school. An experienced teacher of elementary grades describes her methods for children who are deficient in articulation or language:

> A child must hear plenty of correct speech. He must be talked to, talked with, and listened to. Since he learns what he hears, we must give him good patterns to imitate. I can usually tell a lot about a child's speech environment at home, just by noting the standards of speech and language which he brings to school at the kindergarten and first-grade levels. I've noticed that the correctness of a child's

articulation is especially determined as a result of his school experiences. His speech becomes increasingly modified by the corrective influences from teachers and pupils with better standards.

In order to direct my efforts where they are most needed, I have adopted several policies in working with pupils who misarticulate. First, I make a careful survey of how each pupil produces the sounds of his language. For the ones with normal articulation, I try to maintain their achievement through the ordinary school channels of stimulation, practice, and reward. In my conferences with parents, I give evaluations of their children's speech and compliment both the child and parent for the shared credit which they deserve. Parents appreciate this deserved praise for their efforts and, when they receive justifiable credit from their child's teacher, they are more inclined to continue the home practices which are needed to insure the child's speech progress.

Second, in addition to my demonstration of good speech for all of my pupils, I select certain pupils to serve as models for other pupils who are deficient in their articulation or language. For instance, I may pick a child who speaks well to recite to the class the story of the three bears, or to take the lead part in an "Echo" speech exercise, or to read to us a new poem or jingle to be learned. I find that some of the children with faulty articulation will more readily correct themselves through imitating classmates who speak correctly.

My reading of stories to the class is another good opportunity for me to demonstrate good speech patterns. Story reading should provide more than just entertainment. In my reading I try to articulate clearly and correctly. However, in certain of the stories I pointedly make articulatory deviations which are spoken as a part of the story. The Brer Rabbit stories, for example, are used to portray some of the irregularities which I aim to correct in the speech of some of my pupils. In stories containing young children as characters, I sometimes purposely assume "baby talk" and misarticulate, having the pupils listen carefully and signal in some way, like shaking the head or saying the word correctly, whenever they hear me mispronounce a word in the story. They enjoy this element added to the stories and become very perceptive in the process. For a variation I may assign children to the various speaking parts in the stories and let them improvise the speech in these roles and imitate the patterns of Brer Rabbit, "baby talk," and the rest. They become very adept in their impersonations in these creative dramatic settings. They learn to discriminate easily between the correct and incorrect patterns of speech, and I believe that they tend to be more careful in their own natural speech after these impressive sessions of acting.

HOW CAN I GET TO SAY IT EASILY
AND HABITUALLY?

High school students working on their misarticulation expressed this problem in their correction process:

"Sure, I can say the sound all right when I think about it, get set, and take my time. But when I don't think about it, I guess I slip into my old way of saying the sound."

"When I'm here in speech class and you remind me to say the sound right,

I do okay. But when I'm outside on my own and just talking, I get more interested in what I'm saying than how I'm saying it."

"Yes, I know how to say it but I forget, especially when I'm talking fast and am wrapped up in what I'm saying. I guess I need to tie a string around my finger to remind me to keep from lisping."

The preceding complaints by students indicate that this final stage in the therapeutic process is a difficult terminal goal, which speech therapists refer to by such terms as "stabilization," "reinforcement," "effecting a transfer," or "carry-over" of the new skills into everyday speech, "habituating" the new sounds, making them "automatic," etc. It should be remembered, however, that success in this terminal phase of speech correction rests upon critical factors and needs in therapy, such as the client's continuing incentive to change his old speech patterns and to adopt the new ones which we have taught him through the interrelated steps on the therapy route. Before a client can firmly adopt new articulatory patterns through usage, it may become necessary for teachers and therapists to review the earlier therapeutic needs that have been worked on for that client and to strengthen weaknesses which are found. A public school therapist explains how success in the final stage of habituating new articulatory patterns depends upon how well the previous foundations of therapy have been established:

> In my first years of work in the public schools, faced with excessive caseloads and long waiting lists of children needing help, I too often dismissed cases prematurely. I had the tendency to terminate scheduled therapy with a pupil as soon as he could produce the correct sound in words and sentences spoken in therapy sessions under my supervision. In the case of some dismissals, my trust in the ability of the children, their parents, and teacher to carry on was justified. But in other cases I learned that I had dropped my support too soon, that I had not prepared and maintained a strong enough base for their continued progress without me, and that other persons in their lives were needed to provide them with necessary encouragement and practice.
> I still dismiss some cases at the same stage of their incomplete correction, as I did before, but for others I have found it necessary to add extra measures to strengthen their self-reliance and perceptual skills, and to insure for them sufficient opportunities for rewards from practice. For all the pupils who are to be dismissed, I have laid greater stress on cooperation with their parents and teachers to provide this support. If pupils' incentive for improved articulation is too weak or if their rewards for better speech do not sufficiently extend beyond my sessions of direct therapy with them, the old and still strong patterns of articulating may prevail. Classroom teachers are generally my most capable allies in helping a child habituate his new sounds. Parents, too, are important in this phase of therapy, especially with young children who are closely tied to their family influences.

What may be expected of teachers and parents in reinforcing and extending speech therapy for a client? A speech therapist's reliance upon aid from teachers and parents rests upon his faith—what he thinks they can or cannot do to help within the classroom and home settings. Teachers and parents, too, must gain self-confidence and special knowledge for their roles in extending therapy. The therapist should be responsible for their supporting guidance. Therefore, the complete therapist is one who can not only handle his face-to-face work with a client but can also help others to fulfill their rightful responsibilities in insuring that the child's speech gains are not restricted or lost. To work alone with a client may be much more simple and easy than to bring parents and teachers into the therapeutic process. However, if the therapist is acquainted with the everyday roles of parents and teachers and if he invites their appropriate participation throughout the treatment period, their guidance and cooperation will be more helpful than problematical. Black,[8] in her discussion of professional relationships in public school speech correction, advises speech therapists to visit classrooms and observe teachers at work with children at all grade levels. Black also recommends that therapists should invite teachers to observe demonstrations of speech therapy sessions with pupils. Professionals and their clients gain much from this exchange.

Let us consider how some therapists, teachers, and parents have cooperated to insure continued progress for clients whose regularly scheduled therapy has been terminated. A speech therapist explains why the younger pupils of kindergarten, first, and second-grade levels are usually more successful than older pupils in the carry-over of articulatory corrections:

Until I made a follow-up study of my speech cases after their dismissal from my therapy classes, I believed that continued success depended upon the clients themselves. If they failed to progress but had proved before dismissal that they could articulate correctly, I was inclined to blame their relapses upon their lack of motivation, intelligence, maturation, or self-discipline to continue work on the new skills. But after I looked more carefully into the children's environments, I began to see other important determinants of their success or failure. I found that the work of teachers in the first three grades of school held many activities which had close relationship with my therapy work. Teachers and I learned that phonic exercises, oral reading practice, and other speech activities of the classroom could be adapted to help pupils clinch their new skills. In conducting her weekly spelling bees, one second-grade teacher added the requirement that each pupil, after spelling a word, had to speak it carefully in a sentence, thereby giving my speech cases further practice to reinforce newly learned speech patterns. Teachers commonly used oral reading practice as a regular opportunity to remind and encourage a pupil to give due attention to his articulation.

In these speaking situations, teachers were careful not to let their correction of errors interfere with the pupil's fluency and comprehension in reading; they encouraged a child to scan ahead in reading and to monitor himself. If mistakes were made, teachers withheld their corrections of a pupil's misarticulation until he had finished reading the sentence unit. Another first-grade teacher made a special effort to incorporate speech and language practice in such daily chores as collecting milk money. She met each child who filed up for the collection with a clear and correct greeting, such as "Good morning, Jennifer," while the child replied with similar care, "Good morning, Mrs. Schuster." Other teachers made special efforts to teach their pupils to recite carefully and correctly the pronunciation of such memorized recitations as the Pledge of Allegiance, the Declaration of Independence, or the words of *America* and other memorized songs. Special attention and encouragement were given to pupils who had difficulty with certain speech sounds and who had had speech therapy for misarticulated sounds. Two elementary teachers, taking advantage of their ability to speak second languages, stated that their pupils not only enjoyed learning a song or poem spoken in a new foreign language but that the novel experience sharpened the pupils' articulation of their native language. Likewise, another teacher employed her pupils' enjoyment in learning the pronunciation and meaning of new large words, such as the names of dinosaurs, scientific terminology, the names of foreign countries and cities, like *Schenectady* and challenging words like *antidisestablishmentarianism*.

Parents, too, may help to meet the needs of their children in the terminal stages of therapy by appreciating the speech gains, realizing the children's need for practice, and understanding how the new speech skills may be maintained and habituated. Through the satisfying home use of the telephone, for example, children may be given practice in speaking at heightened standards of articulation. Many children have strengthened their new skills by getting extra increments of practice in unhurried conversational speech within the family circle, with occasional compliments appropriately given for good performance or effort. Parents have shown success in providing their children with rewarding speech practice outside the home. For example, one young child was reminded to use good speech by being given the money to make his own transactions for ice cream cones and other purchases. Speech practice has been combined in the many "car games" which are devised for families while touring. Tape recorders have been effectively used to stabilize new articulatory skills by recording speech or self-hearing within the family and by exchanging with friends and relatives carefully taped "speech letters."

It should be emphasized that the terminal stages of speech correction may turn into failure unless constructive interpersonal relationships are maintained between the client and those who attempt to help him. One should be careful in enlisting parental help. If practice at home or in the classroom brings criticism, discouragement, and penalty to the speaker, rather than encouragement and satisfaction, his new skills may deteriorate and the older and stronger patterns of error may regain dominance. For this reason, a speech therapist must be alert for the obstacles which may be met after a client is dismissed from therapy. The therapist's responsibility does not end when he dismisses a client from his therapy sessions; guidance and support must continue for those who must carry onward the responsibility for fixing the client's new usages.

Special Cases of
Misarticulation

When teachers and therapists are confronted with a client whose misarticulation is associated with such organic factors as cleft palate, cerebral palsy, deafness, muscular dystrophy, multiple sclerosis, Parkinson's disease, and loss of the tongue or other speech organs, they may become overly distracted by these organic factors and fail to realize that the client's predominant needs may resemble those of functional cases who misarticulate for nonorganic reasons. Although special problems and techniques may apply to the neurological aspects of a cerebral palsied person's problem of misarticulation, it may be found that much of his therapy regime parallels treatment for cases who do not have cerebral palsy. Similarly, there may be ordinary factors of learning, motivation, and emotional adjustment operating in a speaker with cleft palate, requiring therapy procedures which have much in common with treatment for nonorganic cases. The director of a speech correction program indicated this overlap in the therapies for seemingly distinct cases of misarticulation when he said:

> I have found that the narrowly trained speech therapists may shun work with cleft-palate cases or the cerebral palsied. Or they may not feel justified to group them with children whose misarticulation is purely functional in cause, because they blindly categorize children with these disorders and fail to understand what organic and functional cases often have in common. Of course, one must learn, too, that children with cerebral palsy or cleft palates may also require help from medical specialists, physical therapists, and specific techniques which have been developed within the field of speech correction for the cerebral palsied, for instance. In therapy for severe misarticulation caused by cerebral palsy, a therapist may have to settle for much lower goals of achievement than he can ordinarily expect of functional cases. But a realistic lowering of standards for severely handicapped persons does not necessarily lessen the importance of their therapy and possible achievement. There are times when cases must correct articulation mainly by learning to compensate for their organic faults which cannot be corrected. Sometimes there is a need either for preliminary therapy to prepare a child for surgical correction or for follow-up therapy prescribed by specialists on the rehabilitative team.

As Egland[9] has indicated, speech therapy for the cerebral palsied person must be individualized, based on an understanding of the unique needs and methods which he requires. Therefore, as Mecham, Berko and Berko[10] state in their useful book on speech therapy for the cerebral palsied, teachers must often devise their own teaching techniques to meet special problems faced by these children in the classroom. Nevertheless, they remind teachers that much of the standard school curriculum may be adapted to fit the speech needs of pupils either with or without cerebral palsy. The palsied child needs the same foundation which any child must have in the developmental areas of reading readiness, interests, experience, knowledge, vocabulary, language skills, perceptual training, and emotional adjustment.

Likewise, we find that the articulation of cleft-palate speakers tends to be correlated either with a hypernasality of voice or an escape of oral breath pressure needed for the normal articulation of certain sounds. Books by Westlake and Rutherford[11] and Van Riper and Irwin[12] provide therapists and teachers with some of the unique procedures in therapy for cleft-palate persons. Some of these special measures are not adaptable for classroom practice, but many of them are applicable under the guidance of a speech therapist. Classroom teachers who understand the total therapy program for cleft-palate pupils will be more helpful in their cooperation with the therapist when the children's speech practices need to be extended and strengthened in classroom use. In these special cases of misarticulation where multiple problems hinge upon correlated physical, psychological, and social factors, there is a need for teachers and other members of the therapeutic team to seek a mutual understanding of the total problem and to become acquainted as much as possible with each other's role so as to insure an integrated therapy program. A source of concise and well organized information about special problems and measures related to misarticulation in various types of disorders can be obtained from the *Prentice-Hall Foundations of Speech Pathology Series*.[13]

References

1. R. Milisen, "Articulation Problems," in *Speech Pathology*, ed. R. W. Rieber and R. S. Brubaker. Amsterdam: North-Holland Publishing Co., 1966.

2. Mildred C. Templin and F. L. Darley, "The Templin-Darley Tests of Articulation," *University of Iowa Bureau of Educational Research and Service*, 1960.

3. C. Van Riper, *Speech Correction: Principles and Methods*. Englewood Cliffs, N.J.: Prentice-Hall, Inc., 1963.

4. R. Milisen and associates, "The Disorders of Articulation: A Systematic Clinical and Experimental Approach," *The Journal of Speech and Hearing Disorders*, Monograph Supplement 4, 1954.

5. E. McDonald, *Articulation Testing and Treatment, A Sensory-Motor Approach*. Pittsburgh: Stanwix House, Inc., 1964.

6. Albert J. Harris, *How To Increase Reading Ability*. New York: David McKay Co., Inc., 1961.

7. C. E. Webb and B. M. Siegenthaler, "Comparison of Aural Stimulation Methods for Teaching Speech Sounds," *The Journal of Speech and Hearing Disorders*, 22, No. 2 (June 1957) 264–270.

8. Martha E. Black, *Speech Correction in the Schools*. Englewood Cliffs, N.J.; Prentice-Hall, Inc., 1964.

9. George O. Egland, "Treating 'C.P's' As Persons," *Cerebral Palsy Review*, Vol. XXV (July-August 1964) 10-11.

10. Merlin J. Mecham, Martin J. Berko, and Francis Giden Berko, *Speech Therapy in Cerebral Palsy*. Springfield, Ill.: Charles C. Thomas, Publisher, 1960.

11. Harold Westlake and David Rutherford, *Cleft Palate*. Englewood Cliffs, N.J.: Prentice-Hall, Inc., 1966.

12. Charles Van Riper and John V. Irwin, *Voice and Articulation*. Englewood Cliffs, N.J.: Prentice-Hall, Inc., 1958.

13. *Foundation of Speech Pathology Series*. Englewood Cliffs, N.J.: Prentice-Hall, Inc.

Questions

1. What percentage of speech problems involves misarticulation?

2. After what grade level is there less chance that a child will outgrow misarticulation?

3. If you had to choose between a kindergartner with an unusual type and degree of misarticulation and an older child with a growing problem, which would you select for immediate attention?

4. Of pupils who enter first grade with articulation faults, about what percentage are partly or entirely corrected by the end of first grade?

5. In what forms does misarticulation occur?

6. Name the speech sounds which are most difficult to learn.

7. Give examples of substituted sounds in children's speech, ages when spoken, and prospects for correction.

8. What are speech omissions? Give examples.

9. How do omissions compare with substitutions on the basis of the level of developmental learning to articulate?

10. Define misarticulatory distortion.

11. Why are distortions considered a higher order of mistake than are omissions and substitutions?

12. Are distortions grave handicaps to a speaker?

13. Why are vowels easier to articulate than consonants?

14. Would you consider that an eight-year-old child who misarticulates *th* and *j* has normal speech development?

15. What is the danger in using a language scale which computes single age-points representing the average age for the "average" child?

16. Is misarticulation easily distinguishable from mispronunciation?

17. In what grades is remedial grammar most effective?

18. In the case of Mexican children, what phonemes in English are the most difficult?

19. How do intonation, stress, and rhythm compare in English and in the Latin languages?

20. What is a valid standard for our judgment of pronunciation?

21. Why is a knowledge of a child's background necessary for judging the correctness of his speech?

22. What is dysarthria?

23. What is dyspraxia?

24. How prevalent are dysarthria and dyspraxia? Are they easily diagnosed?

25. What are some anatomical defects which cause misarticulation?

26. What external and internal perceptions are utilized in articulation?

27. Upon what perceptions does the blind person rely?

28. What is Milisen's concept of the inverse process by which speech sounds are learned and self-regulated?

29. Is low intelligence a predictable cause of misarticulation?

30. Why is it more complex to teach a pupil to pronounce phonemes than it is to teach him to sharpen a pencil?

31. Why are the primary grades a critical time in speech therapy?

32. As a speech therapist, would you give more time to an older pupil who fails to improve than to a kindergartner with a mild problem?

33. Discuss the effect of phonic practice on articulation.

34. How may a busy teacher make an adequate survey of articulation?

35. When a pupil realizes that he can say a difficult sound in some words, how may the teacher take advantage of the situation?

36. Which is more important—a teacher's referral at the beginning or at the end of the year?

37. What are the bases of judging the severity of misarticulation?

38. Why do articulation errors vary in difficulty of correction?

39. What is Milisen's *Stimulability Test?*

40. Discuss "deep testing."

41. What must the teacher do when the pupil is unaware of faulty phonemes?

42. Explain: "Diagnosis and therapy go hand in hand."

43. Why must the person and not his defect be the point of reference?

44. How would you answer a second-grader who asks, "Why should I ar-artifilicate better?"

45. Explain: "Therapists have a selling job to do."

46. How may articulation therapy be correlated with hobbies of pupils?

47. Why is heterogeneous grouping effective in therapy?

48. Why is the knowledge of what *not* to do needed in perfecting articulation?

49. Rate hearing and vision on their importance in articulation training.

50. What is the analytic approach to speech correction?

51. Discuss the use of mirrors, large and small, in speech instruction.

52. How effective may the teacher be as a speech model?

53. Why does the use of a tape recorder appeal to children?

54. Why do therapists sometimes err in acting as trainers rather than as helpers and resourcers?

55. Explain the value of joint practice with therapist and children in imitative practice.

56. What were the most effective methods noted by Webb and Siegenthaler?

57. What is the need for "unlearning" in speech therapy?

58. Explain the use of the toothpick in therapy.

59. How do children map their mouth contacts in therapy?

60. How may a puppet become a concrete incentive for work?

61. Explain the use of plastic tape in speech instruction.

62. What is the value of a flashlight for therapy?

63. When a sound cannot be spoken exactly in isolation, how should the teacher say it?

64. Do you consider "Toss the Block" a valuable game? Why?

65. Explain a method of improving middle sounds of words.

Suggested Subjects for
Term Papers

1. Attempt to set up a valid predictive test of articulation to determine whether or not a kindergartner, first- or second-grader will outgrow his difficulty.
2. Analyze the speech of ten fellow students to determine the sections of the country where they learned to talk. Note the percentages who are aware of their peculiarities and are correcting their "errors", the percentage flaunting them, and the percentage who are handicapped in expression.
3. Compare the developmental scales and tests for their degree of agreement on what constitutes articulatory problems and whether they predict by ranges of normality or by single age-points representing the average age for the "average" child. How wide a sampling of children was used as the basis?
4. Examine three novels or short stories by such writers as Joel Chandler Harris, Herbert Best, Mark Twain, Milt Gross, and other writers of dialect, for your analysis of the speech articulation of the characters.
5. Audit the classes of two or three foreign-born professors who will permit you to analyze their production of speech sounds in the form of substitution, omission, distortion or addition.
6. Visit classes from kindergarten to third grade and note instances of misarticulations, attempts by pupils to correct them, pupils showing embarrassment at errors, and the degree of the teacher's control over correction of misarticulation.
7. If you can observe a child of primary grade age daily for two or three weeks, note evidence of his imitation of the teacher's and other pupils' speech mannerisms.
8. Listen to the speakers in radio talk-back conversation shows for a month. Report the prevalence and nature of misarticulation among this segment of the public.
9. Invent three classroom exercises designed to correct misarticulation.

seven

Helping the Child
with a Language Problem

When a child enters school, no developmental skills are more important for adjustment and learning than are his comprehension and use of spoken language. His writing and reading develop upon his foundation of spoken language with its phonetic system, syntax, grammar, and a basic fund of vocabulary. Modern teachers also recognize that a pupil's growth in language must be maintained by integrating its usage in all school subjects. Because language is an important tool for a pupil's adjustment and learning, it is obvious that we should be alert to detect and to diagnose language problems of the schoolchild. Teachers should know what to expect in normal language development when children reach the ages of five, six, seven, and arrive at a fairly stable plateau of language growth. Also, it is important to recognize the symptoms and factors which are associated with language abnormalities, because corrective measures will depend upon this basic understanding.

Understanding Language
Problems

In earlier chapters we examined the nature of spoken language, its course of development, and factors which appear to affect it. We were reminded that language is a social invention. It is socially taught, socially used, and socially maintained. We considered the significance of phonemes, words, the rules of a language's sentence structure, and the growth of vocabulary. Through maturation and learning, the motor skills and the expressive patterns of spoken language are acquired. In Chapter 1 the intricate mental processes and the environmental factors in language development were outlined. In diagnosing language abnormalities, we should remember that the boundaries of normality in language are difficult to determine, partly because of the allowable individuality and variability among normal speakers in their developmental rate and correctness of language achievement. A school diagnostician has stated:

> I am often called upon to assist teachers and speech therapists in their diagnosis of pupils' language problems. We need this team approach not only to make a differential diagnosis but also in the correction of problems. We must consider many aspects of the person if we are to understand his language status. Some of us may not be trained or are not in positions to test and to evaluate some facets of language problems. At times we disagree on our diagnostic labels for a problem. Perhaps a first-grader may be referred to as having "delayed speech" if his misarticulation is so severe that he may hardly be understood. Another person who diagnoses that child may consider his case to be a "language deficit." When we look more analytically into the child's problem, however, we may find that he has not only a normal understanding of spoken language but also has acquired a normal fund of language and expresses it in sentence structures which are normal for his age. The point of his language deficiency may be rather specific or limited —an inability to produce understandable and acceptable speech sounds to convey these spoken units of his inner language.
>
> Let's take another type of language problem. We often find a "culturally deprived" pupil who appears to have a shortage of vocabulary, both in his understanding of what we say to him and in what he says in return. We may verify this lack by giving him formal tests to measure his vocabulary, length of sentences, syntax, and use of the various parts of speech. But we may finally find that he is deficient only in the comprehension and use of our middle-class vocabulary and sentence structure, while he proves to have a well-developed language of his own—a language which adequately and normally fits his particular class of society but which is deficient in school. This discrepancy in our standards of judging him can lead to serious problems. We may make the mistake of thinking that he is mentally deficient or otherwise incapable of meeting normal levels of learning. When we visit this child's home and neighborhood and hear how others speak in his environment, we realize that we may have judged him from entirely different language standards from those we use and test by. If we find these double standards of language in a child's life, we may impatiently expect him to meet our language patterns while we condemn and try to wipe out his own. Actually, this situation is like that of a person's being taught a second language, the second language being his "school language," in which he is taught wider vocabulary, revisions in grammar, and a new set of speech allophones to be used when he speaks his new academic language.

The diagnostician emphasizes proper treatment of a specific language problem through understanding of circumstances which cause, maintain, and may even justify a particular language deviation. Therefore, a team approach is often recommended in making a differential diagnosis to determine the focal points in the cause and treatment of language problems. Teachers, speech therapists, reading specialists, school nurses, psychologists, and social workers may make valuable contributions in this team. Classroom teachers, however, have central positions in work with language because it enters widely into the many daily activities of the classroom.

Types and Degrees of
Language Problems

Perhaps no area in speech correction has accumulated so many poorly defined and loosely classified terms than has the language area. However, Menjuk[1] and Lee[2] and other linguistically oriented researchers in speech pathology are currently building a more sound and disciplined understanding of language structure and its development in normal and abnormal speech. Their research promises that more accurate terms and a more unified system of classification and measurement will be devised as this linguistic investigation continues. As Wood[3] states, to label a pupil with the term *delayed speech* may mean a number of things. It may signify that he is slow or lacking in speech achievement, without specifying whether the problem is mild, moderate, or severe as a permanent disorder or whether it is one which may be helped to clear up with maturation. Too often, *delayed speech* is a vague and loosely used label. It may refer to an inadequacy in one or more of the language components, such as a shortage of vocabulary, poor articulation, faulty structure of language, and other grammatical deficiencies. At times, delayed language may relate to the use of unacceptable colloquialisms or to the adoption of a self-language of gestures or grunts.

Delayed language sometimes refers to a broad category of language disorders which are further classified into subtypes on the basis of causation. One subtype refers to central nervous system impairment which affects the comprehension and use of linguistic symbols for speech. This form of disorder, called *aphasia*, may involve difficulty at one or more of the levels of the communicative process; at the *receptive* level, which functions in the understanding of speech and reading; at the *integrative* level, where language symbols are believed to serve in processes for thinking, appreciation of concepts, and recall; and at the *expressive* level of speech and writing. When brain disorders disrupt reading, the problem is termed *dyslalia*; if writing is affected, it is *dysgraphia*.

The reduction of language disorders into subtypes reminds us not only that one or more of the language forms may be affected but also that each of the forms may be disrupted at different varying and indistinct levels in the behavioral process—the neurological, intellectual, perceptual, experiential, emotional, and learning.

How Teachers Can Recognize and Evaluate Language Problems

As one speech therapist has stated:

It is relatively easy to recognize speech problems of misarticulation, nonfluency, and faulty voice. But the task of testing and evaluating a pupil's language deficit is more complex. There are more levels to test for in the area of language problems. Some of these levels are internal and much more difficult to measure than are the expressed patterns of speech and writing. It is necessary for the examiner to understand the characteristics and degrees which separate language normality from abnormality. The test itself must be a fair one, and testing must be conducted under favorable conditions; otherwise, the client will not reveal the full extent of his language ability or disability. This is one reason that we speech therapists need the cooperation of teachers and other language diagnosticians when we evaluate and work with pupils who are deficient in language. From my conferences with a pupil's teachers and from observations of his spoken and written language in various school situations, I can get a much clearer picture of his language problem than I can by working with him alone.

In her advantageous position for observation, evaluation, and work on language problems of the school child, a teacher may not only determine the nature and the extent of the language deficit at the moment, but she may also forecast its trends by exploring factors which may produce a delayed or an uneven course of development. Teachers who are oriented to teach reading and writing in accordance with the more recently introduced principles which underlie the pupil's basic spoken language are likely to have a more specific understanding of language problems. For the teacher of reading, the *Merrill Linguistic Readers*, by Fries, Wilson, and Rudolph[4] provide regular evaluations of her pupil's comprehension and ability to use language for organizing materials, recalling facts, making conclusions, and following directions. In linguistically oriented programs for teaching reading and English, teachers tend not only to be more alert to language deficiencies but also to be ready with programed materials to correct them. A speech therapist once declared:

I have learned more about delayed speech and language from working with modern teachers of language than I learned from my courses in speech correction. First, I've learned that many of the "delayed speech" cases are in more immediate need of language training than they are in need of the skills of speaking. When I came into the field, fresh from college, I overemphasized the problem of misarticulation which often accompanies the language deficit in delayed speech cases. I found that many of these children need to build their vocabularies, to learn the structure of spoken English which is required of them for reading, recitation, and writing. In the case of the mentally retarded, for example, this need for correlating language learning with speech correction is especially needed. I work closely with classroom teachers. I am helped mostly by teachers who understand and teach the structure of language. Information from these teachers and the objective evidences from their pupils' language workbooks give me the practical guidelines I need in correlating speech correction with language development. In return for their help, I try to give the teachers pointers on how they can facilitate their pupils' speech skills while the language areas are being built.

What is meant by a "fair" test of a pupil's language achievement or of his ability to learn language? There are several features which determine a test's fairness for a particular child. If the test is a "one-shot" affair, it may give a limited picture of his language potential through the narrow scope of test items, the restricted time allotted for the test, or the unfair discrimination against the client's cultural background because the test items lie beyond his experience, needs, or interests. Unless we consider the cultural background of a pupil, we may misjudge not only his language acquisition but even his language-learning ability and perhaps even relegate him to programs geared for the mentally retarded, programs where he is further denied the opportunities to live up to his potentials. In his provocative article dealing with our introduction of middle-class values to disadvantaged children, Lohman[5] advises that we "expose" but "don't impose." He reminds us that a child's patterns of speech and language—however different and nonconforming they may be with respect to ours—are integral parts of *his* culture and that attacks on his differing patterns of speech and language may be attacks on his personal worth, his family heritage, and essentials of his everyday life. This imposition may cause him to resent and to defy our attempts to replace his cultural values with ours.

A kindergarten teacher who taught children predominantly from minority groups with low incomes stated her need for judging and teaching on a double-standard basis:

> When I started to teach in this neighborhood, I referred over half of my pupils to the speech therapist and reading consultant for help in correcting articulation, accents, and limited substandard language. The therapist accepted some of them for work on certain unlearned speech sounds, but she left me with the major responsibility to teach them language generally. At first, I classed them as "culturally deprived" and some of them as mentally subnormal. But after several years of respectful observing, testing, and teaching these children, I have changed my term "culturally deprived" to "culturally different." I've discovered that these children may have learned just as much language in their cultures as middle-class children have in theirs. But the vocabulary lists, which represent the most commonly spoken and understood words, may be very different between these groups of children. Even their syntax of sentences may differ.
>
> These cultural discrepancies in language make a big difference not only in reading readiness and in the selection of suitable readers for beginning reading but also

in pupils' understanding and participation in the everyday communication in the classroom. Pupils with language patterns from the "other side of the tracks" need the teacher's understanding, patience, and extra help when they attend our middle-class schools. We have tried to bridge this language gap, however, by adopting a team-teaching approach in these schools. We have teaching aides who have lived within the cultures of these minority groups and are more capable of helping the children make the cultural transitions, not only in language but in other areas of adjustment. We use special techniques in teaching reading, such as writing our own beginning primers, basing them on experiences and the spoken languages which these children have already acquired.

It is also important to weigh the conditions under which we observe and test a child's language performance. Unless a child is willing to respond through language, he may show up poorly in a test. Distractions, noise, fatigue, or failure to see or to hear in the testing situation may explain low performance in tests of his language perception.

A second-grade teacher gives the following justification for the extra duty which teachers frequently serve in their playground and lunchroom supervision:

> Before I learned that recess and noontime periods were valuable sources of information pertaining to my pupils and their classroom problems, I resented my assignments to them. My viewpoint changed, however, when I overheard a pupil, whom I had mistakenly judged as aphasic, talking a blue streak, using full sentences and communicating normally with the other children in the playground activities. In the classroom he had spoken always in single words or in fragmented sentences, sometimes mixing up his word order. I learned that this child used two systems of language structure: a relatively normal one in conversation with children, and a limited one which had been imposed upon him at home. He was an only child, in a fatherless home, cared for by an elderly grandmother while his mother worked. He spent most of his waking hours playing with children of the neighborhood. For him, language with adults had been a limited one-way reception; he was talked at, mainly to be directed or reprimanded for his actions. But if I had not heard this boy talking with children aside from adults, I might have continued to regard him as brain-injured or aphasic. As it was, I set about to win conversational rapport with this boy and to transfer a more complete use of his language into the classroom. I placed him in small groups, started the group discussion on topics of playground interest and events while I gently entered the conversational ring more and more until he accepted me in conversation alone. It seemed that this boy had never been assured that adults were interested in hearing a full sentence of what he had to say.

Causes of Language Problems

When we consider the complex nature of language, with the development of its related forms of speech, reading, and writing, and when we attempt to fathom the coordinated mental-physical processes involved in its reception, conceptual mechanics, and expressions, it is not surprising that language problems occur. Causal factors underlying language disorders are classified under two broad categories: organic and functional. More specifically, these causal areas include central nervous system impairments, sensory disorders, subnormal intelligence, environmental deprivation, and emotional maladjustment. Since these broad causal areas are interrelated, one or more of them may be operative in a client's language problem.

CENTRAL NERVOUS SYSTEM
IMPAIRMENTS

The language of a brain-injured person may be affected in several ways. At times an incurable form of hearing loss may result from damage to the hearing center in the brain or to the auditory nerve, thereby interfering with the person's reception of spoken language. Even though a brain injury does not damage the sense organs, it may indirectly interfere with perceptions by causing the person to be a poor listener who is easily distracted and who has shorter spans of attention for language learning and communication. If the brain injury lowers the general intelligence, his language learning and usage may be handicapped at the level where the integrative processes of association, generalization, translation, abstraction, and recall occur. Or, if the injury to the brain causes dysarthria, a motor incoordination of the tongue, lips, and jaw, language may be impaired at the expressive level of speech. In *dyspraxia* too, where the uncoordination of the tongue and the jaw interferes in volitionally made speech movements, a speaker may develop apprehensions and evasions which further impede his language development. Under the broad category of *aphasia*, the disruptive use of language symbols may occur at one or more of the levels which we have discussed: reception and comprehension; the integrative level, where symbols are used for associational thinking and translation; and the expressive level, where symbols are communicated through speech, writing, or other special means, such as Braille for the blind and the manual language for the deaf. We should be cautious, however, when we attach the label *aphasia* to a case of impaired language. Difficult to diagnose and to prove, aphasia and "minimal brain damage" too often become wastebasket terms to use when we cannot otherwise readily explain a language disorder. Aphasia is likely to be a misnomer, especially when applied to children. Even if brain injury is found to be a valid cause for language disorder, it is essential to include a thorough search for associated factors in the areas of learning and of emotional and social adjustments. The complexity of making a reliable diagnosis and treatment of aphasia in schoolchildren demands the cooperation of a team of qualified specialists: neurologists, psychologists, audiologists, teachers, and speech therapists.

Language will not be learned unless its symbols are perceived. Furthermore, even after a speaker learns a language, he depends upon perceptual cues and control for the maintenance of his language patterns.

Of the perceptual disorders which interfere with the learning and use of spoken language, hearing impairments are most apparent. Blindness may also handicap reading unless the blind reader can learn to read Braille symbols through the fingertips. Now, with the aid of a device which electronically "sees" and translates ordinary printed language symbols into tonal beep patterns, blind persons may use their auditory perception instead of touch to "read" the written language. When one sense is impaired, other senses must serve extra duty. Carter and McGinnis[6] emphasize that in learning to read, the pupil must integrate linguistic information from all senses: visual, auditory, kinesthetic, and tactile. Although all pupils do not show an equal reliance upon each of these perceptual avenues in learning to read, the experienced teacher is aware that all senses are important. Children who develop problems in reading, for example, may be found to be lacking in one or more of these perceptual areas, not because they are potentially deficient in the senses but because they have had less purpose, exposure, and training in the use of the senses as applied to reading. Chapman,[7] for instance, reports that for perceptually impaired children the regular educational materials and methods in teaching reading, spelling, and writing may not be appropriate. In her observations from two approaches to reading, she concludes that combined perceptual cues are needed in language learning and that the skills and information which are related to these perceptions must be meaningfully integrated. At times, children with language problems of visual or auditory impairment are improperly tagged and dismissed as having poor "self-images" or "body concepts," as being distractible, poor listeners, restless, immature, perverse, deficient in their foreground-background configurations, etc. In the classroom, an unrecognized hearing loss or a visual defect may be the cause of a child's failure to learn language and reading. Because children such as these are perceptually barred from entering into the language instruction of the classroom, they may show symptoms which prove that their learning problem has become more than a perceptual one. Chapter 10 will present a more detailed discussion of how hearing problems, for instance, may spread to include factors which handicap language.

Because of the complexities in diagnosing and meeting special perceptual needs in language instruction, teachers and speech therapists should follow a team approach, similar to that recommended for cases where central nervous system impairment is a *questioned* cause. Ophthalmologists, otologists, audiologists, psychologists, psychiatrists, pediatricians, neurologists, and specialists in the field of speech pathology may have roles in the clinical approach in severe cases of perceptual disorders affecting language. In general, one of the first steps which teachers and therapists should take in the case of language problems is an early examination of the client's hearing and vision. Many schools provide preschool clinics for physical checks on hearing and vision, with audiological tests to follow when pupils attend school. In addition, classroom teachers have the responsibility of being continuously alert for signs in the classroom indicating that pupils have perceptual difficulties.

Intelligence is an important determinant of a person's rate and level of language attainment. In recognition of the fact that language ability and mental ability are closely correlated, intelligence is often rated by the use of tests which are primarily tests of language achievement. It should be remembered, however, that intelligence is but one of the important factors which set the variable limits within the wide range of levels which a person may ultimately master. While it is probable that the child who is mentally subnormal will be slower and more limited in what he may acquire in the realms of language, this likelihood of language retardation in the mentally retarded child does not lessen the importance of language for him and his social environment. Generally, pupils in special education classes for the mentally retarded have special need for extra language training. The director of such a program has commented:

> In our special education program we try to dispel two popular misconceptions of neglects which are often imposed as barriers in the mentally retarded child's development. First, in all areas of our team approach in teaching the child we stress that the language area is one of the most important cores of his curriculum. He needs language not only for personal information, social adjustment, and communication, but also to facilitate his own thinking, his organizational and problem-solving processes. Second, we try to give parents and others a greater confidence in what they may expect of the mentally retarded child's ability to learn language. Too often we find that when people learn that a child is mentally low, they treat him in radically different ways than they treat normal children. Some of these treatments deny him the normal opportunities to learn language and to reap the many returns from its functions. Actually, the social limitations, arising from the ways society reacts to him and his mental retardation, may restrict the retardate more than his lack of brains.

Pinpointing mental retardation as a cause of language problems should be done on the basis of careful, thorough, professional diagnosis. Intelligence is complex and difficult to define and measure. Furthermore, there is a tendency to assume too readily that a person lacks intelligence because he is deficient in language. If we misjudge the factor of intelligence as a cause of a person's language problem, we may wrongly assign that person to a special education program in which he will be more harmed than helped. Wrong diagnoses may be made, filed, and passed along as misinformation. Therefore, teachers and speech therapists and parents should rely upon qualified professionals such as school psychologists or diagnosticians to help in the full evaluations of a pupil's general intelligence.

ENVIRONMENTAL DEPRIVATION

The ideal environment provides initial and continuing incentives for language with sufficient warmth, security, and experiences which are associated with language in a setting where the child is inclined to identify and communicate with others who are important in his life. All of these requisites represent a continuing challenge for parents, teachers, therapists, and others. An experienced speech therapist explains how the high socioeconomic status of a child's home may deceive us into assuming that his environmental conditions are adequate for learning language:

> In our diagnoses of pupils' language problems, we are sometimes misled by our tendency to judge superficially a home's adequacy for promoting good language in its children. If a pupil is clean and well dressed, has acceptable manners, and shows good physical care, we are inclined to assume that his home and parents have provided adequately for his language development too. Our judgment may be unduly influenced by the socioeconomic rank of the child's parents and the outward impressions they create in parent conferences. However, this type of home and parents may be more to blame for children's language problems than a home marked by a low material standard of living and a lack of formal education or sophistication in the parents. We find that some of the children in some of the "better homes" are reared without warmth or good teaching methods. In some well-to-do homes the working parents may have neglected their children by relegating their responsibilities at home to an assortment of ineffective baby-sitters. We must take a careful, objective look into the environments of our speech and language cases.

When a language problem is caused by past deprivations or by poor teaching methods in a child's earlier life at home, the present needs of the child are usually apparent if a careful diagnosis is made. Environmental deprivations are variously revealed in language development, sometimes by restricted vocabulary, sometimes by faulty articulation and grammatical structure. A poor environment may also lead to crippling attitudes and emotional adjustment toward language and group interaction. But teachers and therapists must understand that "culturally deprived" children who represent minority groups may have cultural backgrounds which require of them different language standards from those we require in our middle-class schools. It is important to appreciate that these children who may be problems for us in our society may not be "problem" children or "underachievers" in their own cultural settings. Furthermore, our standards may be as unacceptable to them as their standards are to us. And if we subject them to poor schooling, we may even create additional environmental problems for them.

Substandard programs of education are provided for many of the culturally deprived pupils from minority groups. It is ironic that many children who need the most in the way of special education are getting the least. Compare suburban schools with schools in the low-income areas—in terms of their physical plants, instructional materials, the supply and qualifications of teachers, special services, and general public support. Such a survey may reveal that the greater language problems of low-income groups tend to be compounded by inferior academic environments imposed upon them. As professionals, responsible for our pupils' education, we should be alert to recognize and to campaign for improvement of inferior school programs.

When we look for causal factors in the environment of a child who has language problems, we generally consider such requirements for language learning as motivation and stimulation with adequate language models. We examine his relationship with siblings, parents, and other persons who affect his personal and social life, to get information from a wide picture of his life, through first-hand observations and language tests and from reports and interviews with persons who know him and his environment. A speech therapist summarized the steps in her examination of environmental causes:

> I begin my examination of a language case by having an informal conversation with the child, stimulating him with a variety of objects, pictures, and topics which are designed to tap his interests and show his maximum comprehension and ability to use language. I may follow with more formal tests of language, to get a measure of his vocabulary, his use of the rules of speech governing syntax, his use of nouns, pronouns, verbs, adverbs, adjectives, prepositions, tense, number, gender, use of abstract and concrete concepts, etc. His articulatory skills and fluency with language are observed, too. I note and record how talkative he is and whether he initiates conversation or speaks only when asked to speak. I consider the different ways he uses speech—to ask, to tell, to direct, to provide self-expression of his feelings. His attitudes toward me and our communication usually give me other valuable cues—whether or not he enjoys talking and whether he shows awareness or insecurity toward his language problem.
>
> Having completed this personal session with the child, I contact his classroom teacher and get her picture of the same areas of language I have appraised in my private examination of him. Often the teacher has also talked with one or both of the child's parents. This gives information on the home and family, siblings, parental personalities, speech traits, and attitudes toward the child and his problem. If the child has siblings who are in school at the time, I confer with their teachers too, to get a comparison of the language picture in other members of the family. I also contact teachers who have had the child in previous grades to learn more about the problem's history and changes.
>
> If the child's language problem is serious of if I feel that additional information is needed after having made my personal examination and interviews with teachers, I arrange to visit the child's home. Preferably, I schedule the visit in the

afternoon so that I can have about a half-hour conference with the child's mother before he and his siblings return from school. When the kids come home, I linger a while to get some first-hand information on how the child and his other family members react in this social situation. These home visits give me valuable insights. Parents usually appreciate my personal visits, and it gives me a chance to prepare them for the cooperative roles I may desire of them in my language work with their children.

EMOTIONAL MALADJUSTMENT

Obviously, emotional maladjustment may be a component of other causes of language problems. In the preceding discussion of environmental deprivation, there were frequent suggestions of how various environmental conditions might cause frustration, insecurities, fear, and other maladjustments. It is obvious how parents who reject children and fail to give them proper language stimulation may produce emotional problems which create further barriers to the children's language development. An elementary school principal expressed this causal relationship:

> We have proved that more school failures and emotional behavior problems of all sorts are associated with language problems than with any other problem area. Language problems become critical and complicated when children start to read. A child may enter school shy, socially immature. and poorly equipped with language. When he runs into difficulties in the language parts of the school curriculum, he often develops dislikes of these troublesome subjects, especially if his parents also get upset over his school difficulties. So we may end up with a child who fails grade after grade, becoming a school misfit and finally a school dropout and perhaps a delinquent.

Language may become completely muted by severe emotional conflicts, traumatic shocks associated with accidents, or illnesses. In the case of severe personality aberrations, as in childhood autism and schizophrenia, language patterns reflect the peculiar patterns of the emotionality. The sensitive autistic child, for instance, may isolate himself socially, psychologically, and linguistically. Language for him may be a self-centered monologue, regulated and used as a more safe form of self-stimulation than that which his unbearable environment would impose upon him if he were to join its turmoils of excessive stimulation. Fortunately, these extreme types of emotional disturbances are relatively rare, but when a child is suspected of being autistic or preschizophrenic, he should be referred for qualified psychiatric attention.

Preventing and Correcting Language Problems

Primary emphasis should always be on prevention. Even while efforts are directed toward the correction of a specific language problem, it is important to remain alert to the prevention of further associated problems. Otherwise minor problems may grow into serious ones. A teacher has pointed out this danger:

> I have learned to relax some of the high standards of language which I previously tried to establish in all situations of my young pupils' speech and writing. I would correct them for using slang, improper case, number, tense, etc. I conscientiously pointed out their errors even in such language situations as their creative writing and informal class discussions. But when I noticed that my corrections of their grammatical faults was curbing their willingness to write and to say what they had on their minds, I limited my criticisms to periods devoted principally to language study, when corrections could be made without creating these harmful side effects. Language teaching is a tricky business; one must keep in mind the whole broad front of language and human behavior.

No one ever attains perfection in the language proficiencies—a complete and perfectly discriminative vocabulary or a flawless use of grammar. We recognize that standards of correctness vary. This latitude is evident within the standards of acknowledged dictionaries and linguists. Therefore we must be cautious in judging a pupil's language as being either correct or incorrect. It is more practical to think of individuals having varying degrees of oral and written language proficiency but usually with corresponding possibilities for improvement.

There are, however, persons who are so obviously deficient in one or more areas of their language skills that their problems are critical handicaps in their regular communication. We often find that measures which will correct language problems are the same measures which would have prevented these problems if the actions had been instituted earlier. A child can more easily learn language correctly from the start than he can unlearn and relearn it after faults have been established. There also appear to be optimal periods within language's developmental timetable when language skills are most easily acquired, either initially or correctively. If learning does not occur at these times, later development and correction may become more difficult.

Every section of a pupil's curriculum holds opportunities for teaching and correcting language. Language should be taught and improved in all school subjects while subject matter and other academic skills are being acquired. Generally, language instruction is more effective when it is integrated with the total school program. The importance of a favorable teacher-pupil relationship must again be stressed, as it was in the teacher's work with stuttering, mis-articulation, and other speech deficiencies.

We recognize that teachers do not have a monopoly on opportunities for influencing language. Parents, therapists, janitors, school bus drivers, principals, and the general public also have contributing roles.

Correlating Speech and
Language Arts

While the four language arts—communicative perception, speaking, reading, and writing—are closely related, each of them requires the learning of certain skills, some of which are prerequisites for other abilities. The importance of listening and looking and other perceptions in speech development has been repeatedly stressed. A teacher explains perceptual avenues to facilitate her pupils' reception and expression of language:

I believe that the learning and use of language in all its forms—speaking, reading, and writing—should involve all the inner senses of the pupil, his total imageries of sound, sight, touch, smell, and even taste. That's why I have pupils dramatize some of the stories they are learning to read. I may take a story like "Goldilocks and The Three Bears," for example, a story that easily lends itself to many perceptions while it is being read, told, and acted out. First, I may read the story to the class while they watch and listen. I try to express through my voice, facial expressions, and other body actions as many of the story's perceptual experiences as possible: moving around from room to room of the bears' house, shifting from place to place at their table and chairs, testing as realistically as possible such perceptual qualities as hot, warm, cold, hard, soft, big, little, etc. After the pupils have openly observed my acting of the story, I ask them to rest their faces on their crossed forearms while they just listen to a repetition of my acted-out story. Then I may ask one or more of the pupils to volunteer reading the story while the rest of us listen and try to capture the sensations the reader is trying to portray. Here are some of the returns which I think come from this perceptual training in my language program. Pupils take a more keen personal interest in the stories. They show this interest by volunteering their related experiences and sharing some of the same perceptual sensations which are generated by the stories. Children more quickly learn to speak, read, and spell when the new vocabulary of stories is imbued with personalized values. When pupils read these stories after having "lived" the concepts in them, their oral expressions show that they are reading thoughts, feelings, and actions, not just a series of words. It's one of the best ways I've found to prevent "word-readers." Writing becomes more creative. I believe that even while first-graders are going through the difficulties of learning to read and write, they should not lose sight of the magical powers of language to create and recreate experiences.

In the work schedule of the busy classroom teacher, language may be more economically and effectively taught if reading, writing, spelling, and the basic build-up of spoken language are coordinated instead of being separated into timeslots and separate work projects which fail to take advantage of the common skills which come from an integration of these related subjects. The following third-grade teacher explains why she coordinates these language learning areas:

Everything we learn should be given as much purpose and practice as possible. A skill doesn't amount to much unless it applies to an activity which is important to the person. Better yet, if a skill helps the person in other personalized areas of his life, it's more likely that that skill will be prized and maintained. One way that we teachers may help pupils make this tie-up and carry-over of their language learnings is to coordinate the language art areas of speech, reading, and writing. We teachers may be at fault when we find that our pupils speak with good language but write poorly. Even at the college level we hear many students complain that they do well in oral reports, but when it comes to writing, they have no confidence and do poorly. When they are finally assured that it is usually appropriate to write more as they speak, their written English improves. I'll wager that most of these poor writers have never had teachers who have allowed them to tell stories and then to write up what they told.

Teachers have also learned that language instruction needs to be correlated with all subjects and activities, not only with those which are most clearly based on the language arts. Hahn[8] reports that language ability of first-graders correlates highly with leadership, social success, and willingness to speak in "show-and-tell." This relationship suggests that language may be improved through many classroom activities which will supply these effects from successes, leadership experiences, and general confidence. Dallmann[9] discusses how teachers may guide the language growth of their pupils through various situations of oral communication in the classroom: class reports, conversation, discussion, announcements, riddles, jokes, telling stories, giving explanations and directions, telephoning, making introductions, etc. She believes that teachers should expect first-graders to have learned the wide range of declarative, interrogative, exclamatory, imperative, simple, compound, and complex types of sentences and that special instruction should be given to the pupils who have not learned these forms of language. In guiding the growth of creative written language, and of dramatic expression too, she advises that teachers should be careful not to interfere with the freedom and practice which creativity requires.

Published materials are available to assist teachers in using pupils' speech foundations as a basis for teaching reading. One set of materials by Martin, Weil, and Kohan[10] approaches reading through story-telling, discussion, oral reading, and the use of posters of pictures with figures and magnetic cards. The vocabulary of most modern primers is being closely aligned to the spoken vocabulary which pupils already have learned to understand, pronounce, and use. Accordingly, as Saporta[11] has cautioned, although spoken language should be the basis of reading and writing, the spoken vocabulary which is used in readers should be respectful of language differences between the child's home and school. Furthermore, modern teachers of reading are recognizing that a too rigid control of vocabulary in readers may cause an unnatural language usage within the stories. Stories may be dull in content when they are wrung from a vocabulary of limited and overworked words which are systematically doled out and used repeatedly a set number of times before new words are introduced. The following imaginative and adaptive teacher suggests how to incorporate language in some of these unusual places for language learning:

> I find excellent opportunities for teaching language, tailored to fit the needs of each particular child, in art, music, recreational periods, and in the daily chores which begin and end each pupil's school day. In art, where self-expression is generally encouraged, each child is also encouraged to give his own verbal interpretations of what he draws and makes. Sometimes I use art work for later writing projects, having each child write an interpretation or a story of what he drew in art. In music, where songs are learned, I sometimes have written exercises in which each child is encouraged to write up his own interpretation of a song, the meaning of its words, how the song makes him feel, and perhaps a special spelling lesson based on the words in the song. Poetry, too, may be used in these ways.
>
> When pupils arrive in the morning and are getting ready for school, I make a special effort to help the ones who I know need help in certain aspects of language. I find other opportunities at the end of the day and also at recess times when I am supervising their playground activities. For example, I may stroll over to the monkey-bars to be in a position to give some language stimulation to a young child who has not learned parts of his language or has a lack of vocabulary. While he climbs up and down, swings and slides, and goes through all sorts of antics, I may follow his actions with a running commentary which supplies him with the language models that he lacks. I think that verbalization can be very helpful to all the children who overhear it. They enjoy it. Personal conversation may make a pupil feel that he is respectfully recognized and belongs. I notice that children later repeat some of the improved language patterns I use around them, proving that the words and sentences carry lasting impacts.

Favorable Teacher-Pupil Relationship

One capable elementary teacher gave this description of what she considers to be a warm and secure interpersonal relationship for teaching language:

> Some children need the teacher or other pupils to prime their linguistic pumps, someone whom they like and trust to add to their language source. Usually it's best to be client-centered with children who have language problems. I believe that one must first determine the child's interests, abilities, and limitations in language matters. Then I try to join him where he is, to adopt his interests and even to talk his language for a while, until he feels that I sincerely appreciate him and his interests and can communicate on his level before expecting him to operate at my level. If his language is difficult to understand, we should work to understand him; but if we don't understand what he says, we must be honest and not pretend that we do. If a child knows that a teacher is at least sincerely trying to understand his poor language, he will be more likely to accept his deficiencies and to cooperate in the teacher's work to correct his problem.

A teacher must be careful in giving praise and criticism while working with a child on his language problem. If praise is gushy and indiscriminate, it loses value and even causes the child to lose faith in the teacher's sincerity and judgment. Ordinarily it's more effective to rely upon demonstration rather than criticism to correct a pupil's language problem. If the teacher-pupil relationship is a good one, the pupil will more readily adopt the language usage suggested by the teacher's example without the need for direct criticism or command. When criticism is given, the child should be supplied with an alternative usage which is made reasonable and preferable to him. All of these cautions sound pretty difficult to do, but they really aren't if the teacher is patient and convinces the pupil that she sincerely desires to help him with his problem. The intuitive teacher also learns that pupils prefer to work for teachers whose voices and facial expressions are on the pleasant side. Too many teachers are afraid even to smile for fear they will lose disciplinary power.

Teacher-pupil relationships are also indirectly affected by physical conditions and facilities of the classroom. Learning is generally more difficult in rooms where inadequate ventilation, uncomfortable temperatures, and faulty lighting set a climate which hampers the pupils' perception and application to tasks. A teacher describes her room as follows:

I try to keep a cheerful and stimulating room, both physically and in spirit. Pleasing colors in the room, bouquets of flowers, interesting posters, pictures, and displays all help. One of my room-keeping policies is to have something new in the classroom every day. One corner of the room is reserved for the pupils to bring and display things of their own choice. And I conduct a daily ten- to fifteen-minute discussion about the items they bring, as well as about the new display which I provided for the day. I believe that this policy of encouraging pupils to share in the provision of instructional materials makes them feel closer to me, our room, the instructional materials, and to instruction itself. Incidentally, we teachers also learn that our relationship with pupils is largely governed by the relationship which we establish with our pupils' parents.

Direct Measures for Improving Language

By using methods similar to our suggestions throughout these chapters, teachers and therapists can build pupils' language while correcting other aspects of speech, such as misarticulation and speech maladjustments during the early formative years when speech is developing. The same methods and policies which assist parents in their teaching of language during children's preschool years apply to teachers, who continue with the speech and language development. When language problems arise because parents have failed to meet their responsibilities in language teaching, then teachers and therapists may be handicapped in following the same methods and policies which the parents had failed to fulfill earlier at a more favorable language-learning age.

Some of the following measures for improving pupils' language will resemble the therapeutic procedures which are emphasized throughout this book, indicating that speech and language in all of its forms are not to be isolated in therapy. The speech therapist, the linguist, and the general classroom teacher have much in common when they deal with problems of spoken language.

The following classroom exercises relate principally to the teaching or correction of language. They represent only a few samples of the many projects, methods, and policies which teachers have devised. In considering them, we need to recall some of the language problems which may be corrected by these exercises—deficiencies of vocabulary, unlearned sentence structure, faulty word functions, and grammatical deficiencies.

Dictionaries offer a familiar and direct way to build up a meaningful vocabulary of words and their pronunciations. An elementary school supervisor outlines the sequence followed in building readiness for using the dictionary:

> As a part of the reading program, we teach our youngsters how to use the dictionary, so that when they are third-graders, they can independently look up any words, to find their meanings, spellings, and pronunciations. This takes preparation during their first and second years. They must be taught to find words according to their alphabetical arrangement. Later, when pupils use the dictionary to look up an unknown word in a reading passage and find that it has several meanings, they know that they must go back to the passage and decide which meaning fits.

> In their reading program the pupils are taught to identify root words in inflected and derived forms. They learn the prefixes and suffixes of words and how spelling of the root changes when suffixes are added. They learn the meaning of each diacritical mark and how to derive pronunciations from it. When the children reach the stage, during the third grade, of knowing how to use the dictionary independently, they carry this new independence into their reading. They read more books of personal choice. Several of our P.T.A. groups have a project to buy personal dictionaries for all third-graders.

Word games, dictionary drills, rhymes, and exercises are used by teachers for the main purpose of teaching language. Many of the activities discussed in Chapter 6 when conducted orally may serve other purposes, such as correcting misarticulation, teaching pronunciation together with spelling, and improving the grammatical form of sentences. The following teacher describes some of these games which he favors for children who are deficient in language:

> My pupils in the third grade like word games in the form of crossword puzzles. However, besides using the regular vertical-horizontal crossword puzzles which one can buy ready-made for children, it's possible to simplify the word games so that every child may find at least some words for the blank squares. The pupils are encouraged to think up their own words and to provide the necessary spaces

for them. I may also have them write or speak a complete and meaningful sentence in which the word is used. Our self-made puzzles are submitted to the class. For instance, a child may submit three sentences and spaces such as:

What pet scratches? – – –
What is the biggest animal in the jungle? – – – – – – – –
What rings in the steeple? – – – –

We work on more than vocabulary in this word game. By having each pupil write a complete sentence to give the meaning of a word, I get good opportunities to teach all aspects of language. Besides, when a pupil replies with a word, he is also required to read the sentence that was provided for its meaning. In this way, he gets speech practice and reading practice, and it helps the entire listening class to get extra impacts of the learning involved. At times, I think that we get more all-around language instruction in fifteen minutes of class exercise from these crossword puzzles than we do in other more formal language work which is outlined for the day.

The next teacher tells how she and her pupils make up sentences which call for words that rhyme with clues contained in the sentence:

My children in the third grade enjoy a daily exercise in which they and I compose and write on the board ten questions which call for rhyming words having the meanings indicated by the sentences. For example, three of the questions may be:

What animal rhymes with *house*?
What color rhymes with *jello*?
What part of a car rhymes with *fire*?

We read aloud these sentences when we give their answers. We check the sentences for misspelled words. If anyone thinks of another word that fits the answer to the question, he may propose it, of course. This is a stimulating exercise. It makes the children think and share their knowledge. In this exercise, I believe that the children do more teaching of each other than I do. And it reveals to me the areas of interest and vocabulary weaknesses in pupils.

Teachers have devised various exercises for dictionary practice. The next teacher describes two of her methods:

My fifth-graders like to be challenged in their search and selection of words. One game they like is called "Same or Different." I put a list of word-pairs on the board; the pupils are to write *same* or *different* in the blank after each pair, indicating whether the two words are similar or different in meaning. They are encouraged to use their dictionaries or the thesaurus in the process. For example, the pairs may be

rough · · · uneven ....
accept · · · refuse ....
exaggerate · · · minimize ....
scatter · · · collect ....

Another popular game requires the pupils to look in their dictionaries and find synonyms for a given list of words or meanings—their synonyms to start with a given prefix or beginning syllable, such as *com* in the following list:

praise ....
to start or begin ....
to force or make someone do something ....
to agree or to obey ....
to put together ....
to fight against ....
a friend or companion ....

We save these lists and review them occasionally, and it's surprising how many of the new words are remembered. Pupils learn to put the words in sentences, and occasionally I hear some of the words being used in their conversational speech. Parents, too, have proudly commented on some of the "big words" their children bring home.

Teachers have invented many exercises which not only build vocabulary but also teach children the proper syntax and grammatical uses of words in sentences. The next teacher describes a sentence-building game which she calls "Make the Sentence Grow":

In some of our language games, a child starts by saying a word. Then, each consecutive child repeats what had been said and adds one word of his own to keep the sentence building in correct fashion. I may put the sentence on the board to help children remember what had been said. Then when the sentence has reached a child who decides to finish it, or if the child cannot continue to build it in a correct fashion, that sentence is considered built.

We play another question-answer game called "Ask Your Dictionary." I write a word on the board and make an oral statement which contains a right and wrong usage of that word. The children are asked to consult their dictionaries to help them decide which choice of statements is correct. For instance, I may put the word *fatigue* on the board and ask, "If you were fatigued, would you be sleepy or rested?" The pupils read the definitions of the word and reply with the answer in a complete sentence, such as, "If I were fatigued, I should be sleepy."

My pupils enjoy another game called "Sentence Bee." This is conducted like a spelling bee except that each pupil speaks up and selects a sentence in which the word is meaningfully used.

We also make good use of pictures cut from magazines, showing interesting actions and a number of subjects. As a class, we compose a story around a picture, using correct sentences and descriptive language.

Pictures are also collected by the children to make language scrapbooks around personal interests. Boys may pick topics like the space program, life on the seashore, collecting, or boy scouting. Girls often choose the subject of pets, an area of fashions, or girl scouting. In connection with their pictures, they keep a glossary of terms which they come across in their reading and experience in these areas of interest. The terms are not only defined as a dictionary would do but are also used in sentences to give the pupils practice in sharing these interesting concepts in readable form.

Our school is fortunate to have access to a good supply of movies and film strips covering almost any field of interest. I find that film strips are especially adaptable for language instruction. Each classroom has its own projector, and these films may be checked out like library books. Some of the films come with resource information and are programed with questions and topics for discussion. There are endless ways these colorful film strips can be used for language learning while, of course, valuable information is being learned too. I prefer film strips to regular movies because one can stop at any frame of a film strip, discuss it, and use the informative scenes in connection with speech and language exercises.

Teachers and speech therapists may take advantage of the growing availability of movies, film strips, and transparencies for all levels of education, including preschool ages. Informative catalogues like that of Stanley Bowmar Co., Inc., Valhalla, N.Y., 10595, offer wide selections of audio-visual materials, arranged alphabetically by subject area and with grade level coding. Films cover the language arts, social studies, teacher education, science, mathematics, health education, driver education, home economics, guidance, foreign languages, music, arts, and crafts. The teaching transparencies with their overlays are professionally planned to give teachers step-by-step help in teaching and illustrating certain concepts. A teaching guide and suggestions are included with each transparency. Pupils may effectively use some of these transparencies by themselves in the fashion of programed learning by individualized self-study. Students who read and trace from transparencies which show the parts of an airplane or of the human body, for example, not only learn the names, locations, and functions of these parts but are also equipped with an excellent organization of this information for giving oral or written reports about these topics. Visual teaching or learning aids, like transparencies and film strips, are especially helpful for pupils with language problems which cause insecurity and difficulty in the organization and expression of thought.

Indirect and Cooperative Measures

It is difficult to distinguish between the direct and indirect measures which influence and shape a schoolchild's language development. From our positions in the classroom or therapy room, we may arbitrarily judge the role of a child's parents and his other nonschool influences as being secondary, supplementary, or indirect. While it is probable that language development for most schoolchildren depends chiefly upon what happens at school, teachers are justified in giving more attention to outside influences when language is inadequate upon school entrance or when problems persist through the school years. Teachers commonly depend upon the pupil's foundation of spoken language, which has been built normally during his preschool years, from his limitless potential for linguistic patterns into the beginnings of a grammatical system required by his society and the school.

Although the school is formally charged with much of the direct responsibility for building and shaping a schoolchild's language, it is important for teachers and parents to realize that a pupil's continued language growth demands their mutual cooperation. Perhaps much of the existing mediocrity in the skills and uses of language would be prevented or corrected with closer cooperation between schools and their supporting public.

Recent surveys have estimated that about one-third of the U.S. population are not active readers in the sense that they read daily either for information or for recreational pleasure. With the increase of leisure time and the reorientation needed for modern life, there is growing emphasis on language skills and their everyday usage beyond our school years. If the majority of parents and the general public fail to maintain and use the language skills of their schooldays, it is unlikely that children will be influenced and given full opportunities to do so—even while they are under the jurisdiction of teachers in the language arts programs at school. Schools tend to be neglectful of this area of public education. A director of special education summarized this lack of cooperation between education and the public when he stated:

> I believe that our school staffs should be as aware of and well trained in the art of public relations as people are in the most successful businesses, in the field of advertising, and in politics. We school people complain when we get a shameful turnout in voting on important school issues. In campaigning to build new schools or add to library services and special education facilities, we remind the public that their costs will be less than what is spent on cigarettes and booze. Parents are blamed for having poor attendance at our P.T.A.'s, and yet we as teachers and administrators may privately admit that we would not attend our poorly planned P.T.A. programs if we weren't compelled to do so.
>
> We find fault with our public, our school boards, superintendents, and other elected officials, and yet we fail to take part in elections, may never attend public meetings concerning schools, or even read about school matters in the local newspaper. As teachers or therapists, we may not really give parents a genuine and warm welcome when they visit our classroom and open-house events. When parents ask us how they can help their children with homework, or how they can correct a problem of school adjustment, of language, arithmetic, etc., we are too often inclined to make the parents feel that they should stand aside and let us handle the matter. I'm afraid that we are partly to blame for the weak cooperation which generally exists between education and the public.

The opinion expressed by this director would apply to many areas which affect a pupil's language growth, whether we classify these influences upon language as direct or indirect, major or minor, primary or secondary. Whether or not we as teachers and therapists assume responsibility for these charges under our already crowded list of duties depends primarily upon our educational philosophy. From a practical standpoint, our actions are limited by the factors of time, energy, and facilities. But if greater community resources could be developed for language instruction beyond the realm of schools, teachers would be spared some of the problems and burdens in their present work to build and maintain the language arts.

Language Support from
Parents and Home

A coordinator of elementary education in a large school system has stated:

> Every day our teachers are asked by eager parents, "How can I help my children learn to read?" Many parents who should be asking this question do not do so because they do not feel responsible for this parental help. But when parents realize that language skills must be taught and that language serves as the most important of all skills needed for success in school and in later life, we find that many parents would like to know how to help. This is a question that requires careful answers. We have conducted workshops on how we can safely counsel parents on these matters. We know that there may be as much danger in what parents wrongly do in their concern to help children as there may be in what unconcerned parents fail to do at all.
>
> In counseling parents who want to know how they can help their children read, we point out that reading is a highly complicated process, not primarily a mechanical skill. We emphasize that parental influences and the child's experiences at home consist of creative forces and resources of language which must continue or else the child may lack the desire and ingredients to master the intricate mechanics of language in reading and writing.
>
> We advise parents to allow teachers to teach the mechanical aspects of reading and writing. However, we try to impress parents with the fact that they make the teacher's task a relatively easy one if the child's home and outer environment have provided him with an adequate resource of spoken language and if he has been imbued with a pleasurable desire to read.
>
> We have prepared a list of practical suggestions for parents to follow in helping preschoolers to meet the language standards needed for school. They include such pointers as:
>
> 1. Spend plenty of time with your child. Enthusiastically share all types of experiences with him. Talk with him about these experiences you share. Keep in mind that experiences which may be commonplace and dull for you may well be exciting and full of new knowledge for him. Of course, fathers should realize that their companionship with children is needed too.
>
> 2. Pick your baby-sitters with care—ones who like children and can set favorable examples of constructive learning and behavior for your child. Likewise, if you place your child in a private preschool day nursery, select one where your child's language development will be favorably stimulated and enriched. Remember, too, that you may need to do some social maneuvering to insure that your child's spoken language is helped rather than hindered by his regular neighborhood playmates.

3. Encourage your child to develop self-interests. Invite his adoption of these interests from a sampling of subjects which may later lend themselves to resources of contributing information from pictures, books, maps for travel, directions and diagrams for model-making, and records and charts for hobbies of collecting, for instance.

4. As parents, you should set personal examples of being interested readers who read not only for information and enjoyment but also by reading to your child for his enjoyment and information. Librarians and teachers will gladly help you in the selection of suitable stories. Libraries and educational TV programs which offer story-reading periods for preschool children may also guide you in the art of reading and telling stories to children. You have an important responsibility to select TV programs which are educationally constructive. And a higher quality of TV programs would be available for children if more parents would write TV networks and sponsors to express their likes or dislikes of what is offered.

5. Although we do not recommend that parents should take the initiative in teaching a preschooler his A-B-C's in preparation for school, neither do we discourage parents from answering a child's inquiries about letters, words and numbers which he may voluntarily point out on signboards, labels, posters, his dad's newspaper, etc. The danger in this prereading period may arise either if a child is forced to memorize language symbols prematurely or if a parent fails to respond with any shared interest when his child makes inquiries about the symbols and the mysteries of meanings which he has begun to associate with them. After a child enters school and has begun to read, our counseling of parents includes some additional pointers:

1. Take an active interest in your child's steps in learning to read and write. Be appreciative of his efforts and accomplishments. When he brings home pages from his reading-readiness workbook, for instance, or shows you lists of his word-spellings, show your appreciation.

2. Avoid being critical of flaws in his work. In his learning of language skills he needs encouragement and confidence which comes from success; a child who respects his parents may well measure his successes by the way they react to his steps in learning. Remember that each child is an individual with a certain profile of abilities and limitations; therefore, he should not be burdened with feelings of comparison with other children. Your child will meet the many difficulties in speech, reading, and writing if he has the security of knowing that his parents have patient and unbroken faith in his ability to meet tasks.

3. Your child's interest and skill in oral reading may be strengthened by your genuine interest in having him read to you. But when he reads to you, make him feel that you are interested mainly in the content of what he is reading, not in how well he can perform the mechanics of the reading. While he is reading, give him your sincere and undivided attention, without hurrying or prompting or interrupting him with corrections unless he asks for help. It is likely that there are established periods at school when his corrections will be duly handled.

4. Provide him with plenty of suitable materials for both recreational and informative reading. Books, magazines, and encyclopedias make valuable gifts. The public library and bookmobile should be patronized.

5. In your parent-teacher conferences, teachers will appreciate your views, questions, and reports concerning your child's language progress. Our teachers

solicit your cooperation because they realize that an important share of each child's educational growth depends upon his parents and his experiences outside school.

A mother gave the following explanations of her children's precocity in language and their unusual successes in school:

My husband and I have always catered to our children's language needs, but we have done so without making them feel that we are pushing language itself. We have made language serve useful and satisfying purposes which were built into our experiences. When the children were too young to read for themselves, we read enjoyable stories to them and discussed the pictures and thoughts of the stories. And, of course, through everyday conversation we gave them all sorts of chances to learn and use speech. When the children learned to read, they had access to plenty of books and magazines. We make regular use of public libraries, and each child has had his or her library card to make the use of books as personalized as possible. Too many parents neglect their children by not using the public libraries. Every family can afford this wide source of learning, especially when bookmobiles may bring books conveniently into one's neighborhood.

We have also made it a point to have ample family-centered activities, although we have also tried to let each child exercise his individuality. We have always done a lot of family camping, travel, and picnicking. These excursions invite the use of language. In our car travels we have collected and devised many car games which not only counteract the weariness of long miles but also incidentally teach language as we roll along. Each of us has developed hobbies from family camping, and these interests entail reading and writing as well as speech. There are economical ways to have these valuable experiences. In fact, out of necessity we learned that rustic, do-it-yourself tent-camping is likely to be more rewarding for a family than is most camping with modernized equipment in the commercialized and highly developed campgrounds. Personally, we believe that families with young children should at least start with tent-camping and leave the modern homelike conveniences of travel trailers and motorhomes, etc., for later periods of life.

When our children started school and learned to read, all of their teachers remarked about their unusually wide vocabularies, a factor which helped in their reading, writing, class contributions, and over-all learning.

Other Special Aids to Language

Many new developments have facilitated the teaching of language and the correction of its problems. Audio-visual equipment and programed courses of language instruction have made the learning of foreign languages more efficient and individualized. Aphasic patients, with impaired language resulting from brain damage, may also gain help from a similar programing of language materials electronically recorded and played back in a planned and systematic way. Young children may benefit from language recordings on tapes and records designed for special problems. In cases of perceptual impairments, new equipment is being developed to compensate for a loss of sight or hearing. Special materials and methods are being used by teachers and therapists in their work to correct some of the unique language problems. One of the achievements in the Head Start program, for example, has been the development of better approaches in teaching new language patterns to the "culturally deprived" pupil who may not be deprived in the language of his different culture but who may require learning principally through physical, visual, and action-centered avenues in order to attain the language standards required at school. Egland[12] suggests the needs for greater cooperation with parents in the Head Start programs. Chapel,[13] in a special program designed to give migrant farm children help in learning to read and to adjust to regular school life, found that the experiential training and adjustment of the Mexican, Negro, and "Anglo" children were obviously helped by incorporating their families and community interests into the program.

Teachers may learn of these special aids to language by consulting departments of special education. A second-grade teacher has voiced the following appreciation of a specialist who served as a resource person in the field of language instruction:

> Our county provides a full-time reading consultant who works solely with teachers in our various schools, to supply information and special materials and equipment to supplement our work in the language areas. She is trained not only to teach language at every level but is also informed and equipped with the latest books, manuals, charts, and other materials for teaching. She may lend or requisition materials for us when she feels that we need the added facilities. Sometimes she introduces new audio-visual equipment and teaches us how to use it. Or she may conduct an in-service workshop in which she uses her special materials and procedures with a group or a roomful of our pupils. In certain special cases of language difficulty, she may help us diagnostically by conducting intensive tests. She is hopeful that more schools will adopt progressive steps to include language learning and other educational experiences into previously uncharted areas like the school bus program, while pupils are being transported to and from school.

This teacher's attitude is representative of the convictions of the other classroom teachers and the therapists quoted on language problems. From the one-room rural school to the newest city complex, other conscientious teachers would agree with them that the primary emphasis should always be on the prevention of speech problems, whether in the initial or in the secondary stages of development. The teacher's capabilities of sound language knowledge, sympathetic understanding, and experience combine in a positive evaluation of therapy methods for successful solutions to speech problems.

References

1. P. Menjuk, "Comparison of Grammar of Children with Functionally Deviant and Normal Speech," *Journal of Speech and Hearing Research*, 7 (1967), 109–21.

2. Laura Lee, "Developmental Sentence Types: A Method for Comparing Normal and Deviant Syntactic Development," *Journal of Speech and Hearing Disorders*, 31 (November 1966), 311–30.

3. Nancy E. Wood, *Delayed Speech and Language Development*. Englewood Cliffs, N.J.: Prentice-Hall, Inc., 1964.

4. Charles C. Fries, Rosemary G. Wilson, and Mildred K. Rudolph, *Merrill Linguistic Readers*. Columbus, O.: Charles E. Merrill Books, Inc., 1966.

5. Joseph D. Lohman, "Expose—Don't Impose," *N.E.A. Journal*, 55, No. 1 (January 1966), 24–26.

6. Homer L. Carter and Dorothy J. McGinnis, *Teaching Individuals to Read*. Boston: D. C. Heath and Co., 1962.

7. Joan Chapman, "Some Observations of Perceptually Impaired Children in Two Approaches to Reading," *Reading Horizons* 4, No. 2 (1964), 41–50. (Published by Psycho-Educational Clinic and Western Michigan University Chapter of the International Reading Association, Kalamazoo, Michigan), 41–50.

8. Elise Hahn, "Analysis of the Content and Form of the Speech of First Grade Children," *Quarterly Journal of Speech*, 34 (1948), 361–66.

9. Martha Dallmann, *Teaching the Language Arts in the Elementary School*. Dubuque, Iowa: William C. Brown Co., 1966.

10. Bill Martin, Jr., Trudy T. Weil, Frances H. Kohan, *Sounds and Patterns of Language: Talking Our Way to Reading*. New York: Holt, Rinehart and Winston, Inc., 1966.

11. Sol Saporta, *Psycholinguistics: A Book of Readings*. New York: Holt, Rinehart and Winston, Inc., 1966.

12. George O. Egland, "Parents in Head Start Programs," *Young Children*, XXI, No. 5 (May 1966), 292–97.

13. Joe R. Chapel, "And It Happened to Me," *Reading Horizons*, 8, No. 3 (1968), 117–22.

Questions

1. Is language growth a skill learned in isolation from studies other than grammar and language study?

2. Why are boundaries of language normality difficult to determine?

3. Describe the responsibility of the school nurse in diagnosing speech problems.

4. Define "delayed" speech and its subtypes.

5. Why is it difficult to test and to evaluate a pupil's language deficit?

6. What are the values of using aids like the *Merrill Linguistic Readers*?

7. What is required of a "fair" test of language achievement?

8. Explain Lohman's advice of "expose, don't impose."

9. Name some organic causal factors in language disorders.

10. What perceptual disorders interfere with language?

11. Should we ignore language training for the mentally retarded?

12. How does language reveal environmental deprivations?

13. What is the effect of emotional maladjustment on language?

14. Should the teacher always correct language errors immediately?

15. Explain: Measures which correct language problems are often the same measures which would have prevented these problems if action had been taken earlier.

16. Explain the value of perceptual training in language development.

17. Contrast primers of a generation ago with modern primers and language and reading materials.

18. Describe the teacher-pupil relationship favorable for learning.

19. What is the value of the dictionary in language development?

20. Explain the popularity of word games and puzzles.

21. How may pictures and films aid language growth?

22. What is the significance for teachers of the fact that one-third of the U.S. population are not active readers?

23. What are two ways by which parents can help children learn to read?

24. How may hobbies encourage language development?

25. Should parents take the initiative in teaching a preschooler his A-B-C's when he shows lack of interest?

26. Should the parent show more interest in content or in the manner of reading by his children?

27. Can you suggest utilizing some other "wasted" opportunity, such as the school bus program, for using headphones for language and music training?

Suggested Subjects for
Term Papers

1. Write a modern primer on one of the following themes: (a) Kindness to Animals; (b) How I Help Mom and Dad; (c) My Garden; (d) The Kind of Kids I Like; (e) Why I'd Like to Be Grown-up.
2. How would you deal with: (a) the overtalkative child; (b) the shy, withdrawn child; (c) the compulsive "story teller"; (d) the tattle-tale?
3. How would you handle a situation in which your children have begun to speak like the children next door, who are "from the other side of the tracks"?
4. A nation gets the type of entertainment it deserves. Do you agreee?
5. Write out a fifteen-minute speech which you would give to your school's P.T.A. meeting on the subject "How Parents May Help Children Learn to Read."
6. If you were assigned to teach first grade in a ghetto district, what special language problems would you anticipate and how would you handle them?

eight

Helping the Nonfluent Child

A lucky 95 per cent of us are fluent speakers. The ideal of fluency may restrict the classroom teacher in rating pupils not only in recitation and in oral reading but also in general school achievement. Despite the fact that approximately 1 per cent of schoolchildren stutter as compared with 4 per cent who have other types of speech defects, the major emphasis on stuttering research and therapy indicates our great concern with this disorder.

There is a growing realization that help for the school stutterer will be more successful if our therapy extends and adapts to his regular schoolwork and experiences. However, this increasing need for cooperation between the therapist and the classroom teacher in helping the stuttering child, for example, should not impose unreasonable duties or burdens upon teachers. In the case of a stuttering pupil, the speech therapist should take the lead in this cooperative work with the teacher, to fit the corrective measures into the activities of the classroom. This requires that speech therapists should be acquainted with the classroom teacher's role and the activities and opportunities where the teacher may contribute in speech correction. It is also important for therapists to be acquainted with the complications that often arise in school for the child who stutters, because if we can recognize and anticipate these complications, we may prevent the development of problems. When school problems have already arisen to aggravate stuttering, speech therapists should be ready and willing to give all possible assistance to the classroom teacher in handling them. A disorder as complicated and insidious as stuttering demands the best combined efforts of teacher, speech therapist, and parents.

Types, Labels, and Degrees
of Nonfluency

From their experience with children in a wide range of speech situations, teachers can appreciate the way speakers vary in their fluency and flow of speech. Furthermore, teachers are in good positions to observe that fluency not only varies from speaker to speaker but that each speaker's fluency also fluctuates from situation to situation as favorable or unfavorable factors influence

171

it. Some of these factors are obvious; others are insidious and subtle. The latter are often the ones we need most to know and to control. And it will be as important to understand positive factors that allow and facilitate fluency as it is to know the conditions which deny and undermine it.

A first-grade teacher says of a pupil:

I wouldn't say that Milton stutters, but his speech is so hesitant and full of pauses. In reading he's not bad, but in recitation or show-and-tell he makes us impatient and fidgety by his many pauses. He gets worse when we try to help him by saying words for him. But he hardly ever has this trouble in informal conversation outside the classroom. Why? As a teacher, I feel that my influence and control should make his speech more fluent around me.

Another teacher describes what she thinks may be stuttering:

Ralph has the habit of repeating words and phrases here and there in his sentences. It doesn't seem to bother him at all, though. In fact, he's a regular chatterbox, at times talking more than he should. He's worse when trying to get his words in edgewise. At first, he had repetitions while reading in class, especially when he came to words he didn't know. Then he'd repeat the preceding word until either he or the rest of the class could figure out the questionable word. However, Ralph doesn't repeat so many words in reading since I stopped letting his classmates prompt him on stuck-words. He likes to do things his way.

A third teacher describes *cluttering*, another kind of speech nonfluency:

Frances runs her words together and talks so fast that at times we can hardly understand what she says. She tries to say so much all at once that she ends up by leaving out sounds, syllables, and even whole words in her spurts of rapid speech. She doesn't talk at a smooth rate either. I've told her to slow down and speak more carefully, but it seems to help her for only a sentence or two. Then she's back at her breakneck course. It doesn't seem to bother her, though.

This classroom teacher in a children's hospital school describes nonfluency as a part of a larger speech disorder resulting from cerebral palsy:

Stella is continually struggling word by word when she speaks. Sometimes she can say several words at once, but often she works on a word, syllable by syllable. Her lack of breath control wrecks her pace too, slowing her down, causing her to split words and to pause and get ready for the next utterance. Her broken speech is very hard to understand, but we've learned to understand her better. I've noticed that her control and fluency have improved since I've found ways to allow her to speak with less hurry and impatience.

The following type of nonfluency is reported by a high school pupil:

One of our high school teachers has an awful habit of saying "ah" when he talks, especially in class. He says so many "ahs'" that it really becomes funny. It's distracting too, when you need to keep your mind on the lecture. Some of the kids keep count of the times he says "ah" during a single class period. One kid marked 187 in one hour. My mother had this same teacher when she was here in school. She said he talked the same way then.

The Nature of Stuttering

Nonfluency that is labeled as *stuttering* or *stammering* reveals exceptionally wide variations in symptoms as the disorder develops. It is not surprising to find that teachers and others often differ in their judgments of stuttering. This confusion over differences among stutterers is further complicated by the fact that "stuttering" has accumulated a variety of related terms, some based on symptoms, some on causation, and some on different stages in its development.

In America speech therapists rarely use the term *stammering*. When they do, they mean *stuttering*. However, European speech therapists and a diminishing segment of the American lay-public still use the two words. *Stammering* may mean that the nonfluencies are characterized by speech hesitations or prolongations, while *stuttering* refers in this narrowed sense to a speaker who repeats a sound, syllable, word, or phrase. The terms *tonic* and *clonic* are sometimes used to indicate the above mentioned symptoms of "stammerers" and "stutterers" respectively.

Symptoms of stuttering are sometimes classified by the terms *overt* and *covert*. In overt stuttering the nonfluency is "externalized", or expressed openly so that the stutterers' audience can plainly see and hear that he stutters. Covert stuttering is hidden, covered up, and "internalized" in its form. Therefore, teachers must be alert to recognize the covert type of stutterer who may camouflage his secretive fears, limited speech, and repressed symptoms of stuttering. Unless these subtle forms of stuttering are detected, covert stutterers will be ignored, and their camouflages may deny them help and may even add complications to their problems.

The terms *primary stuttering*, *transitional stuttering* and *secondary stuttering* reflect the general belief that stuttering is developmental and that its course of growth is marked by rather distinguishable steps or stages unless its development is halted. Later, this chapter will emphasize how dangerous it is to treat a primary stutterer as a secondary one. It should be pointed out, however, that *primary* and *secondary* in the case of stuttering do not refer to the stutterer's chronological age nor his grade level. Stutterers in every stage can be found at every age level, from preschool to adulthood.

The following puzzled teacher is telling about a primary stutterer:

Peter, a pupil in my kindergarten class, seems to have a tendency to stutter. I'm not sure that it is stuttering. It's not bad and it doesn't seem to bother him at all. He talks as much as anyone in class. The other children don't seem to be aware of his speech difference either. But in comparison with other kindergartners, he does repeat more, perhaps one repetition per twenty-five spoken words. And when he repeats, his repetitions last longer, from one to six times before he goes on. Usually his repetitions are of phrases, words, and syllables. Sometimes he repeats the first sound of a word before saying the word. However, these repetitions don't seem to hold up his speech much. They more or less just bubble out spontaneously without apparent tension or forcing on his part. The stuttering is not consistent either. Samples of Peter's stuttering-like symptoms are as follows:

"I saw it in the—in the—in the supermarket." (Repetition of phrase)

"He—he—he—hit me first!" (Repetition of word)

"Glen-Glen-Glendale Avenue." (Repetition of syllable)

"I t-t-t-told him to stop." (Repetition of a speech sound)

"MMMMMMMMMMMMMary, come here!" (Prolongation of a sound).

The following kindergarten teacher describes some developmental changes in her pupil, Steve, a stutterer who had been in the primary stage but who is now showing symptoms of the transitional stage, with signs of becoming secondary. Steve is beginning to show signs of self-awareness and self-concern over his nonfluencies. Although his repetitions and prolongations are still fairly free and uncomplicated, associated symptoms of tension, forcing, and complications are beginning to develop.

> Steve and his speech are beginning to concern me, partly because I think his stuttering may be getting worse since he started to school last fall and partly because I know his mother is getting worried over it. Some changes are beginning to show in his speech as well as in his attitudes toward his speaking. Lately, his speech repetitions and prolongations appear more noticeable, perhaps because he now seems to be trying to do something about them. Occasionally when he is blocked on one of his prolongations of a sound, his voice will rise in pitch and he'll squint as if he's impatient and trying to get the word out.
> But I'm worried most by Steve's changing attitude. He's not as ready and willing to recite and volunteer in show-and-tell as he was. I don't think that the other children have reacted unfavorably toward his speech, though. The problem appears to be mostly in Steve's mouth and mind. Another problem facing me, however, is what to advise Steve's mother when we have our next conference. I know that she'll bring up the subject of Steve's stuttering.

The following teacher describes a stutterer in the secondary stage, characterized by symptoms definitely indicating that this stutterer is personally and socially concerned over her speech problem.

> In my 9 o'clock section of English, I have an eighth-grade girl, Marion, who stutters. I hadn't known about her problem until I gave assignments for oral book reports. Then she came to me after class and asked to be excused from giving her report before the class. Before that, she had never recited orally, even when I had called on her. At those times she either said "I don't know" or simply waited until

I called on someone else. But I knew from her written work that she was intelligent and a good student, except for her lack of oral participation.

Anyway, in that private conference it was easy to see why she would be reluctant to stand up before the class and give an oral report. In nearly every sentence she got completely stuck on one or more words, often on the beginning of a sentence. Sometimes she hesitated or repeated a sound before saying the rest of the word. During her blocks she strained and worked hard to get the word out. Obviously it was an unpleasant struggle for her. Sometimes her jaw dropped open and seemed to lock. At times she lowered and even closed her eyes. It was pitiful to watch, and I found myself looking away from her. I'm afraid that I was almost as tense and embarrassed as she was. At least, I didn't have the heart to refuse her request, even though I know that we're supposed to treat stutterers like anyone else. What else could I have done? What good would have come from making a miserable spectacle of herself? In fact, I doubt that she would have done it.

Speech therapists have termed and classified these reactions preliminary to the moment of blockage as *anticipations*, *postponements*, and *avoidances*. Reactions which occur during the moment of block have been variously referred to as the *block pattern* or *spasm pattern*, *release reactions*, *control pattern*, *struggle reactions*, and *interruption devices*. It is also important for teachers to know that these reactions in stuttering tend to become stubbornly fixed habits that characterize each secondary stutterer.

The various fears and attitudes which breed these reactions of the secondary stage include emotional states which have been analyzed and labeled by Van Riper[1] and others as *anxiety*, *frustration*, *guilt*, *shame*, *hostility*, etc. More will be said about these emotions in later discussion.

In summary, the array of terms describing the nature and development of stuttering reminds the classroom teacher of the following important facts:

1. Stuttering takes many forms, depending upon its level of development and the unique pattern of reactions that each stutterer tends to build around his problem.
2. As stuttering develops from primary to secondary stages, it tends to become more habitual, consistent, and individualized, because of the unique combination of attitudes and reactions that tend to be patterned and habituated in each person who stutters.
3. Some types of stuttering are easy to detect; others are hard to identify because of their mildness, their secrecy, or, perhaps, their unusual and bizarre characteristics, suggestive of other disorders.
4. There are many degrees of difficulty and handicap among secondary stutterers. The wide range of severity and specific handicaps in stuttering will be discussed later in this chapter.

Causes of Poor Fluency

If we are to prevent and to correct poor fluency, such as stuttering, we must understand, recognize, and control its causal and contributing factors. Stuttering usually begins when the child is two to four years of age, with another lesser peak of incidence when the child starts school. A knowledge of causes and effects is necessary for all who deal with children during this formative period while speech and language are relatively susceptible to influences and change. Parents need to know what may precipitate nonfluency and lead to stuttering, and a teacher may be the only informed person who can give parents information and counseling. Now that school programs are being extended to "preschool" children as young as two years of age, teachers in these programs become more directly responsible for insuring good speech fluency in its earliest stages of development. A teacher's role brings her into contact with many factors which affect the flow and rhythm of children's speech.

Speech is a highly intricate neuro-muscular act, basically dependent upon the maturation of structures, muscles, and neurological control. The teacher who has a brain-injured pupil with cerebral palsy more easily understands that the flow of speech may be irregular and halting when nerve damage prevents the synchronized control of muscles for breathing, articulation, and voice. Then, too, the cerebral-palsied child's fluency may also be lowered by the same conditions and factors that lower fluency in anyone, brain-injured or not. This is important for us to keep in mind to avoid putting too much blame upon the more obvious factor of brain injury in the cerebral palsied person and neglecting to see other factors—causes which are more open to correction.

The child with cleft palate, too, may have poor fluency, not because of any impairment of the nervous system but perhaps because of faulty palatal structures that require him to take extra time in making the special compensatory controls needed for certain of his speech sounds. Later, after attaining greater speed in these skills, his fluency may improve. It is well to remember that in the case of a multiple disorder, where more than one cause and skill are involved, it may be wise to work on a limited front rather than on all areas of the problem at once. The speech therapist can give assistance to the classroom teacher in determining what segments of the problem should be worked on and in what order.

However, the more common causes of nonfluency do not rest upon faulty organic structure or neurological injury. There are many of these ordinary factors, and teachers come into contact with most of them. Let us examine what some of them may be.

Even before two years of age, the average child has started the intricate process of talking in sentences, complete and incomplete as they are. This marvelous accomplishment occurs at a physical and maturational age when it is reasonable to expect that the child will have some awkwardness and difficulty in executing many of his motor skills. At this age when the child is not yet smoothly coordinated in most of his physical acts, he should not be expected to meet the adult's polished proficiencies, especially in the finer physical and mental skills of speech.

At about eighteen months of age, the average child will go through a speech practice period of several months in which his babbling and single "word" utterances are intermingled with strings of sentence-like, conversation-like jabber called *jargon*, often carried on while the child is alone. It is believed that this stage of jargon is an essential period of learning and practice of the basic patterns of stress, inflection, and tempo which are required in connected speech. If for some reason a child is prevented from getting enough of this playful practice of pretending to converse in adult-like styles of rhythm, his fluency may suffer in the next stages when he is faced with the necessity of putting thoughts into real words, phrases, and sentences within these same but unlearned frameworks of stress, inflection, and tempo.

Fluency in oral communication depends upon a combination of related elements: the choice of correct words, with their correct articulation, inflection, and placement in sentences; and the prosodic qualities comprising the melody, accent, or rhythm of speech. This melody pattern of speech depends upon the correct placing of stress upon syllables and words within the sentence, the shifting of pitch from one part of speech to another, and the variable effects upon language-meanings which depend upon the speaker's use of pauses, sound prolongations, emphasis, and changes in pitch and in timing.

Classroom teachers are often made aware of how the speech fluency of pupils varies under emotions, tensions, and insecurities. Some pupils are affected more than others by these disrupters of fluency. One pupil, hurriedly relating his observations of an exciting playground accident, may clutter his speech with hesitations, repetitions, and fragments of unfinished utterances; another child in the same communicative spot may speak with more smoothness and organization. But if these two pupils in this situation feel unjustly blamed and threatened with punishment for their part in the accident, their fluencies may suffer more than when they are merely reporting it impersonally. A wise teacher in this case would judge fluency in the light of its situational setting. A schoolchild's life has many speech situations where fluency is lowered because of these "pressures" upon it. And it is doubly important for a teacher to recognize the less obvious school "pressures" which may arise to nag at and to undermine a pupil's speech fluency. Some of these more subtle and insidious classroom pressures upon fluency will be analyzed later in this chapter.

Besides the foregoing factors that are common in the development and life of every speaker, child and adult, there are special factors which have been blamed as special causes of stuttering. One of these theories has to do with the shift of a child's handedness. Research has tried to prove whether or not stuttering is caused by a shift; yet the issue is still unsettled, though less popular than it was. Nevertheless, present-day speech correctionists and classroom teachers generally agree that the safer policy is to allow a young child to develop his naturally preferred handedness in all activities, including writing. This policy of being permissive toward handedness rests partly upon the belief that the child, his personal adjustment, and fluency may be harmed chiefly by the forceful tactics and the emotional conflicts that parents and teachers may produce in their enforcement of the shift. However, the well informed kindergarten or first grade teacher should be ready to give the young southpaw writer special instruction on how to place his paper and to hold his pencil, so that he will not adopt by himself the faulty slant and cramped positions that handicap some left-handed writers.

Research on the causes of stuttering has also delved into hereditary factors. This complex area, too, is uncharted. The fact that stuttering does have a tendency to "run in families" has led some people to suspect that heredity may operate in a predisposing way, if not directly. Other authorities have pointed out that stuttering may run in a family line because of psychological, social, and environmental factors which are commonly imposed upon members of a household or passed from one family circle to another via sociological links. Regardless of the questions concerning heredity, we are justified and obligated to adopt the philosophy that stuttering in a child may be prevented, cleared up, or at least altered—for better or for worse.

Another rather commonly suspected cause of stuttering, one that research has proved to be more fanciful than factual, stems from the idea that mouth structures or breathing are directly faulty and responsible. Years ago many stutterers were taken to physicians and had tongues clipped or tonsils and adenoids removed in the popular belief that these structures were causing stuttering. Remnants of this groundless belief still exist, although modern doctors are no longer likely to use surgery to cure stuttering.

The Start and Growth of Stuttering

Our discussion of how stuttering starts and grows will follow a case history approach, describing and tracing stuttering in two children, Jimmy and Helen. Although Jimmy's history of stuttering will be given in more detail, Helen's characteristics, together with excerpts from other stutterers' case histories, will be brought into the discussion to remind us not to generalize too much on the basis of Jimmy, who is no more typical than Helen. No two stutterers follow identical paths in their stuttering development. In the beginning stage of stuttering there is a stronger similarity among stutterers than when they advance into secondary stages. Jimmy and Helen might have resembled each other in their early types of speech nonfluencies and in the causal factors for their early symptoms. But since Helen and Jimmy led different lives, their experiences of causes and effects were not identical. They diverged in their attitudes and reactions toward their stuttering according to their differing experiences and the multitudes of influences associated with their stuttering. There are many degrees of Jimmy's characteristics and many of Helen's. Then too, there are stutterers who do not appear to possess any of

Jimmy's or Helen's characteristics. At times these outward differences may obscure what they have in common. Despite the variations, there are similar stages and basic types of behavior common among secondary stutterers, and it is important to learn to recognize and to understand these signposts in their development.

While we consider Jimmy and Helen, it will be especially important to note the cause-and-effect elements in their behavior. Much of this conduct occurs at school with teachers and pupils. Unless a teacher can read these signs, she will be unable to locate the pupil along the stuttering route, unable to tell whether he is getting better or worse, and unable to help him.

JIMMY

Jimmy's parents reported that he began to "stammer or stutter" at the age of three. For about a year, his nonfluencies were relatively simple, with no apparent self-awareness nor self-concern. During this period his nonfluencies were mostly repetitions of first sounds of words, l-l-like this, and repetitions of whole words, such as, "Where-where-where are you going?" Jimmy was freely talkative in this preliminary stage of his stuttering and did not show that his repetitions were socially bothersome to him.

After he had been repeating in this manner for about nine months, his parents admitted that they began to be concerned. He was approaching school age, and they did not want a speech problem to stand in his way. They asked him to repeat words and sentences in which they had noticed his repetitions. They said words and sentences for him, to give him models of how to speak correctly. They tried to help him by telling him to speak more slowly, to be more careful, and to think about what he was going to say.

Jimmy was described by his parents as conscientious and obedient, sensitive to criticism and punishment, indecisive, and inclined to worry about problems of the past, present, and future. A child with these personality traits may not only have more of the ordinary nonfluencies in his early speech development but may also be more susceptible and reactive to the pressures imposed upon him by others in their well meant but futile efforts to correct his speech faults.

According to his parents, Jimmy did not fit comfortably into his family circle of two older brothers and a sister two years younger. His brothers had more advanced interests and standards and often did not include Jimmy in their activities. However, Jimmy idolized his brothers and sought their favor, companionship, and approval. Although none of Jimmy's family had ever teased him or made fun of his nonfluencies, his brothers were inclined to interrupt him and to monopolize speech in their conversations with him.

Jimmy's repetitions became noticeable to his parents soon after his sister was born. Some jealousy of the new baby was noted at this time, but the dutiful and conscientious Jimmy soon fell into the family's cooperative roles to give care and attention to the baby.

At five years, a series of new changes occurred in Jimmy's stuttering as he began to exhibit new attitudes and reactions toward his speech and speech situations when his parents were trying hard in various ways to help him stop his stuttering. Jimmy began to reveal by frowns and pauses that he was now aware of his moments of repetitions. His awareness of nonfluencies included growing signs that repetitions were bothering him, both by themselves and as undesirable obstacles in his social relationships. Jimmy had started to show some reluctance to talk. Sometimes he paused after a nonfluency and shrugged his shoulders as if to say that he was through talking. At this stage, some of his repetitions were ending in prolongations and tight blocks, and he began to force on them.

Next, Jimmy's stuttering increased as he became impatient and even resentful toward the corrective efforts of his parents. He avoided speech situations more and more. Tension, forcing, and struggle appeared to surround his moments of stuttering and began to invade even his anticipation of having to speak. Finally, just before the age of six, Jimmy's patterns of attitudes and reactions expressed the elements of shame, social withdrawal, and a sense of helplessness.

In view of Jimmy's serious speech problem, his parents decided that he should postpone school for a year in the hope that by then his stuttering might be "outgrown," as the family doctor had earlier predicted that it would. Hopeful assurances were offered, together with suggestions that his stuttering might be cured by self-practice in talking and through prayer.

That sixth year was filled with growing anxieties, fading hopes, and new dreads as Jimmy tried an array of ways to avoid, minimize, and wipe out this devil stuttering—something that he now knew was serious enough to exclude him from school. From now on, the subject of his stuttering was not discussed, except on infrequent occasions when he appealed for special help in some unusual dilemma. Otherwise, he worked alone and secretly prayed to be cured of his stuttering in time for school.

Shortly before the start of the next school year, Jimmy, now seven and stuttering worse than ever, was told that he must begin school. His parents offered to speak to his first-grade teacher and to give him written excuses to take to his future teachers, requesting that he be excused from all recitation and oral reading. Jimmy readily accepted this offer, and the dreaded uncertainties of school were somewhat reduced.

From that point on through high school, Jimmy carried these notes from home to each of his teachers. Every regular teacher during his first eight grades accepted his requests without question. As one teacher explained: "I knew about Jimmy and his inability to speak long before he came to my grade. Since he was a very good pupil except for speaking, I thought he could afford to be excused from talking." Occasionally substitute teachers called on him to read or to recite, but at these critical times Jimmy's classmates explained that "Jimmy isn't supposed to read."

In high school several teachers invited verbal responses from him in a few informal situations, in laboratory periods, and in occasional short conferences over schoolwork. However, except for a speech teacher, who shared with the teaching of oral English in Jimmy's junior year, no teacher ever openly discussed the subject of his stuttering. This speech teacher, prompted by the fact that Jimmy would not fulfill the public speaking requirements for the year, held a private conference with him, telling him in a frank and respectful way that she believed he should try to face his speech responsibilities in life, stuttering or not. As Jimmy later stated in speech therapy, which began in his college years, "That speech teacher in my junior year of high school did more to help me face my problem and to start to work on it than all the rest of the teachers combined. She didn't tell me anything I didn't already know or suspect, but it was such a relief to know that a teacher could understand and be openly honest with me. She gave me some good practical suggestions too, even though she wasn't a regular speech therapist."

Jimmy quit school because a history teacher kept calling on him for recitation. After being a determined dropout for two weeks, Jimmy agreed to be reinstated, following his parents' conference with the principal, who again reminded his teachers not to call on Jimmy. In view of the fact that he was a conscientious pupil who graduated as valedictorian, teachers were not inclined to object to excusing him from oral work. Throughout his school life, Jimmy had worked hard to excel in written work, and his deportment had always been appreciated.

Although he was well liked and respected by his fellow pupils in the small grade school, in informal conversation outside the classroom Jimmy spoke sparingly and cautiously, under constant guard to conceal his stuttering as much as possible. He learned to avoid children who had been known to tease him.

During twelve years of extremely unhappy school years, he counted the days when the school year would end and then began to worry when school would begin again. He worried about substitute teachers and the likelihood of their calling on him to read or to recite. He felt humiliated by being excluded from spell-downs and school programs. When his third-grade teacher once enticed him into a school program on the grounds that it would be easy for him to speak several memorized lines behind a large cardboard face of Humpty Dumpty, he got stuck in shameful silence halfway through this public performance and was obliged to quit the embarrassed, whispering audience of pupils and their parents.

In present-day education it is more likely that classroom teachers would have earlier contact with Jimmy and his parents. Educational services are now being extended into preschool years, when Jimmy's problems began and could have been corrected. Later in this chapter we shall suggest specific ways by which Jimmy and his parents could have been helped, how his fluency problems might have been prevented, and how Jimmy might have "outgrown" stuttering and not seen it mushroom into miserably fixed and ingrown complexes. Teachers can have important roles in these preventive and corrective programs. With their aides, teachers have opportunities to provide this help in nursery schools, day-care centers, preschool clinics, and public education. Speech therapists have a leading role in the counseling of parents and in the management of stutterers in these educational situations; and teachers, therefore, should know where speech therapists are located, how to secure their services, and what to expect from therapists.

But there are times when speech therapists are unavailable. And the work-and-time schedules of speech therapists may be filled with children having other problems and of later age levels. For instance, even if Jimmy's school had had a speech therapist, her work requirements might have been an honest excuse for not attempting to treat Jimmy's difficult and advanced stage of stuttering, a case in which speech therapy should have been started three or four years before he entered school. State laws which regulate school therapists may not allow them enough time for parent counseling and individualized work on problems like Jimmy's. Speech therapy provided in speech clinics and in child guidance centers may be better situated to give this help. Speech therapists, teachers, and parents should know of these agencies and how to refer speech problems to them.

As a classroom teacher, you have been wondering how you would have handled Jimmy's stuttering problem. What would you have said to his mother when she gave you the excusal note? How would you have advised Jimmy at times of spell-downs, class programs, and taking rollcall? How would you have personally felt and behaved in the rare situations when Jimmy had to talk with you and became almost speechless with long blocks? Would you have made any efforts to help him? How? If you had been the speech teacher in his junior year, what would you have said in the private conference with him? These are some of the thoughts to consider also in Helen's case.

HELEN

Helen's earliest symptoms of speech nonfluency resembled Jimmy's. Her mother, a remedial reading teacher, described Helen's speech problem and offered the following explanations:

> Since the age of three or three and a half years, Helen had been a rather rattled, careless, and excitable speaker; but I didn't regard it as a problem until she started kindergarten. She was precocious in her speech and language development, perhaps because she was an only child and was around adults so much. As I look back on it, I'm afraid I may have been too critical of her grammar and pronunciation. But at that time Helen was under day-care in a neighbor's home while I taught school, and I thought that she deserved all the extra attention and help I could give her in the limited time I could be with her. Besides, speech standards were not very good in that neighbor's home, and I was afraid that Helen would pick up some careless speech habits.

Nevertheless, Helen's tendency to stutter was not very noticeable during her pre-school years. She didn't seem to be bothered by it. She talked readily. Her non-fluency consisted of occasional repetitions of syllables and words. However, we didn't do anything to bring the problem to her attention, and I do not recall that anyone else made an issue of it during her preschool years. But, as I said, when she started kindergarten I felt that her speech deserved attention, partly because I was afraid the kids might notice her repetitions and tease her, and partly because, as a teacher, I know how important good speech was for reading and other school achievements. During this year and a half, her speech didn't seem to be getting any smoother.

Shortly after Helen started kindergarten, her mother arranged a con-ference with the teacher to discuss Helen's readiness for school, including her "careless" speech habits. Her teacher agreed that Helen did appear to have a hurried and jerky manner of speaking, with more than the usual amount of speech nonfluencies, namely, repetitions of initial sounds, words, and phrases, the use of "um" and "ah," and a few prolongations of the initial sounds of words. Helen's mother was assured, however, that other kindergarten children spoke with variable degrees of similar nonfluencies and that Helen's speech was noticeably more fluent in some speech situations than in others. The teacher reported the fortunate facts that Helen was willing to talk in school, that she was being given sufficient favorable opportunities to do so, and that classmates had not yet shown any specific reactions toward her nonfluency.

After this initial parent-teacher conference, the kindergarten teacher referred the problem to the speech therapist, who arranged a conference with Helen's teacher to set up a two-week program in which the therapist observed Helen in various speech situations at school, gathered further information from parents and teacher, and arranged a joint conference with Helen's parents and teacher. At this conference, the therapist presented her diagnosis with specific recommendations for helping the child through a cooperative program and assumed primary responsibility and leadership in coordinating team efforts with Helen's parents and teacher.

At the end of Helen's kindergarten year, her mother summarized progress:

Helen is much less hurried, impatient, and indecisive in her speech around home and is more confident, individualistic, and independent in all areas of behavior, not only in speech. She enjoys talking, and we try to give her plenty of chances to feel satisfactions from conversation. We've curbed our former tendencies to interrupt her and to correct her faults in pronunciation and grammar. We have become appreciative and respectful listeners in our home. We have tried to strengthen her ego and self-respect outside the realm of speech too, by supplying her with the means and encouragement to develop personal interests and activities that lead to successful achievements. School life has become a new life for Helen, a satisfying life that more truly belongs to her, a life in which speech is satisfying and useful. In fact, she told me the other day that she wants to be a teacher when she gets big.

At any rate, Helen rarely repeats or falters in her speech anymore. We are no longer concerned over the question of her stuttering. Thank goodness that our school had a teacher and a speech therapist who could help us correct this problem before it really became serious!

Helen's teacher gives another version of progress:

When Helen started kindergarten I soon observed that she was a rather nervous, high-strung child who sought attention and affection. In informal conversation she was about as talkative as the average kindergartner, both in the classroom and on the playground; but in class she was somewhat shy to recite unless she was interested in a subject and felt confident of answers. Her tendency to stutter was characterized mostly by word and syllable repetitions, especially when she felt insecure and hurried.

Within several weeks after Helen's parents and I had started our unified speech program, I began to see signs of improvement in Helen's speech. She became more confident and relaxed in all school activities. Her rhythm, rate, and tone of voice correspondingly improved. She expressed thoughts with better organization too. In recitation and in show-and-tell she no longer gives the impression that she feels threatened or hurried by something. At present I believe that we have Helen safely on the road toward normal speech fluency.

The speech therapist, who had worked mainly through the teacher and the parents, described Helen's progress at midyear in the following terms, reiterating essentially what Helen's mother and teacher had said:

Helen, who was in the primary stage of stuttering as she entered kindergarten, is definitely improving. The frequency and nature of her nonfluencies, repetitions, hesitations, and prolongations are reducing to a point safely within the range of normality. Helen is freely talkative and has not shown any self-concern or secondary reactions toward her nonfluency, nor have social penalties from her stuttering been reported. Thanks to the excellent cooperation by Helen's teacher and parents in fulfilling our goals and policies, it appears that this case of primary stuttering will be "outgrown" rather than become secondary. However, I intend to follow Helen for the rest of this year, next summer, and during her transition into the first grade, to insure that favorable influences and policies are maintained at home and in school.

We shall return to Jimmy and Helen from time to time to illustrate in a limited fashion how stuttering may originate and grow, and to relate various aspects of stuttering to them in discussing how stuttering handicaps the school child.

COMPARISONS

Helen and Jimmy might have been predisposed toward nonfluent speech because of a common, inherent, constitutional make-up. Perhaps future research will show that such children enter life with a similar pattern in their neuro-chemical make-up, a programing which conceivably could direct behavioral patterns, including those of speech fluency. But until such discoveries and curative "pills" for stuttering are found, we must diagnose and treat stuttering on the basis of our best substantiated present knowledge.

Both Jimmy and Helen had parents who were conscientiously concerned with their children's welfare. Perhaps Jimmy's parents were moved by stronger sympathy and conviction that nonfluency in early ages was a serious problem and that it required direct parental action. Perhaps Helen's mother had learned in her professional training that parents should be cautious in their well-meant efforts to correct such speech faults, especially ones dependent upon immaturities. At any rate, Helen remained in the "primary" stage of stuttering and "outgrew" her speech problem in her kindergarten year; but Jimmy soon advanced into a complicated "secondary" form of stuttering years before he started school. Consequently, we should expect differences in their school lives, in the extent of their handicaps, and in the policies and measures of helping them. Teachers were sympathetic and cooperative for both Jimmy and Helen, but the teachers' philosophies and methods varied for the two children. Jimmy's teachers not only lacked in their understanding of stuttering but were without the cooperative support and guidance of a speech therapist. Helen's success, contrasted with Jimmy's mounting failure and fixations as a stutterer, illustrates how important it is that teachers and speech therapists be informed and work together in matters that involve both general and special education. To meet this need, requirements for graduation and certification are being increased for both regular teachers and speech therapists. But our training must be correspondingly expanded and upgraded beyond restrictions of present professional boundaries.

How Stuttering Handicaps
the Schoolchild

Why should we be so concerned about stuttering when it represents only about 5 per cent of all speech disorders? Other speech problems may appear far more serious than the outward symptoms of many cases of stuttering seem to be. We differ in our judgments of how stuttering generally handicaps a person; and in evaluating the seriousness of a particular case of stuttering, we also vary in our concerns and judgments of its handicapping effects. Why is this? In the case of Jimmy, a severe stutterer throughout his school life, perhaps the majority of teachers lacked concern over his many school problems related to stuttering because, despite his silent role in the classroom, he satisfied them academically through his written evidence of learning, together with his harmonious deportment in the classroom. If he had openly and aggressively rebelled in the face of his frustrations and hatred of school, caused by his stuttering, his teachers might or might not have regarded such behavior as symptoms of stuttering and considered it a more serious handicap. We tend to judge the seriousness of children's behavior problems in terms of values dictated by the framework of our professional work and philosophy. If teachers consider behavior problems to be more critical when they disrupt the law and the social order of the classroom, hall, or playground, then they may appreciate without question a shy, withdrawn, meek, but cooperative stutterer like Jimmy, who presents no problems for a teacher with a large group of active, talkative children to manage on a tight schedule—plus hallways, lunchroom, and playground to keep in prescribed order.

If the handicap of stuttering is judged on the basis of its effects upon the stutterer rather than upon the way it affects others, then we might find that the silently suffering, unobtrusive stutterer is more of a problem than the one who openly exhibits his stuttering, gets into fights over it, and induces sympathy, embarrassment, and other unsettling emotions in his teachers and others. Recognizing that a teacher has responsibility for the group as well as for an individual within the group, we must neither overlook nor exaggerate the position and the welfare of the handicapped individual. This does not mean, however, that an individual may not be helped by a teacher who also pays attention to the group and utilizes its cause-and-effect dynamics upon the individual. In addition, the other members of the group are likely to gain when the individual receives therapy in a group setting.

Stuttering often handicaps the schoolchild in many subtle ways. Because of his fear and reluctance to stutter, a child may not even attempt to join school activities which strongly interest him. The threat and difficulty in speaking may cause a dislike and avoidance of speaking and school subjects requiring speech. Lowered achievements and grades, and a sense of frustration and failure, often result. He may withdraw from extracurricular activities, drop out of school, or select a course of study primarily aimed at speech avoidance and leading into vocations where his basic interests and potentials cannot be fulfilled.

Stutterers may be misjudged and penalized if they follow unwise compensatory paths and openly rebel in the face of their speech threats and failures. If a stutterer cannot find recognition through the important role of speech, he may resort to tactics that overshadow his stuttering and identify him as being lazy, unfriendly, belligerent, domineering, uncooperative, uninterested, etc. The stutterer may pay a double price for these undesirable social traits that stem from his stuttering. Besides suffering from various forms of social penalty, he often finds that his stuttering gets worse under adverse social climates which he and others may create if people do not understand the true cause of his negative social behavior.

Besides handicapping a stutterer's outward social life and achievements, stuttering may also affect his personality and inner life. Stuttering often leads to personal maladjustment, with gnawing states of anxiety, frustration, shame, embarrassment, hopelessness, fear, loss of self-respect, and so on. The worries and strains associated with stuttering may lead to ulcers and other physical ills that further handicap the person. This unhappiness and inner turmoil is difficult to detect and to measure and is often misinterpreted and attributed to other causes. The stutterer may also falsely blame stuttering for some of his failures, frustrations, and unhappiness. But whether the blame for this inner conflict is based upon fact or fancy, its destructive effects upon the person may be just as severe and difficult to treat.

Although Jimmy received excellent grades throughout his school career because of his extra compensatory efforts through written work, his lack of oral participation probably led to other deficiencies in his education. Excused from all recitation and oral reading, Jimmy was limited to being a silent absorber, a lonely thinker, a pupil who was a classroom spectator with no intention to volunteer and with only a rare and dreaded expectation of being called upon to talk. As a recluse, with no responsibility or likelihood of having to speak, Jimmy had difficulty in maintaining interest in classroom recitations. Daydreaming became a much more satisfying pastime than being a mere spectator in the tabooed activities of oral reading, recitation, reports by pupils, and class discussion. Besides, to identify with his speaking and reading classmates was an unpleasant reminder that he could not speak or read orally, that he should not speak, that he was not really a member of the group. As Jimmy's third-grade teacher reported to his mother at a parent-teacher conference: "I used to think that Jimmy was a poor listener, not at all interested in school subjects, and was not learning things that we covered in class. He had that faraway look. But his written work proves that he's getting it, all right."

Nevertheless, it is likely that Jimmy did miss certain personal, social, and academic values by being psychologically apart from classroom discussion and recitation. With limited speech practice and under lessened identification with others who spoke normally, it was apparent that Jimmy had difficulty in developing good patterns of organization and flow of language, even in written English. Language patterns which tend to become automatic with practice in speaking and listening to normal speech remained longer on the level of voluntary deliberation for Jimmy. In his later years, when speech therapy had given him relative freedom from stuttering, his difficulty in language fluency, oral and written, still suggested that his earlier years of limited talking and poor listening to normal speech and language in conversation and in recitation might have retarded him in the basic skills of language formulation and expression. Handicaps from stuttering may spread in cancerous ways.

Jimmy's social development was also handicapped by his widespread avoidance of speech situations, ranging from everyday conversation to invitational parties and their feared speech games. The establishment of new friendships was a risk and ordeal for Jimmy, usually precipitating an increase in stuttering, along with the necessity for new adjustments on the part of himself and his associates. Consequently, he limited his friendships to a few who accepted him, stuttering and all, without question, ridicule, humor, pity, rejection, or efforts to help. Just as he avoided most extracurricular activities at school, he refused to join scouting and other organizations, fearing not only the adjustments in making new friendships but the anticipated need to speak at initiation ceremonies and in fulfilling other speech requirements.

Incidents in Jimmy's religious training illustrate how the handicap of stuttering may permeate other areas of a child's life, having a cause-and-effect relationship with the fears and avoidances at school and elsewhere—and even threatening a child's faith in religion itself. He was excused from reading and recitation in Sunday school classes, never volunteered, and was never asked to speak. He willingly participated in singing and in the choral recital of prayers, since Jimmy, like most stutterers, could sing and speak in unison without stuttering. But trouble increased when he reached the age of fourteen and faced the requirement of "meeting the minister" for a year's memorization of answers to the church's catechism in preparation for his formal entry into the church on Confirmation Sunday.

Jimmy agreed to recite the memorized answers each week before the minister and the several other pupils in training, under the provision that he be excused from the final recitation on Confirmation Sunday before the congregation. However, the Sunday arrived with altered plans: confirmands were directed to face the minister, with their backs to the congregation, and Jimmy was called upon to recite in rotation with the other children. Struggling with his stuttering, as usual, he was dismayed at the minister's failure to keep his promise but grateful, at least, for the slight compassion in thus preventing his contorted face from being seen by the audience behind him.

The foregoing incident may seem to be a rare and extreme one in the lives of stutterers. It is not. There are many Jimmys, and even nonstutterers, who suffer unduly in speech situations contrived by adults without sufficient thought or preparation to make the situations profitable instead of destructive for the children. The old cliché "Honesty is the best policy" certainly holds true for the way we treat stutterers; otherwise, deceit and subterfuge may worsen stuttering and its handicaps.

Encouraged by a scholarship, Jim went to a university and enrolled in engineering, a field which not only suited his interests and academic background but also gave more assurance of success for a stutterer. He learned that the university had a speech clinic offering reputable help for stutterers, but he shunned the clinic during his freshman year. His faith in therapy had been shaken by the years of fruitless efforts to correct his stuttering, ranging from countless self-experimentations and ineffective counsel from parents and teachers to the impressive failure to get promised help at the age of twelve when he was sent to an expensive commercial school for stutterers, a school which unethically guaranteed to "cure" stuttering.

So, primarily because of his stuttering, Jim's freshman year was a routine of hard and lonely study of tough courses, with a continuation of his old policy of not speaking in classes and with little fun from the limited recreation of going to a weekly movie by himself. Under the anxiety and the strain of this unhealthful college life, he developed ulcers. But the handicap of his stuttering came to a focus during his third quarter of college when his chemistry professor told him that unless he sought clinical help and improved his speech, he could expect no chance of success as a future engineer. Jim believed him. Although the real intent of this counseling was probably to prompt Jim to seek clinical help rather than to discourage him from engineering, Jim accepted the latter alternative and lost hope in the future of engineering. After finishing the year, he quit engineering and the university.

In several ways Jim's stuttering handicapped his college life. In general, his maladjusted, speech-restricted life at the university was a continuation of the same policies and patterns of maladjustments which had been established and repeatedly reinforced throughout his earlier school years.

Counseling, unless sound, may add to a stutterer's handicap, just as an absence of necessary counseling may also perpetuate a handicap. As teachers and therapists, we must realize that counseling a stutterer or otherwise handicapped person on vocational matters, for example, places a serious responsibility and requirement upon the counselor. *Qualified* school counselors should be sought in these matters. Otherwise, unsound guidance will compound the handicaps from stuttering.

It may seem that Jim's life as a stutterer is an unusual one, extreme in the nature and extent of its handicaps. It is not. In the face of their handicaps and despair, stutterers have committed suicide. At times Jim considered suicide, even while he was undergoing speech therapy later at the university. Some stutterers turn to alcohol or drugs and become further handicapped by addiction. Many of them become school dropouts and take jobs that do not fulfill their interests and abilities.

We should be cautious, however, in judging the handicaps of a particular stutterer. In our sympathy and limited experience with stutterers we should be careful neither to assume handicaps when they do not exist nor to exaggerate the extent of a handicap. In evaluating handicaps, past, present, and future, we often can make only educated guesses. Many handicapped persons have fooled the "experts" in what they can or cannot do. Various factors need to be taken into account if we are to judge handicaps correctly. Often our counseling should be limited to providing the handicapped person with the opportunity and encouragement to prove for himself what he can or cannot do. In counseling we must be well informed, realistic, and democratic.

Helen, as a primary stutterer, had not developed a problematical frame of mind around her stuttering. Handicapping effects were either prevented or counteracted before they could establish themselves in her self-concept and speech patterns. She was given favorable conditions under which her fluency improved through learning, maturation, and practice. Consequently, Helen outgrew her stuttering and escaped the growth of handicaps such as Jim's. As we indicate elsewhere in this chapter, the credit for Helen's lack of handicap in stuttering and the blame for Jim's condition rest in important part upon their succession of teachers throughout school—from Sunday school to first grade to college.

Why Stutterers Should be
Helped by Teachers

In a broad sense, it is likely that stuttering is affected in various degrees, favorably or unfavorably by everything that affects speech and language generally, and particularly by everything that affects the stutterer personally and socially. Certainly many of these influences are indirect and limited in degree; many are highly potent, direct, and observable. Some influences create immediate effects upon stuttering; others, equally important, produce effects that are slow-acting, cumulative, and not immediately apparent in the person who stutters. If we take this broad view and consider the *person* who stutters, rather than only the *stuttering act*, we must admit that teachers are important in the lives of schoolchildren who stutter. This is true whether or not teachers have access to help from speech therapists, speech clinics, etc. There are times when the classroom teacher is left with the job of dealing with the school stutterer, even though the school has a speech therapist. For several reasons, a speech therapist may bypass or neglect a school stutterer. Crowded therapy schedules and excessive numbers of cases needing therapy may explain, justifiably or not, why some stutterers do not get deserved attention. Some therapists may be reluctant, insecure, or inadequately trained to work with stutterers, primary or secondary. As one therapist agreed:

> I'm ashamed to admit that in my professional training I failed to learn how to handle secondary-type stutterers of the younger age levels. My clinical training in stuttering has been largely with adult stutterers on a one-to-one basis. I find that it pretty well fits the high school stutterer when I can afford or arrange the time in my required schedule to work with him alone. But it is something else to adapt this therapy to a younger stutterer, especially when it must be done in a group of children having other problems. So, I admit that I tend to omit stutterers from my therapy schedule; but I do try to help them through parents and teachers as much as I can. Next summer I hope to attend a postgraduate seminar workshop on stuttering.

How Stutterers Can Be
Helped by Teachers

Speech corrective measures must be possible and suitable within the regular roles of classroom teachers, who are not expected to duplicate the work of therapists, though teachers have an advantage over therapists in their classroom setting. But if the teacher and the therapist are to work together effectively, there is a need for *both* to become acquainted with each other's work-setting and corrective measures, however separate they may appear to be. One speech therapist expressed the importance of keeping in touch with all the branches of therapy:

> I am working with a group of stutterers, two from different third grades, one from a fourth grade, with differences in their problems and in their therapy procedures. My information for this diagnosis and guidance in the therapy comes from several sources: from my examination and trial therapy, from observational visits to the classrooms, from information given by the classroom teachers, and from interviews with the parents. Furthermore, we really have three cooperative branches of therapy going on at once for each of these children, under my principal direction: my twice-a-week therapy sessions with the three boys; a program of helpful policies and practices conducted by each of their teachers; and a program of parental counseling, which I hope will provide help at home. But each of these three-way programs is a matter of teamwork, even though I am responsible for directing them. It's pretty much up to each teacher to figure out when, where, and how to carry out the things that will be therapeutic for her pupil. The more I learn about the teacher's role and the conditions under which she works, the more I can be of help to her in suggesting how she can integrate therapy smoothly into her program.

Recognizing and Judging Stutterers

How do we begin? The first step in any corrective program is to recognize problems that really are problems and to diagnose them correctly, through a knowledge of the differences between the ordinary nonfluencies of normal speakers and the abnormal ones of stutterers and a knowledge of the danger signs indicating that a child's nonfluencies are exceeding normal boundaries. Nonfluency may be evaluated more correctly if we recognize that it normally decreases as a child's maturation, learning, and adjustment increase; that various personal and social conditions cause fluctuations in the fluency curve; and that nonfluency may be correctly or incorrectly judged as stuttering, depending upon various qualitative and quantitative features. In the advanced stages of stuttering, the bases for judging it are usually more obvious; in the nonfluent speaker and in the primary stutterer the points of difference are less distinct.

Of the different kinds of repetitions in nonfluency, some kinds attract our attention as apparent stuttering. For instance, if a speaker has *single* repetitions on *each* of four words in a total of one hundred words, the repetitions may be overlooked or, if noticed, considered normal enough. But, if that speaker has *several* repetitions on *each* of those same four words, he may be judged a stutterer even though repetitions occurred on only 4 per cent of the total words in each sample of speech.

Speech repetitions and prolongations may go unnoticed or they may be more readily tolerated on some words or in some positions than in others. For example, would the repetitions be likely to sound more abnormal to you in the sentence "Well—well—well, why didn't you go?" than in the sentence "Well, why didn't you—you—you go?" Why? Or, what would be the more stuttering-like series of repetitions in the sentence "My—my—my name is Mi-Mi-Mike"? Why would there be a greater tendency to overlook the repetitions in the sentence "Well, what if—what if—what if I can't?" than the ones in "Well, what if I—if I—if I can't?" In the following sentence, why would the first series of repetitions seem more abnormal? "Ah—ah—ah, I—I—I don't know." Inquiring of the Pledge of Allegiance, a kindergarten child's question "What is in—in—indebisable?" is noticeable but ordinarily would not be regarded as stuttering. Would repetition arouse attention in the following report made by a sobbing child on the playground—"He—he—he—he hit me first"? Would a four-year-old appear to be a stutterer if he declared: "I—I—I—I—— Me wanta go too"? Perhaps not.

The preceding illustrations show how nonfluencies act variably to affect speech and communication. Some create discord by breaking up the units of articulation, the language structures, and the thought. Some nonfluencies spoil the sentence's over-all pattern of melody or its profile of accent and timing. Like mushrooms that show differently against different backgrounds, the signs of stuttering must be perceived against various total backgrounds of speech. For instance, the hesitations and the repetitions in the oral reading of a first-grader, speaking in an expressionless monotone and with regularity of rate and stress, may attract little attention. However, in that same child's conversation, conveying interesting and communicative units of thought, similar nonfluencies might stand out to interfere and to produce different effects upon listeners.

As in all perceptions, our prejudices and mental sets underlie, and often overlie, our recognition and judgments of stuttering. We tend to hear what we want to hear, what we expect to hear, or what we are afraid we might hear. Likewise, we often see what our mental sets prepare us to see. For example, a stuttering parent who apprehensively expects that his child will become a stutterer may wrongly see and hear and judge his child's symptoms to be stuttering, just as a teacher who admires and expects high standards of speech in her pupils may perceive those nonfluencies more readily and critically than a teacher who is not so mindful of them.

Johnson[2] has coined the term *diagnosogenic* to emphasize the belief that one of the causes of stuttering stems from faulty diagnosis, usually by parents, who, of course, are not ordinarily trained in speech pathology. Since this faulty diagnosis of stuttering may also lead to its aggravation, speech therapists and teachers—especially at the kindergarten and the first grade levels—are often faced with the need to correct faulty diagnosis and its resulting mistreatment. The therapeutic importance of our ability to help parents and others make a correct diagnosis of stuttering has been reported by Johnson and others. Trends of nonfluency in young children, wrongly classified by their parents as "stutterers," have been cleared up principally through timely counseling which convinced parents of their misdiagnosis. This counseling need is not surprising in view of the fact that misdiagnosis often leads to mistreatment.

In the cases of Jimmy and Helen we recall how their nonfluency patterns at age three were at first similar. Their so-called stuttering began with relatively simple, tension-free, carefree repetitions. In both cases their parents soon recognized their nonfluencies and judged them as symptoms of "stuttering" or "stammering." Perhaps Jimmy's and Helen's symptoms of nonfluency really were somewhat different, qualitatively or quantitatively, from those of most children. But the different ways these parents acted upon their divergent diagnostic thoughts may well have brought success in one case and failure in the other.

As teachers and therapists, we have an increasing need to learn how to discriminate between the normal and the not-so-normal patterns of nonfluency in children of preschool years—not only for informing and counseling parents of these children, but also for extending more and more of our education and therapy into programs for two-, three-, and four-year-olds. The Head Start movement and the extension of day nurseries and other preschool programs require that parents and teachers share responsibility for recognizing and handling many problems found in "preschool" years, including that of stuttering. The following excerpts from parental interviews suggest why teachers and speech therapists must be able to recognize danger signs in stuttering behavior and to deal with them.

Jimmy's mother spoke of her early recognition and judgments of his nonfluency in this way:

> We first noticed Jimmy's stuttering several weeks after his sister was born. He was three at the time. As I recollect, I took notice of his stuttering tendency when he repeated sounds and words as many as three times or more before going on to finish the word or sentence. At first the stuttering itself didn't seem to bother Jimmy, although it did occur mostly when he was excited, hurried, or trying to get something said when others were trying to talk too. But, I'm sorry to say, it soon began to bother me. If I had known then what I've learned since, I certainly would not have regarded it as a careless habit demanding attention on Jimmy's part, which would be an added burden for him at his tender age. Instead, I should have taken responsibility for his repetitions, as symptoms of home conditions which could be putting too much pressure upon the little fellow's speech. If I had understood Jimmy's early signs of stuttering as signs of tensions rather than only signs of poor ability in his speech, I wouldn't have made matters worse by telling him such things as: "Talk slower, Jimmy," "Think carefully before you start to talk, Jimmy," "Just take it easy and don't hurry, Jimmy," "You don't have to say a word over and over like that," "Say it once. That's enough," "Be careful, Jimmy, and then you won't stutter like that," "When you start to stutter,

just stop, relax, and start over," "If you have trouble on a word, Jimmy, just stop and think what you're going to say and then say it." But, after several months of trying to help him with these reminders, I realized there were new problems coming in his stuttering. He began to be touchy about stuttering. I see now that my efforts to help him must have irritated him. Unknowingly I actually spread his problem rather than helped it. But here again, I must admit that at the time I felt that Jimmy's problem was mainly a matter of retraining his tongue and breathing instead of building him up and improving his whole life. When I did understand this, after he had become an adult, his stuttering had already reached a serious and chronic state.

It is important to recognize danger signs which indicate that a speaker is developing negative feelings and reactions toward his nonfluency. The following descriptions are some of Jimmy's behavioral reactions whose impressions accumulated to make his mother definitely realize that he was passing from the primary stage into the more seriously complicated secondary stages of the disorder:

When Jimmy approached five years of age, we noticed certain changes that worried us because they showed that he also was getting disturbed about his stuttering. He began to do more than just repeat or prolong sounds or words. At times he'd frown or look away during stuttering. Before this, his repetitions were almost a connected part of his sentences, but now he began to pause before he came out with a repetition. Long drawn-out blocks appeared, and some of them turned into completely silent blocks with his lips clammed shut for a while before the word came out. He might repeat a sound or syllable several times, pause and then go through the repetitions again before he'd get out the word. After these changes had gone on for a while, we noticed that Jimmy began to get choosy about when to talk, what to say, how much to say, and even with whom to talk. He became shy in talking with strangers or visitors and finally began to cut out talking with everyone except his family members and closest friends. He'd often keep mum or let us do the talking for him, which I now realize we did far too often. At the time, we felt it was a kind thing to do.
I didn't notice that anyone ever teased Jimmy about his stuttering in those preschool years, but he began to act as if people had made fun of his speech. Perhaps his embarrassment and sensitivity came from our painful expressions of sympathy and our futile efforts to cure him. After the age of five he seemed to lose faith in our ability to help. When we saw that he resented our direct efforts, instead of appreciating them, we quit our direct measures and began the equally unwise policy of encouraging him to avoid stuttering. We even discouraged him from speaking at all in certain situations, such as getting him excused from reciting at school.

Tendencies to avoid speech are critical danger signs in the development of stuttering. The warning signs indicating unwholesome avoidance of stuttering and its feared consequences may be subtle, overlooked, and misinterpreted.

Some of these danger signs are expressed in the following observations made by Jimmy's various classroom teachers. His first-grade teacher stated:

> When Jimmy brought that note to me on the first day of school, asking me to excuse him from speaking in class, it didn't take me long to realize how terribly anxious he was to be excused. At first, I thought that his shyness was temporary. This was not the case. But he became more and more tense and on guard as he learned of the many school situations in which pupils were ordinarily expected to speak. I know that Jimmy's sober manner and silence could easily have been interpreted by some to be simply shyness and reluctance to talk, not necessarily based on stuttering. When one of the teachers who substituted for me, and whom I forgot to tell about Jimmy's excusal, called on him to recite in a word drill, he remained silent, eyes downcast, in an oppressed, fearful manner. She thought he either didn't know the answers or else was merely shy generally. Since he didn't do any speaking, she didn't have much reason to suspect stuttering. But later in the day, when she again called on Jimmy and he again refused, one of his classmates piped up with the information, "Jimmy isn't supposed to talk." The teacher wondered whether this was more than ordinary shyness.
>
> I made it a point to watch Jimmy on the playground and in the halls. In his informal exchanges, interjections, and bits of spontaneous speech during play, he was relatively fluent. But several times I observed him in the act of asking someone a question or replying to a direct question. Then he really had some long blocks. In one of these stuttering episodes on the playground, one of the older children made a grinning remark to him. It obviously hurt Jimmy's feelings. After that, he seemed to be more careful not to talk or even play around the older children. But for the most part, his classmates accepted both his stuttering and nontalkative nature.

Jimmy's second-grade teacher reported similar signs of his fearful avoidance of speech and stuttering, although she rather inadvertently called on him twice daily to respond with single words: "present" in roll call, and stating his grade from the daily class-corrected spelling test. When Jimmy finally responded in these two situations of limited speech, she regarded them as successes even though achieved in violation of the no-speech agreement. But the teacher failed to realize the price Jimmy paid for these partial answers, with a harmful strategy of avoidances and substitutions being contrived behind those two words. Consequently, by the end of the second grade, the words *present*, *here*, *hundred*, and similar words were more feared and difficult than ever. An analysis of these situations in detail will illustrate how a stutterer's fears and unwholesome mechanisms of stuttering may intensify and develop and yet be unrecognized by others who are not trained to detect these detrimental mechanisms.

Each morning Jimmy's second-grade teacher took oral roll, calling out his name along with the rest. After two weeks of failure to respond at all, he began to answer with *here*, the only child in the room to use that substitute for *present*. His teacher accepted this substitute without question, glad that he was at least beginning to talk. He continued to answer roll with *here* for about a month, then returned to his policy of not answering the roll at all. His teacher made no issue of this refusal.

In the second daily open invitation for Jimmy to speak, the teacher called on him, along with the others, to state his grade in the daily spelling test over a list of ten words that were corrected in class. Because Jimmy had already begun his school policy of trying to make up for his lack of recitation by doing good written work, he felt a strong necessity to get good grades and to be credited with them. Since spelling was easy for him, its attainable grade of "100" was one of the few sources of measurable satisfaction which Jimmy had found in the classroom. Therefore, being reluctant to sacrifice these good grades, Jimmy made an appraisal of his ability to say the words *one hundred, ninety, eighty*, etc. And wanting to earn and to be able to report as high a grade as possible, he focused first upon a way to escape the fear and difficulty that threatened him in saying *one hundred*. Since the saying of *one* began with a feared lip posture that seemed to trigger long, tight blocks, he decided to leave off the *one* and say only *hundred*. This solution seemed more possible at the time because he was saying *here* fairly successfully in rollcall, realizing that word began with an *h* also.

For a month he carefully worked on spelling, to be certain of getting and reporting this particular grade. Then, when greater fear developed around saying *here* in rollcall, Jimmy also lost confidence in his ability to say *hundred*, which he knew began with that new bugaboo "h" sound. So he switched to the serious job of being able to learn and say *ninety*, a word which fortunately had not yet accumulated too much anticipation and fear of stuttering. Then, believing that by dropping the feared *hu* of *hundred* and saying only "ndred," he felt that it should be as easy to say as the grade *ninety*, since both began with the less feared "n" sound. For the rest of that year, he regularly managed to get and report *ndreds*, despite the situation's continual tension and its jeopardy to his no-speech policy in school.

As Jimmy continued through elementary grades and high school, his teachers and associates generally did not realize that his stuttering and maladjustments were becoming increasingly fixed and serious. Teachers generally looked upon Jimmy as a "good pupil," "cooperative," "interested," a "high achiever," etc. None realized that Jimmy hated school intensely because of the irreconcilable dilemmas it forced upon him as a maladjusted stutterer: either to speak and to suffer the dreaded penalties of his stuttering, or to avoid speech and deny himself the many daily benefits which only speech could provide. Nobody knew that his humiliation from stuttering kept him at home on days when substitutes were to teach or when all but him had speaking parts in school programs. His third- and fourth-grade teachers, who included Jimmy in the weekly team-chosen spelling games, and had him write the words on the blackboard rather than spell them orally, may not have realized that he purposely misspelled the first word each time, in order that he might be seated and escape the continued shame of being the only one who could not speak. But by so doing, he ruined his reputation as a spelling contestant and suffered the added shame of being the last one chosen on the teams.

Perhaps teachers who reported that Jimmy was "exceptionally attentive and seriously interested in classwork" did not understand that much of this close attention was prompted by his special need to be vigilant, since he could not rely on asking for any restatement or clarification of what teachers said the first time. With purchase orders written by his mother in conventional shopping lists, Jimmy developed ways of submitting notes to store clerks so that stuttering would not be suspected. But he did this shameful avoidance at the price of self-respect, undermining his faith in being able to speak for himself.

It is also doubtful that most of his teachers knew that stuttering kept Jimmy from school parties and even from associating freely with children other than proven friends from his grade. He avoided everyone until he could be more sure of the person's reactions to his stuttering—if he must disclose it.

In contrast, the primary-type stutterer Helen had not yet developed self-concern and avoidances around stuttering at kindergarten age. She was willing to participate in speech situations; her nonfluency symptoms were relatively simple and free of the facial grimaces, tension, struggles, and other odd behavioral reactions that characterized Jimmy's secondary stages. Although Helen's nonfluencies were unsuppressed and out in the open, her kindergarten teacher suggests why her stuttering did not attract significant notice or reactions from classmates and others:

> As I look back on Helen's speech during that kindergarten year, I find it rather hard to think of her as a real stutterer. I don't think that her schoolmates gave her speech much thought either. Why? Well, in the first place it's natural to expect more of such nonfluencies in children of kindergarten age. Young children may notice unusual differences and may be quick and frank in their curiosity and questions concerning the differences, but they are more adaptable and willing to go along with their teacher's expressed judgments—to feel and act the way she does toward differences. But I think there's another reason why Helen's stuttering tendencies were generally accepted without further thought by me or by the children. Her moments of stuttering really didn't have much of a spoiling effect upon her behavior, speech or otherwise. She didn't appear to avoid any situations because of it; her repetitions didn't seem to dampen her spirit or cramp her style in anything she did. The repetitions just popped out in a spontaneous and unpredictable manner, interrupted her communication for a moment or two, and that's all. Her stuttering really didn't chop up the flow of her speech much. If one didn't notice that her repetitions were of the same sound, syllable, or word, he might easily have overlooked them because of the way they blended into the tempo of the rest of her sentence. Of course, when Helen strung out too many repetitions in a series, then I, for one, found that I began to notice her nonfluency more.

The foregoing patterns and judgments reported in Jimmy's and Helen's stuttering are only suggestive of what teachers must learn to recognize and to interpret in the unique expression of other stutterers.

Referral

In the prevention and the treatment of stuttering, we cannot over-emphasize the importance of timely and judicious use of referral. Unless the early symptoms are identified and given early referral for accurate diagnosis and appropriate treatment, stuttering may advance into complicated and incurable stages. We cannot afford to allow parents, teachers, or anyone else responsible for a stuttering child to feel guilty or unwilling to refer their suspicions about the case. Authoritative referral will determine whether or not suspicions and concerns are groundless. Parental suspicions and worries over stuttering are justifiable reasons in themselves for making referral. But if we understand the types and degrees of nonfluency and can truly recognize the danger signs of stuttering in young children, then our referrals will more likely bring timely help for success.

A kindergarten teacher reported to her school's speech therapist:

> Since Ralph started school five months ago, I have noticed that he stuttered some, but I hesitated to report it as a problem, either to you or to his parents. I wasn't sure it was a problem serious enough to refer for speech therapy—crowded as your program already is. I knew that stuttering can become worse if one makes more of an issue of it than it deserves. In fact, I held off in the first conference with Ralph's mother, hoping that she would bring it up, but she didn't. In later conferences I avoided the subject because I thought that if Ralph should be having these stuttering tendencies only at school, I might spread the problem homeward if I made his folks alarmed over what was only a school problem. Recently, though, when my substitute teacher asked me about Ralph's stuttering, I thought I'd better ask you to look into this problem.

Later, Ralph's teacher made these comments to a fellow teacher:

> I'm glad I referred Ralph to our speech therapist. She was glad that I brought her in on it too, although she admitted that she could appreciate why I was slow in referring his problem to anyone. She found out that his parents knew that he stuttered, all right but were reluctant to mention it to me for the same reason that I hesitated to mention it to them. Anyway, the therapist has opened our lines of communication, and we're getting organized on some policies that should help Ralph at school as well as at home. I'm telling you this because you'll be having Ralph in your room next year.

The following explanation given by parents to a kindergarten teacher reveals a rather common reason for failure to refer stutterers for therapeutic help:

Jeff began to stutter at about three. We didn't think much about it until he was about three and a half. When we saw it wasn't getting any better, we got worried and made an appointment with our family doctor. He told us not to worry, that "all children go through this stage" and that it would very likely clear up by the time he started school. Well, we took him at his word and tried to forget it, but we couldn't. We had more doubts when we saw that Jeff was getting worse, not better. Understand, we have a good family doctor and have faith in him, but one can't expect doctors to know everything, I guess. Dr. Spock's book doesn't have much in it about stuttering either. Now that Jeff is starting school, though, and still stuttering, we're turning to you for help.

In the foregoing conference, Jeff's teacher informed his parents that she would promptly refer the matter to the school's speech therapist and that she and the therapist would confer and give them a report of their findings and recommendations. This was done as promised, after observational visits to the classroom, followed by interviews and a joint conference with Jeff's parents and teachers. In this conference the speech therapist gave basic information and outlined goals and guidelines designed to insure cooperative work upon his speech in three areas: at home, in the classroom, and in the twice-a-week speech therapy sessions which she had scheduled. Jeff's experience proves not only that help may be needed and given when a preschool stutterer starts school, but that authoritative professional help should be sought and received *whenever it is needed*—before the problem spreads and hardens.

The next experience reveals that another parent put off referring a stuttering problem to her school's speech therapist because she believed a neighborly bit of misinformation.

Barbara had stuttered for about a year before my husband and I decided to check with our school therapist to find out if therapy was needed. But first I mentioned this to my neighbor, who has a child in therapy in school, and was told that our school has a policy that no kids below first grade are allowed to get therapy— not even kindergartners who are already in school. So we gave up the idea. Later, we learned that our school's therapist is anxious to know about any pre- school stutterer whose parents are concerned or should be concerned. She can't schedule a preschooler for regular therapy sessions, as she does for the children in school, but she has conferences with the parents, examines the child's speech, and gives the parents helpful suggestions. That's what we had wanted and needed at that time. We have also learned that most universities have a speech and hearing clinic and that child guidance centers in our community can help with such problems. We have two such service centers but didn't know about them at the time we needed them the most.

The following case of a high school stutterer indicates why a teacher may not refer an older pupil for therapy:

Frank transferred into our school this year. Came from a small parochial school where they've never had any speech therapy. He really had a bad case of stuttering. He's very shy about it—most of the time, he won't even answer when I call on him to recite. Early in the year when the therapist sent around a referral form, asking us to write down names of pupils we thought needed help, I decided to leave Frank off the list. In the first place, I thought he had enough to adjust to, being so shy and coming in as a stranger from a little school like that. He wasn't a very good student either. Missing classwork on account of therapy wouldn't help his scholastics any. Besides, when I asked him if he wanted to have therapy, he shook his head and acted resentful.

Later in the year the speech therapist personally recognized Frank's problem when she gave routine speech screening tests to all transfer pupils. After conferring with him and his teacher, she scheduled him for therapy. The following comments by the therapist reflect some of the original problems in his referral:

> At first, Frank didn't want speech therapy. But he agreed to give it a try when I gave him a picture of what it would be like. Now he comes willingly and is making progress. I think he feared it because it was something new and unknown. It eased him to learn that his teachers are all for it and are cooperative in helping him make up any classwork he misses.

Parents have many other reasons for not seeking professional help for problems of stuttering. Some parents do not know that help exists in many of our publicly supported agencies, such as schools, universities, speech and hearing centers, child guidance centers, and special education programs. Other parents hesitate to seek speech help from agencies because of their mistaken ideas about cost, not knowing that these public agencies give services that are usually free or inexpensive. Occasionally, parents may be reluctant to take children to child guidance centers because they feel that these places are only for parents who have shamefully failed as parents, whose children have been neglected and who are delinquent. Other parents hesitate to arrange for outside therapeutic services because of practical everyday reasons: transportation may be difficult; baby-sitting for other children in the family may be a need and a problem; and on top of everything else, parents may not know how to go about making a referral when they should.

What can we, as teachers and speech therapists, do in this tangle of issues surrounding referral? We should know *whether, when, where,* and *how* parents should refer, to seek outside professional information and counseling concerning stuttering. We should realize that parental anxiety can breed stuttering and is, therefore, a justifiable criterion for referral. Application for professional help is indicated also if we, as teachers or therapists, are concerned over danger signs which we see in a child's speech, whether or not his parents are likewise concerned. However, this means that we must truly know these danger signs; otherwise, his parents may become unduly concerned. Knowing where to send a child for the extra professional help requires that we keep informed on community resources and their referral procedures, requirements, and costs, if any.

The following outline condenses some of the behavioral signs and information that may help a teacher decide *whether* or *when* to refer a child for stuttering diagnosis and treatment. It also summarizes *where* and *how* a teacher should make a referral. The summary does not attempt to rate the seriousness of items. While some items may be indicative of problems other than stuttering, we may expect that a child's need and urgency for referral will depend upon the number and the spread of the danger signs, as well as upon their depth or their strength.

The Question of Referral

WHETHER OR WHEN TO REFER

Danger Signals in the Child

Unusual frequency and nature of his speech repetitions
Unusual number of speech prolongations or hesitations
"The kids tease me 'cause I don't talk right."
His nonfluencies make him shy, impatient, irritated, or unwilling to talk.
"Teacher says I'm not a stutterer, but Mom says I am."
"I'm *not* stuttering! I was just pretending!"
He is trying to do something about his moments of speech nonfluency—either before, during, or after their occurrence.
His nonfluencies show signs of interfering with the over-all rate and melody of his speech.
"You—you—you say it. I can't."
His nonfluencies cause him to make special efforts in speaking.
His stuttering-like moments seem to dampen his spirit and affect his interests, choices of friends, and activities.

Signs of Danger Recognized by the Child's Associates

"He's beginning to stutter."
"He talks funny."
"He's beginning to make hard work of stuttering."
"His stuttering seems to be getting worse, not better."
"He doesn't stutter so much, but he doesn't talk so much either."
"His stuttering is just carelessness. I tell him to slow up and think."
"When he stutters, I tell him to stop and say it over."
"When he stutters, I scold him and have even tried swatting him over the mouth, whipping him, and have threatened to put soap in his mouth if he stutters. He's stubborn."
"He's beginning to resent our efforts to correct his stutter."
"Several of our friends think our child stutters."

"He stutters now and then but not all the time."

"Our doctor says he'll outgrow his stuttering in time, without any help."

"His stuttering is beginning to change his personality and interests."

WHERE TO REFER

Local Level. Speech therapy services for stuttering, as well as for other speech and language problems, are usually available within a local public school system through local administrators, superintendents, special education directors, or the speech therapist. If this assistance at the local level is not available, the inquiries and requests by parents and teachers may provide the impetus required to obtain it.

County Level. If the local school lacks speech therapy services, the superintendent or director of special education of the county may have information on special education programs which are administered and tax-supported at the county level to provide speech therapy that local schools do not offer.

Universities and Colleges. Most state-supported universities and colleges offer diagnosis and therapy for speech and language problems. Information will be available from the Director of the Speech Clinic at the University.

State Level. If you wish further information on services and agencies relative to speech and language problems, contact your state's department of special education.

National Level. Anyone wishing reliable information provided on a national scope may write to the national headquarters of The American Speech and Hearing Association, 9030 Old Georgetown Road, Washington, D.C.

HOW TO REFER

Speech therapists have the responsibility of acquainting teachers and parents with the referral procedures for obtaining speech therapy at local levels. To chart the individual needs of a pupil with a speech problem will demand the conscientious consideration of all available and qualified professional aid and a clear analysis of the parents' interest and financial ability to cooperate in their child's project.

The Need for Careful
Diagnosis

We should enlist the aid of the most qualified professionals to help in this first step of correcting a stuttering problem. This requires that teachers and parents should look to their school's speech therapist for help in making every initial diagnosis—the basis for determining the course of therapy. Perhaps in some difficult cases the speech therapist in turn will also seek further diagnostic help.

It is not enough for a diagnostician to make a careful and correct assessment of a child's speech problem and then to come forth simply with a term to categorize the problem: "stuttering," "not stuttering," "cluttering," "normal nonfluency," "primary stuttering," "transitional stuttering," "secondary stuttering," "mild stuttering," "severe stuttering," etc. Careful and thorough diagnosis may be wasted, and may even lead to harm, unless we define our use of labels and terms, unless we show how the child in question fits the framework of our definition, and unless we help to make diagnosis relevant to therapy.

We must also keep in mind that diagnosis is not an end in itself. The results of tests, observations, interviews, and our concluding summary should aim to answer the questions "What?" and "So what?" If a teacher, for example, receives a diagnostic report, oral or written, and cannot understand it, she has an ethical duty to request a clarification of the report, not only for her own use but also for insuring that the diagnostic report will be understood by the client, his parents, and others who are cooperating on the problem. In this age of specialization and departmentalism when clients are sent around to clinics and divided services where diagnosis is done jointly, on a collective team basis, there are times when final reports leave the teacher, her client's parents, and others in ignorance because of inexcusably vague and uncoordinated piecemeal reports that sometimes collect from the professional merry-go-round.

If this problem occurs, the speech therapist may help to coordinate the several reports—ones that may be received from referrals to psychologists, social workers, physicians, psychiatrists, neurologists, audiologists, and other speech therapists or speech pathologists. Even if each of several joint reports is sincerely meant to be clearly understood for what it alone is worth, a broadly informed professional may be needed to interpret, analyze, and coordinate the various subreports and finally to convey the most substantiated answers to the questions "What?" and "So what?" Diagnostic reports would improve all along the professional line, however, if we for whom diagnoses and recommendations are intended would openly demand that all professionals working for us would aim to make their information and communiques more understandable and translatable into corrective action.

"Primary" vs. "Secondary" Stages of Stuttering

In discussion of the origin and the growth of stuttering, we considered the terms *primary, transitional,* and *secondary* stages and how the characteristics and treatment of each stage differ. Both Jimmy and Helen began as primary stutterers, but when they started school Jimmy had advanced into secondary stages while Helen remained in primary. She "outgrew" her primary stage and attained normal speech; Jimmy continued to be a secondary stutterer. Why did Helen remain in the relatively unaffected and carefree primary stage while Jimmy advanced to levels where his speech became increasingly marked by self-concern, anxiety, fears, avoidance, shame, guilts, tensions, compensatory mechanisms, and other handicapping effects? The causes, nature, and remedies of stuttering are still largely theoretical, in spite of thousands of research studies.

We do know, however, that stuttering is a developmental disorder and that its course may be checked, improved, or made worse. In stressing the need for careful diagnosis, we emphasized that a stutterer in the primary stage requires treatment different from that given at secondary stages. Consequently, in the following section on goals and guidelines for teachers, we continue to discuss Jimmy and Helen.

Goals and Guidelines for
the Teacher

Objectives for helping a stutterer must be determined by the particular problems that pertain to that stutterer, and the process of solving his problems follows the steps generally found in any problem-solving situation. Successful experience has proved that a problem is often half solved once it has been duly sensed, carefully evaluated, and clearly stated in a solvable form.

The following speech therapist's report of a kindergartner's speech problem and excerpts from her conferences with a teacher reveal how an actual problem was sensed, formulated, researched, "brainstormed," and finally solved:

> Carl, given a speech test soon after entering kindergarten, was found to be a primary stutterer and to have misarticulation on several sounds. Partly because of limited time, I scheduled him in a therapy group with three other classmates who had similar articulatory errors. I arranged it this way to keep a careful watch over his nonfluency and to give him a socially controlled opportunity to improve his articulation. For six weeks all went well: Carl spoke readily, was interested in therapy, showed no awareness or concern over his infrequent non-fluencies, and progressed in his articulatory skills. Then signs of problems appeared. He began to lose interest in certain activities during therapy, and he even refused to reply to some of my direct requests to say words and sentences. Along with these behavioral changes, his nonfluency increased, together with beginning signs of anxiety over his nonfluencies. I promptly arranged a conference with his teacher, who reported similar speech resistance in the classroom. She and I exchanged information and views and sought the core of his problem—where to focus our efforts.

The following quotations from Carl's therapist and teacher illustrate the trends of their thoughts while gathering facts, analyzing his problem, and formulating it for solution.

> THERAPIST: In therapy sessions I've recently noticed that Carl's stuttering is on the increase. I consider this to be more immediately important than his misarticulation. But that's a pretty broad order to tackle until we gather more information on him and compare our findings, pool our ideas, and thereby figure out more specifically where and how our cooperative efforts should be directed.

TEACHER: Yes, I am more concerned about his increased stuttering and tension than I am over his misarticulation. Perhaps, if we could find means of lessening his tension and making him feel at ease while speaking, he'd stutter less.

THERAPIST: That's the hard core of the problem. But have you any ideas on what is causing this stepped-up tension? Especially tensions that are directly associated with his speech and stuttering?

TEACHER: Well, when I take a closer look at these emotional signs of uneasiness and reluctance to talk, I think that they usually mount when Carl is in a situation that requires him to recite, not in informal conversation and in spontaneous speaking or in show-and-tell where he says what he wants to.

THERAPIST: I've noticed that this particular type of reluctance has occurred in therapy sessions too and have been trying to find out what may be precipitating it. I've wondered whether my work upon his articulation could be having negative effects upon him. I've wondered whether I made a mistake by starting work on his articulation in the face of his stuttering. However, Carl is willing to attend therapy sessions. He appears to like all of us in the group, is cooperative, attentive, and generally interested in therapy, except when he is asked to say certain things.

TEACHER: Well, it's obvious he's more tense when on the spot in recitation, without the confidence and leeway he has in ordinary conversation and in discussion of a subject based on his everyday interests and self-choice.

THERAPIST: Let's meet again next Friday, after we've made further observations, especially on this aspect of Carl's problem, to see if we can locate the key-log that may be jamming his peace of mind and fluency.

In the next conference, the teacher and the therapist continued their exchange of information and the clarification of the problem:

THERAPIST: What have you learned about Carl's reluctance to recite in the past week?

TEACHER: Well, he told me something that may be at the root of his resistance. This noon I had a good opportunity to have an informal, private, friendly chat with him about how he liked school, speech class, recess time, the children, you, me, and his classroom activities. He told me that he didn't like to have people ask him to say things because he's afraid he'll get spanked. He cried when he told me how his dad scolds him and spanks him when he can't say his a-b-c's "right." Anyway, if this situation is true, it could be a basic source of his increased tension and stuttering at school too.

THERAPIST: Yes, preposterous as this claim is, you may have found the source of Carl's reluctance. I've known other children who have been scolded, spanked, shamed, and have had their mouths soaped or slapped for making speech mistakes that they can't help. Ironically, these measures are more often meted out by strict and conscientious parents who mean to be helpful, not vengeful. If it is true that Carl's dad is punishing him for being nonfluent, this may be the key to his problem for us to try to solve.

Having decided upon this immediate and specific goal, the teacher and the therapist continued to exchange information and ideas directed toward its solution.

THERAPIST: When I began therapy with Carl, I invited his parents for a conference. His father did not come, but his mother was given the information and general counseling that I regularly give all parents of stutterers, primary or secondary. She gave no indications at that time that she or her husband punished Carl for faulty speaking or that they even made any direct attempts to correct him. She did state, however, that both of them were fearful that his defective speech would hold him back in school. Now I wish that I had spent more time investigating and counseling on this parental angle. Perhaps I mistakenly assumed that home conditions were better than they were. We'll see.

TEACHER: Well, I admit that I may have assumed too much too, in my preschool conference with his mother. She expressed this same concern to me. But she seemed to accept my assurance that speech faults are relatively common in kindergarten and that they ordinarily improve. But now to get on with our ideas for settling this open conflict between Carl and his father.

THERAPIST: Yes, if Carl's father needs counseling and if he's mostly concerned about the educational handicaps of his son's speech faults, then he may heed you more than he does me. In my conference with Carl's mother, I have already emphasized that you and I work cooperatively, that we share information unless it is given in confidence, and that many speech problems must be mutually solved by us.

TEACHER: It should be evident to Carl's father that you work with me in his son's whole school program. Besides, if you conducted the conference, I can see that you'd have some good chances to give your specific professional information and pointers on how the father should handle this and other matters related to Carl's stuttering and misarticulation. You may never have a better chance to do this. Another possibility would be for both of us to meet with Carl's father. But that may not be necessary. Might turn the tables on the poor guy and make him too tense and defensive if he's confronted by too many females. But would you include the mother in the conference? How about sending the parents a letter, stating the problem and giving them hints on what to do and what not to do? Would it be better to have a conference at school or to go to their home? What if the father won't or can't come to school for a conference? And how are you going to open the subject of the father's reported punishment of Carl's speech? I presume you'll have to treat confidentially what Carl told me and protect him from repercussions from squealing on his dad. But listen to me—telling a therapist what to do!

THERAPIST: Well, I know that if I were not here to assume the responsibility, you'd do it and devise strategy to solve the problem too. And for that extra work, you teachers certainly deserve extra professional allowances and credit. Your questions are good ones. Yes, I think my chances would be better if both parents came for the conference. You can see why. As for sending them a letter to try to explain everything, instead of having a face-to-face confab, I think I'd have a much more difficult time in communicating my thoughts in writing and in gauging their understanding and acceptance of points. Our ready-made pamphlets and books are not concise and specific enough to pinpoint and handle this problem; its point could get lost in all the rest of the *Do*'s and *Don't*'s to be read. I've found that pamphlets and mimeographed sheets too often are either laid aside or are not carefully read and digested by those who need the information the most—assuming, of course, that the information is written in a form that they can understand in the first place.

I think I'll try to hold the conference at school, where the professional setting can support me and help the parents maintain objectivity and a better intellectual-emotional balance than they might have if I were being received as a guest in their home. But if the father cannot get off work to come to school, I'll request a conference at their home, at a time when Carl won't be present to overhear the discussion. And, of course, as you say, I'll be careful not to put Carl on the spot by letting his parents know that he specifically told of getting spanked for stuttering. And it's important, as you know, to keep the parents from becoming defensive and shamefully guilty when their mistakes are pointed out. Otherwise, they cannot respond rationally to counseling. I know that parents find it much easier to accept our criticism and guidelines if we can make it clear to them that their child's welfare is the most important thing at stake and that we, as well as they, are primarily interested in his welfare—even at the minor expense of admitting our ignorance and unintentional mistakes.

The foregoing problem was solved when the therapist met both parents at school. She opened the conference by giving them a report of Carl's progress in articulation therapy and followed with a clear picture of the special problem and the reasons that it necessitated the conference. She suggested some of the ways such problems have been known to develop in other children. She pointed out how this problem could have damaging effects upon stuttering and educational achievements unless it were solved. Without being told, Carl's father perceived his error in the issue and voluntarily admitted that he had been following a "too harsh and impatient" policy with his boy for not saying his a-b-c's rightly, believing that the child was "just being careless and stubborn." The parents were appreciatively wiser, and their son's home tensions over stuttering were gradually relieved.

As in the teaching of reading and other complex processes requiring a network of learnings and skills, we find that the goals and the solving of stuttering problems become a continuous process, requiring our constant appraisals and adjustments along the child's developmental route. Certain general needs and policies apply to most stutterers; but, as emphasized throughout this chapter, each stutterer has certain differences which need to be met individually, even in the case of a primary stutterer whose problems have not yet significantly diverged.

We must be careful not to harm a stutterer by assuming that he has problems which he does not have and by applying procedures that do not fit him. There is danger in our memorizing definite sequences of rules for stuttering therapy. Students of speech correction are sometimes taught that stuttering and its treatment may be reduced to nicely established sets of "rules," "keys," or "ladders" of certain fixed steps to be taken in a definite sequential order. Formulae, diagrams, and various analogies have been devised by authors and lecturers in attempts to impress students and to aid their memories—only to find later that these devices have been learned and applied too literally and blindly. The problems of every stutterer will not be unlocked by the same set of "keys." Not every stutterer needs to start at the bottom rung of our therapeutic ladders or to proceed up each and every rung. Therefore, we shall not use numbers or letters in listing therapeutic goals and procedures, in order that unintended sequences will not be implied.

To illustrate how a speech therapist or teacher may go astray in therapy and may even harm a stutterer if procedures and sequences are indiscriminately fixed, suppose that a therapist has inferred from a formula or from a set of cardinal "rules" that every secondary stutterer may be expected to have certain component feelings of guilt, anxiety, hostility, shame, nonacceptance, and avoidance toward his stuttering. Furthermore, suppose that this therapist, who believes that every secondary stutterer will have this definite mixture of speech maladjustments, has also mistakenly assumed that every secondary stutterer must adhere to the following therapy sequence: *first*, to get the stutterer to admit openly and to tell others that he is a stutterer; *second*, to keep the stutterer from hiding or avoiding his stuttering—a rule that may be too narrowly translated into a commandment to maintain constant eye-contact with his audiences; *third*, to teach him to imitate his way of stuttering; *fourth*, to teach him to stutter in a new and "better" way, to be dictated by the therapist; *fifth*, . . . etc.

A therapist equipped with the above goals and philosophy may go astray in various ways. In one instance, a misguided therapist held the rigid conviction that the first necessary step which had to be fulfilled was to convince and to force her high school stutterer to admit to her verbally: "I stutter." The ensuing battle, waged over the therapist's determined attempts to force this verbal admission from her equally stubborn client, ended their cooperation and harmed the student's morale. In another instance, a therapist worked with a stutterer so long and so exclusively on step two, the rigid control of eye-contact in a stutterer whose eye-contact was already adequate, that the child wanted to quit therapy because of his dislike for this undue and obnoxious control over him.

Our goals and procedures for stutterers may be classified in other ways, too. Some goals are general; others are specific. Some are long-range or ultimate; others are immediate, temporary, or operational. It is important to keep in mind that the effectiveness of what we do for a child is often determined by our recognition that some goals have priority over others and that some goals need to be met before others may be fulfilled. For example, suppose a teacher has the aim of making a third-grader more willing to stutter in class. This goal could become a long-range one, to be temporarily replaced by one which is more urgent to reach if it is found that the child is unwilling even to *speak* in class, stuttering or not. Furthermore, if it is found that his reluctance to speak stems from class pressures in oral reading, a still more specific and immediate goal may be set for him: how to increase his willingness to read orally. Analysis of this last goal may reveal that the reading pressures come from his classmates' nagging practice of prompting each other for mistakes in reading. By solving this immediate problem in reading, the stutterer may gain willingness not only to read but also to speak, and even to stutter, in other situations.

In our consideration of goals that are generally recommended either for primary or secondary stutterers and of goals that are applicable to both types, we should not be misled by the reference to "direct" versus "indirect" goals. "Direct" goals and "direct" therapy often refer to work focused upon the act of stuttering itself. "Indirect" therapy applies to work upon background factors of environment, the stutterer's adequacy of language, his physical condition, his social or emotional life. But this distinction should not imply that "indirect" therapy is less important and requires less professional direction and know-how. What we may regard as an "indirect" cause may really be a "direct" one, as far as the cause and the solution of the problem are concerned.

For instance, if a young child is beginning to stutter because of his inadequate vocabulary and shaky language skills, we may tend to minimize these causes as being "indirect" and to exclude them from our realm of professional responsibility. "Indirect" causes and therapy may be more direct and important than we realize. This fact is an argument against any tendency of allied professions to isolate themselves from each other. Important goals in stuttering therapy may also be found within the roles of teachers, the remedial reading specialist, social workers, psychologists, physicians, counselors, and others. We professionals should also remember that we often need the cooperative efforts of parents and other laymen if problems of stuttering are to be solved.

General Goal: Earn and Maintain Good Interpersonal Relationships

The following recommendations generally apply to both primary and secondary stutterers. Most of them do not have a definite priority of importance or of procedure. For example, it is important not only to establish good rapport with a child in your early contacts with him but also to maintain it throughout therapy. If you do not realize this elemental fact, you may win rapport but later lose it.

Let the child realize that you are interested in him as an individual. Let him know from the first that you can accept him as he is, faults and all. Show him that you have faith and kindly interest in him and his welfare.

The speech of any stutterer is likely to improve under a teacher who can strengthen the pupil's self-respect, self-confidence, sense of self-worth, and faith in the support that he may desire and need from others. One highly effective first-grade teacher describes this relationship:

In general, I try to treat stutterers the same as I treat pupils who don't stutter. I try to be a calm, patient, and appreciative listener when they speak. I have learned to accept and to remain calm and unflustered during their moments of stuttering —not making them feel that their stuttering bothers me in any way. I want them to know that I can easily accept them as persons and as speakers without batting an eye or making them feel apologetic for stuttering. However, without making an issue of my efforts, I see to it that stutterers are encouraged to talk often and that they get genuine satisfaction from talking in all sorts of situations. But if stutterers are hesitant to talk, I don't force them. I try to figure out what makes them reluctant and to correct that factor or factors. But in general, I try to make shy stutterers feel that I have more confidence in them than they have in themselves. By having successes first on easier levels, stutterers generally gain this self-confidence.

Because our relationships with a stutterer's parents are important too, we must convince them that we, as teachers and therapists, are aligned with them and that their child is the main object of our mutual efforts to help. One of the most effective ways to win this respect and cooperation from parents is to let them observe us at work with their child in actual therapeutic situations. One perceptive mother of a secondary stutterer has reported:

> When I visited Kenneth in his classroom, I realized why he likes his teacher and school better this year than before. I can also understand why he no longer complains about stuttering at school. His teacher has ways of making him feel more calm, confident, and unhurried in talking. It's hard to explain in words, but I could sense these same traits in her friendly manner and calmness. The whole classroom atmosphere reflected it. She gave due consideration to each individual in that room, and yet she created a family feeling for the whole group. Teaching becomes an art when you teach like that. In fact, from that classroom visit, I think I learned a few important things that may explain why my boy's stuttering gets pretty rough sometimes at home. Now I can see that our family conversations too often get jammed with excessive hurry, all sorts of interruptions, and disrespect for what is said—especially by certain members of the family.

A teacher's professional relationship with the speech therapist often determines the course of therapy. This is true whether the pupil's stuttering is of primary or of secondary nature. A fifth-grade teacher put it this way:

> In my eleven years of teaching, I have known five speech therapists and have referred to them seven pupils who stuttered. I've relied upon the speech therapists to direct and coordinate our mutual work with these cases. As a result, these pupils made more gains than they would have if each of us had had to work separately with them. Cooperatively our work was much easier too. In the process, I know I gained knowledge and confidence in dealing with stuttering. Now, if I had a stutterer to manage in my classroom without help from a speech therapist, I feel that there are plenty of safe and helpful things I could do.

The next teacher describes how a speech therapist changed her attitudes toward stuttering:

> In the insecurity of my first year of teaching, I was confronted with a girl who stuttered very severely. I felt dreadfully sorry for her and wanted to help her but didn't know what to do. So I began to ignore her in recitation and reading —at least that was one way to spare both of us from dealing with the dilemma. But, of course, this evasive policy created new problems for her. When the speech therapist found out about the case, though, and came to our rescue, all this turmoil began to change. I learned to look upon stuttering in the same spirit I'd been taught to look upon problems in reading—as an intellectual challenge to be met with my understanding and skill, not with prejudice and mere sentiment.

To help any stutterer generally, a safe guideline will allow and encourage frequent selected opportunities for speaking *where* and *when* he can take satisfying advantage of his current level of fluency. If every stutterer were to be judged on the basis of his personally established standards, we should find that even for the most severe and maladjusted stutterer there are periods and speech situations in which *his* fluency level is relatively high, when he is comparatively more willing to talk and even to stutter, and where personal satisfactions and successes from speaking are relatively greater *for him.*

Each stutterer, according to his personal problem and needs, should have speech opportunities that are planned to allow more success than failure. For instance, it would have been better to arrange for Jimmy's oral participation in classroom discussions and recitations, however limited his first steps in communication may have been. Instead of sentencing him to years of fixed and unpardonable silence in the classroom, he might have been given some alternative ways to work toward achieving more normal verbal interaction. As a first step, he might have been allowed to respond in nonspeech ways: to reply to questions with a nod or a shake of the head, perhaps with grunts to signify approval or disapproval, perhaps with a higher level of responses— saying *yes* or *no* to accompany a nod or headshake. It is likely that stutterers might be given attainable entries into previously forbidden speech areas, by judicious regulation of conditions that would fit their current confidence levels and allow room for success. Primary-type stutterers are especially in need of this "indirect" therapy to reinforce their fluency patterns under favorable conditions that allow optimal fluency. With primary-type stutterers, however, our work to regulate their speech situations is not yet complicated by the speech maladjustments that later handicap them as secondary stutterers.

Any stutterer will tend to be helped by any influence or experience that adds to his nonspeech assets and strengthens his ego, self-respect, and sense of self-worth from achievements. Teachers are often helpful in providing the child with many opportunities to bolster him in such areas as athletics, music, art, writing, friendships, physical attractiveness, crafts, and favored schoolroom chores. If a stutterer gains enough personal security, he may feel that he can afford to stutter and to work openly upon it. Even with the primary-type stutterer, one who is relatively naive, unaware, and unconcerned over his nonfluency, this policy of building up the person's total assets is important.

Special Guidelines for
Primary Stutterers

We must aid the primary stutterer to avoid developing self-awareness and concern and insecurity over his speech nonfluency and his reluctance to talk. These guidelines are summarized in the following series:

Try to protect the child from anything that will make his stuttering an unpleasant issue for him and will focus his attention upon nonfluency as something that is wrong and to be avoided. The speech life of a primary stutterer should be kept as uncluttered, as satisfactory, and as free of speech anxieties as possible.

If the primary stutterer should voluntarily discuss the subject of his non-fluency, react to him and answer his queries with truthful, factual, and clearly stated information, conveyed with calm and friendly attitudes. There is no virtue in trying to conceal the obvious or in creating a Pollyanna attitude on the one hand or in threatening him into a state of over-caution on the other. Even a young child can gain reassurance and peace from knowing true information on the causes and significance of nonfluencies which begin to cause him to question. The mother of a second-grade primary stutterer answered his query, "Mom, a girl at school told me that I stutter. Do I?" as follows:

Well, perhaps you did sound like you stuttered when you talked with her, Billy. All of us sometimes sound like we stutter. Your dad and I sometimes get mixed up and say our words over and over a few times, especially when we get excited or are in a hurry. But try not to let it bother you, Billy. As children get older, their talking usually gets easier. The more we talk, the easier we talk. Just go ahead and talk, and if anyone says anything about it, just smile and say, "Yep, sometimes I get mixed up a little."

In this commentary the mother's over-all manner of reacting to her son's query is as important as her choice of words. Her manner should convey the fact that she understands his concern about his speech and the statement made about it at school. It should indicate in a calm and frank way the facts of his speech defect and the facts of society's attitudes on stuttering. She should encourage his acceptance of these facts without inciting him to feel resentment toward those who may question or even tease him for stuttering.

Every primary stutterer needs frequent speech experiences that are satisfying to him. As teachers, parents, and therapists we exert strong influence over his attitudes and the conditions which determine the fluency of his performances.

We should analyze and reduce environmental pressures, language deficiencies, and other factors that cause extraordinary nonfluencies in the primary stutterer.

We should help to improve the primary stutterer's total skills—a goal which generally improves communicative fluency. This requirement is especially applicable to young children who are not yet proficient in the skills of *how* to speak. Whatever we can do to improve the child's language skills, helping him to find and to assemble words correctly, will tend to make for better fluency.

Specific Goals and Guidelines
for Secondary Stutterers

Most of the foregoing guides for primary stutterers will be likely to facilitate the fluency of *any speaker*—of the secondary stutterer too. The differentiating factor that calls for special care in the management of a secondary stutterer stems from the fact that extra measures are needed to deal with the complications resulting from his handicapping attitudes and reactions.

Our relationships with the secondary stutterer demand from us a greater degree of face-to-face honesty with unemotional acceptance and adjustment. In dealing with his problems, it is important that we prove to him that we can truly understand, accept, and work with his problems objectively. He must know that we can bear the grotesque sight of his facial contortions and that we do not get upset and distracted over the odd-sounding distortions which wreck his sentences.

We may help the secondary stutterer to develop realistic attitudes and adjustments toward his stuttering if we, as teachers, parents, and therapists, face his problem honestly. Since a secondary stutterer already knows that he stutters, we are guilty of deceit and folly if we try to convince him otherwise. If his judgment and views of stuttering are distorted, we should help him to gain more realistic perspectives of it. This insight usually may be developed more readily through arranging his experience rather than through giving him pep talks and lectures. If the person's problem has become overlaid with fears, anxieties, hopelessness, avoidances, and unwise compensations, we should try to replace these complications with constructive attitudes and behavior patterns —attitudes which would encourage him to face present problems and make him want to improve and learn not to fight and to make hard work of stuttering. A secondary stutterer should learn that his progress depends largely upon himself and that his gains will come from meeting challenges that are real to him. These advances, although they may be gradual, difficult, partial, and marred by temporary reversals, are still encouraging and constitute real gains.

Controlling Conditions that
Hinder Fluency

The fluency of every speaker, child or adult, stutterer or non-stutterer, deteriorates from time to time, depending upon a complexity of stresses that affect his communication and disrupt the flow and organization of thoughts which he formulates into language. We learn to expect and to accept the fact that under certain conditions we characteristically hem and haw, hesitate, "stutter," or "stammer." Actors, for example, adopt these nonfluencies to portray a speaker's stressful state of mind, such as that which threatens a suitor in proposing marriage or that which indicates the inner conflict of a person who is cornered under verbal inquisition. Experienced classroom teachers know that school situations also have widely variable effects upon pupils' fluency. Teachers can also observe that conditions which ordinarily reduce the fluency of the average pupil tend especially to provoke the nonfluencies of pupils who have a tendency to stutter. Therefore if pupils are to develop better fluency patterns, we must recognize and regulate the conditions which will permit a favorable ratio of fluency over nonfluency.

In the following discussion of teachers and their classroom policies, our emphasis upon the unfavorable influences which affect the fluency of pupils may create the impression that we are not granting teachers due credit for the help which they ordinarily give to stutterers. Certainly, in the work of every good teacher or therapist, we find far more favorable influences than unfavorable ones. But everyone can improve.

It should be kept in mind that the following categories of nonfluency overlap each other. Poor listening on the part of an audience, involving restlessness, whispering, and other evidences of boredom, may interrupt the speaker and also may hurry and discourage him. Yet we should not infer that factors which hurry speech are necessarily more harmful, or less harmful, than those which discourage or disorganize it. We must observe and discover from experience what conditions undermine each pupil's fluency. The following categories and samples represent some of the common conditions and practices which have been found to hamper fluency in the classroom.

Situations That Discourage
and Threaten Speech Fluency

A relatively common and thoughtless way of discouraging speech in pupils is to criticize, challenge, and penalize what is said rather than to compliment, accept, and reward their speech contributions. In the following directions given by a school principal, the fluency of pupils may be lowered when they are faced with penalties for what they may say: "As you know, this morning we had serious trouble on the school bus. I have reason to believe that several of you were responsible for it. I'll hold all of you here until I get at the bottom of this. I expect all of you to tell me what you know—whether you were involved or not. Let's hear from you first, John."

In his investigation of this incident, the principal could have reduced pressures upon the pupil's speech if he had conducted the interrogations and testimony with each child privately instead of subjecting each pupil to the combined stresses from testifying openly.

The following kindergarten teacher increased a pupil's stuttering tendency in show-and-tell by challenging the credibility of what he was about to say: "Lenny, this time be sure to tell us only the truth—just what happened and nothing else. Last time, you remember, you said that you and your dad went hunting mushrooms, found some that were poisonous, and that all of your family ate them and died except you. So this time you tell us only the truth. Remember."

Here the teacher could have reduced pressure on Lenny's fluency in this later show-and-tell situation if she had made a brief comment to Lenny and the class at the close of his mushroom fantasy, telling how we must learn to separate fact from fiction in both the telling and the reception of events. If Lenny persisted in stretching the truth into tall tales, his teacher could help him through private counseling to reconcile his handling of reality with his personal need to exploit unreality.

During a period of free conversation, a primary stutterer began to stutter more when his kindergarten teacher criticized him for making some disparaging but factual statements about his parents, concerning an incident in which the police were called to quell a drunken brawl between his parents: "Joseph, we don't talk like that about our mothers and fathers. Let's say only nice things about them. You can go on and tell us about what happened at home, but tell us only the nice things about your father and mother."

Here, too, a teacher must realize the dangers in her decision to restrict or to suppress the act of speech in a child who may justifiably lack the moral standards and prejudices of the teacher, a child who may need an outlet for such expressions in situations where free speech is appropriately authorized. The speaker's mental health, as well as his development of fluency, may require a certain freedom of expression. Audiences, too, need an opportunity to learn that black and white are opposites and are separated by shades of gray.

Early nonfluencies in young children are sometimes focused around conflicts in language usage. The repetitions of a young primary stutterer in saying, "I—I—I—I—me did not mean to do it!" may be indicating a compromise between what he has been told to say linguistically and what he personally feels is yet more natural and correct to say. Parents and teachers who have the responsibility of teaching the correct rules of grammar must recognize that our language rules are often arbitrary and without logic or reason. Therefore, if a child is told that he must not use a certain language form—

one which he has already learned in good faith from the poor example of others or from his own faulty logic—his confidence and fluency in speech may unduly suffer. A speaker cannot be expected to use the correct rules of his language until he has developed a built-in feeling for them, gained from repeatedly hearing and saying them in a variety of meaningful experiences. As adults, we know how difficult it is to correct an established grammatical mistake which persists into our mature language usage, despite corrective reminders along the way.

An aura of threat to speech may be imposed upon a child in oral reading if his teacher is too quick merely to pounce upon each misread word before he has a chance to catch and cancel his mistake and before he has had time to evaluate the word's meaning within its sentence framework. Cautious and hesitant reading and poor comprehension often result from this word-pecking practice. Sometimes teachers even enlist a reader's classmates to police and to maintain vigilance by their participation in the nagging correction of his reading mistakes. In oral reading, a pupil deserves the same listening etiquette that he should expect in conversation.

Fluency may suffer when pupils are pressed to recite memorized material in word-perfect manner. In reciting poetry or memorable passages such as the Gettysburg Address, there is more justification for accurate memorization and recitation than there is in portraying roles in plays and in skits, when pupils may exercise a greater degree of self-involvement and freedom of personal expression. In the former type of recitation, the pressure upon fluency may be reduced by providing judicious prompting when needed, without creating a sense of stigma and urgency. Whether a pupil converses, reads, or recites extemporaneously or from memory, he has the right to pause and to use and endure silence when it is needed. Pupils are less likely to acquire the cluttering habit of using *um*, *er*, and *ah* to fill their gaps in speech when teachers help them to cultivate a calm tolerance and an effective use of speech pauses. If pupils who speak memorized lines in dramatic roles are allowed the freedom to improvise appropriately when they forget the exact wording, their confidence, fluency, and dramatic expression in speech are usually heightened.

Teachers sometimes find themselves in difficult situations with young children who have not yet learned to inhibit the classroom use of profanity and unacceptable "four-letter" words. In such instances, a speech conflict may develop in children who have not yet learned to discriminate between acceptable and forbidden word usage if their teachers do not handle the situation with understanding and care. The following speech therapist's report suggests how shyness and nonfluency in the classroom may have sprung from a child's uncertainty and fear over his saying of "bad" words:

> David's kindergarten teacher referred the problem to me soon after he started school. The issue developed from his "foul language." When he started school, he was freely talkative, but his language was peppered with words that would

make even the legendary sailor take notice. However, he did not show any signs that he felt it was wrong to say these words. But evidently some of his classmates were acquainted with these words and had learned that such words were not to be spoken, at least in school. His teacher was prompted, of course, to correct this language problem. She arranged a private talk with David, telling him that there were some words that we shouldn't say in school because they are "not nice." She admitted that she might have been too hasty and stern in rejecting what he said, creating in him a general sense of wariness in his talking to her or to the class and without letting him clearly know and learn what words and phrases were to be avoided and substituted. His teacher, feeling that David's problem should be handled in a private manner instead of running the risk of managing it openly in the classroom, had held several personal conferences with him before she had referred the matter to me. David was scheduled for twenty-minute sessions with me, twice a week for six weeks, before he recovered his former confidence in talking—with most of the offending words cleaned from his language. Aided by the teacher's list of improper phrases and words, I worked toward three goals: to remove his feelings of self-blame and guilt for having learned and used these words; to point out clearly what usages were improper and why they were objectionable; and to suggest for him and to practice with him alternative improved language expressions. Because our sessions were built around conversation that was pleasantly satisfying for David, he gained security in talking. This talkativeness and fluency then spread to other speech situations as well.

Earlier this chapter explained how stuttering is intensified by anything that induces a stutterer to fear and to avoid stuttering. This aggravating condition may be unintentionally created by a teacher who notices that a stutterer falters on certain sounds or words and who suggests to the stutterer that he should avoid them and that he should try to use other words in place of the difficult ones. This practice not only places stuttering in a negative light but also restricts the speaker's facility of language, forcing him to scan ahead and to communicate in a language crippled by these omitted symbols. Instead, a stutterer should be expected and encouraged to say what he wants to say, whether he stutters or not, because stuttering becomes worse when it becomes the dictator of what is or what is not to be said.

Then, too, we may discourage a pupil in speaking and cause heightened nonfluency in his speech if we criticize, challenge, or penalize *how* he speaks. This focus upon *how* he speaks may concern his articulation, his patterns of fluency, his rate, voice, attitudes, and speech mannerisms.

With good intentions, the following teacher reminds one of her first grade pupils to be on the alert and to avoid his habit of substituting *f* for *th* in his speech: "Harold, I know that when you are careful and think about it, you can say good "th" sounds in your words. Try to speak more carefully so that you won't make these mistakes."

This teacher created such a rigid attitude of caution and apprehension in her pupil that his speech became hesitant and mixed with repetitions in his attempt to scan, monitor, and to keep from making the mistakes which were being penalized. At times the pressures created from unresolved concern over misarticulation have led to the more serious problems of stuttering, reluctance to talk, and a distaste for further work on the misarticulation. We must be careful in corrective work on articulation to keep the child motivated to correct his errors and yet to be constructively tolerant of a reasonable balance between success and failure that may be expected along the way.

We sometimes unknowingly err by praising a stutterer for speaking without stuttering or for stuttering less often. This practice often defeats our good intentions because it tends to increase stuttering by inducing the person to avoid stuttering. Consider how the following statement by his teacher would affect the pupil in giving future oral reports: "Frank, do you realize that you stuttered only a few times in giving this last report? I think that you definitely stuttered on fewer words than you did in previous reports. I knew that you could do it. Perhaps next time you may stutter on even fewer words. You are improving!"

Praising a stutterer for having fewer stuttering moments in a situation like this tends to make him want to live up to similar or higher standards in the future, to please the teacher by not "letting her down." Ironically, a stutterer who feels this way is likely to stutter more because of these implanted desires to stutter less. Instead of praising him for having fewer moments of stuttering in a recitation or oral report, a teacher would be helpful to praise what he said. In the case of a secondary stutterer who is learning to face and to control his stuttering, she could help by giving him justifiable credit for handling his moments of stuttering in improved ways.

For example, the following compliment would encourage a secondary stutterer who shows evidence of learning how to reduce the unnecessary force and accessory reactions that complicate his moments of stuttering: "Frank, in your last oral report I was glad to see that you were working to stutter more easily and cleanly, in the way your speech therapist is teaching you. As you know, it's more important right now for you to keep blocks easy, smooth, and simple, not necessarily to have fewer of them. You're doing well, Frank. Recitation gives you a good chance to practice on speech. I'm glad that you're taking advantage of it."

A variety of reactions by audiences may discourage or threaten speaking by pupils. Under these conditions, a mild stutterer may have serious difficulty; a moderate or severe stutterer may be made almost speechless. However, any pupil, whether he stutters or not, will be more fluent when his speech experiences are relatively free of audience reactions like the following which discourage and threaten speaking.

One seventh-grade pupil with an inconsistent tendency to stutter made the following complaint about recitation in class: "The thing that bugs me most in recitation is when my teacher keeps at me to answer a question that I don't know. I'll answer as much as I know, but she sometimes wants more than that, or something else, and then I don't know what to say. It gets me bothered, and then I really stutter."

An eleventh-grade girl criticized her history teacher's handling of recitations: "I find it hard to win in history class. If I know an answer to his question and show that I want to answer it, he's not likely to call on me at all; if I don't know an answer and let it show, I end up either admitting I don't know or trying to bluff my way through. But when I bluff, some of my old stuttering returns. The other kids in class don't like to play this game of cat and mouse with the teacher either."

Another high school student describes why tensions are created in social science class when the teacher asks a broad or vague question but demands a specific answer to it: "She will ask us a question that could be answered in several ways, or at least we think it could. But until someone comes up with the certain answer that she wants, she keeps asking around. Often we could have given the right answer if we'd understood the question. That makes us look as if we hadn't studied the lesson. We feel on needles and pins when we recite in that class."

Pupils with obvious abnormalities, such as stuttering, tend to be discouraged from talking when they observe that their abnormalities arouse pity, embarrassment, irritation, impatience, and other undesirable reactions in their audiences—especially when those audiences are teachers, parents, friends, and others whom pupils respect and want to please. One pupil explained to his speech therapist: "I know that I should volunteer to recite more, but whenever I do and stutter, my teacher feels so sorry for me that she can't even look at me. When other kids recite, the teacher will sometimes smile and show interest in what they say. But when I stutter, she gets only worried and serious—doesn't seem to be interested in what I say. It makes me feel that I'm bothering her."

Another pupil gave the following reason for failing to do a therapy assignment in which he was to try to work on five stuttered words in recitation and to handle them by smoothly prolonging each block at least three seconds without exerting excessive force and without reverting to his habitual devices for releasing the block: "I handled two words by holding their blocks for about four seconds but my teacher began to get uneasy and tried to guess what my stuck-word was. On the third block I didn't hold it long enough because she guessed the word and said it before I finished holding it. Then, on the fourth block I didn't handle it smoothly at all. I guess I was thinking too much about what the teacher would do about it." The therapist controlled the impulse to tell this pupil that she would confer with his teacher and secure a better reaction from her. Instead, realizing that the teacher's response is a rather common audience error when stutterers have long blocks, she told her client that he would gain more in therapy from learning to control his stuttering in the face of such reactions, which would often be met.

Although not a stutterer, the following college student blames an experience in the third grade for her extreme shyness and hesitant speech in recitation since that time.

> During my first three years in school, I spoke in class more than anyone else. I volunteered the most, was usually the first to talk, and the one to talk the longest. But the third-grade teacher really cracked down on me. She warned me that if I didn't stop talking so much, she'd seat me in the far corner of the classroom and not call on me. By the time I was in high school, I was so shy and uneasy that I hardly spoke at all. If I did talk, I usually had trouble thinking about what I was going to say. I realize that in these early grades I talked too much and that it was a classroom problem for the teacher, but I don't think that my teacher handled the problem very well so far as I was concerned.

A first-grade teacher once gave this reason for her reluctance to call on a pupil who had very grotesque symptoms of stuttering: "Until I learned that stuttering was not contagious, that it was not learned from merely being around and imitating others who stutter, I ignored and did not let this child recite for fear that his stuttering would cause other classmates to stutter too."

A shy high school pupil points out several classroom policies that cause a build-up of tension in students when they recite:

> You ask me how teachers could encourage pupils to recite and still help them to feel at ease in reciting. Well, here are some things that have bothered me. Too often I've felt that my grades depended upon what I said in class. But this isn't the only thing that has made recitation unpleasant. In the early grades, especially, I recall the rough competition among classmates to gain the teacher's attention and to get her permission to speak. We'd wave hands, utter gasps of breath, assume eager expressions—only to find that our bids to speak were often useless. Too often the teacher seemed to call on a few pets or to want something that wasn't exactly what I had to say. Some of the teachers went right down the line, calling on pupils in the alphabetical order of their names or according to their seating. This really put the heat on me. The teachers who called on us at random made it easier for me not only to answer but also to maintain my interest throughout the class period. Why don't teachers realize this?

Pupils are, of course, discouraged and threatened in their speaking at times by humor reactions of giggling, teasing, mocking, joking, and nick-naming—reactions which may occur even during recitation in the classroom, with or without the teacher's knowledge. Teachers vary in their views and methods of handling teasing and humor responses directed at stuttering. Focusing their concern upon the classmates who express these reactions, some teachers may take a punitive stand, to threaten the offenders with shame and punishment if they continue the teasing, giggling, etc. This policy often defeats its purpose by alienating the stutterer from his classmates and making him feel and appear like a teacher's pet. Furthermore, this policy may create in the pupils an exaggerated sense of awareness and significance surrounding the pupil's stuttering, to invite more attention than would occur if they were allowed greater freedom in evaluating his problem. This policy may also lead to a double standard in the treatment given to the pupil by his classmates. On the playground, on the bus, and in other situations beyond the teacher's surveillance and enforcement, classmates may resort to tactics that are temptingly inspired by the fact that the issue had been emphasized and marked as taboo by the teacher.

Other teachers follow a more moderate policy in handling situations in which classmates express thoughtless amusement at pupils with odd differences, such as stuttering. These teachers openly acknowledge that there is novelty in stuttering behavior, as the public taste has been conditioned by Porky Pig and other entertainers; but they recommend that listeners should express their humor reactions only if it is obvious to them that the stutterer is likewise capable of admitting the primitive humor in his own behavior. In connection with this policy, these teachers may privately suggest and encourage the stutterer not only to accept the fact that some persons will feel amusement and react humorously toward stuttering but also to realize that the stutterer bears the primary responsibility of accepting and even joining in their expression of humor. Even young stutterers can be shown that it is better to try to roll with the punch in a good-humored fashion than to bear the brunt in serious defensiveness, since they themselves largely determine the nature and course of audience reactions to their stuttering. One fourth-grader explained: "At first, I fought with every kid who teased or laughed at my stuttering. But this made it all the worse. More and more kids began to tease me, especially the ones who could lick me or who could outrun me. Then my teacher found out what was happening on the playground. She told me that they'd stop it if I'd just smile and try to be a good sport when they teased me. It worked too. Once in a while a kid will still joke about my stuttering, but I don't mind it like I did before."

It will take time for a sensitive stutterer to cultivate this saving sense of humor toward the novel aspects of stuttering—especially toward his own stuttering. But he will never recognize the shoddy claims of "genuine" humor to be found in stuttering. He must develop a realistic sense of humor, for ready use. He will learn that most children and adults who laugh at stuttering fail to understand the nature and the seriousness of the handicap. When he discovers that bullies focus upon his stuttering in their teasing, he must learn that a social strategy like joining in the laughter against him spoils the fun of the pack.

However, the most effective safeguard against uncontrolled teasing of a stutterer by classmates comes from the teacher's own example of adjustment to him and to his stuttering. We know that classmates are inclined to look to their teacher and to follow her patterns of interpretation, appreciation, acceptance, rejection, prejudice, and mannerisms. If classmates see that their teacher is calm, comfortable, and respectful toward a stutterer and his stuttering, they will tend to imitate her attitude. On the other hand, if children see that their teacher is uneasy, pained, troubled, overly sympathetic and "helpful" toward a child's stuttering, they will tend to react similarly and to play up the handicap for more than it is worth.

There are times when a pupil is unwillingly called upon by his teacher to display reading or recitation before his visiting parents. A speech therapist who asked a fourth-grader to pick one of his most difficult speech situations received this reply: "I don't mind reading or talking in school except when Mother comes to visit. Then the teacher calls on me most. I don't like to show off, and besides it makes me stutter more. I don't know why. At home I don't stutter much talking with Mom."

When a teacher notices that a child's stuttering has had discouraging, threatening, and deteriorating effects upon him in the classroom, it is generally a good policy to insure that the pupil can close his performance on some positive note. If a child has struggled through an oral report but has told some interesting information, his teacher might well conclude his ordeal by acknowledging some point which she regarded as being informative and interesting in his talk. A third-grade teacher commented on a severe stutterer's struggling account of how a tornado had wrecked a cottage: "You gave a good description of that tornado, Larry. I could almost see that cottage being smashed and scattered about by the twisting wind. Even though you had difficulty in talking, you went ahead and gave us an exciting picture of what a tornado can do." Deserved credit, such as this, may not only cancel some of the unpleasant effects of stuttering for the speaker, but may also encourage attitudes of acceptance and respect by classmates.

Nonfluency from Interruption, Indecision, and Distraction

Normal speech requires the organization of several mental and physical functions. As Bluemel[3] explains, nonfluency results either when developing speech has not yet gained sufficient organization or when stresses act upon the speaker to disrupt his flow of thoughts, his language patterns, and the physical skills which enable the speech act to function as a smoothly flowing and integrated sequence. We are aware of the disorganizing effects which may be produced by sudden acute stresses, "shocks," or emotional traumas from accidents and experiences which threaten life. But, as Bluemel points out, we are less likely to notice the gradual and prolonged stresses that gnaw at a person's security in a cumulative manner through worry, anxiety, fear, frustration, and failure. Although stress is an inescapable part of life, it may become seriously disorganizing in a child's developing speech life if the stress mounts too high, if it continues too long without relief, or if the child has not yet gained a normal adjustment or resistance to even the ordinary stresses of life.

We have mentioned some of these disorganizing stresses upon speech behavior in the previous discussion of the conditions which discourage and threaten speech. In the following section we shall consider situations which discourage speech in ways that are often overlooked.

This third-grader complains how his fluency is hampered by his teacher's habit of interrupting him: "Every time I start to stutter on a word, my teacher tries to say the word before I say it. I guess she's trying to help me, but I don't like it. Sometimes she doesn't know at all what I'm trying to say, and when she says a wrong word I get all mixed up and even forget what I was going to say."

A kindergarten teacher explains her policy of allowing her pupils greater fluency when they retell stories they have learned:

> When I began teaching, I was too particular in wanting the children to recite stories with all details correct and in proper sequence—stories like "Goldilocks and the Three Bears," you know. But when I noticed that some of the children got rattled, bothered, and lost confidence when I interrupted their stories with my corrections, I quit it. After all, there are other things more important than keeping a child straight on the original version of "Goldilocks"—whether or not Goldilocks sat on the chairs before she tried the bears' porridge, etc. However, if I find that a child is making errors or changes that go too far astray from a given story, I may call attention to the fact, but I do so after he has concluded the story. Then it doesn't interfere with his talking.

Another teacher explains:

> From my experience with all grade levels, kindergarten through high school, I've found that children often need some props in giving oral reports and lengthy recitations. Strip films which illustrate stories, like "The Three Pigs" or "Jack and the Beanstalk," can be used by young children to accompany their telling of these stories, to give them confidence, remove some of the burden from the act of speaking, and organize their thoughts. I find that an opaque projector is especially adaptable to the same purpose—to train children and adults to think on their feet with greater confidence, fluency, and effectiveness. Some children have gained a lot from using the blackboard to supplement their talk with an outline, tables, or sketches. These visual aids help me, so why shouldn't they help my pupils?

Stutterers may be hampered by the policies of teachers, parents, and others to give advice and "help." These "helps" may not only become habituated abnormalities in themselves, but in the process they may also have the effects of interrupting and distracting the speaker. A sixth-grader made this complaint to her speech therapist:

> It's hard for me to remember to do all the things I'm supposed to do when I talk. At home Mom tells me to talk slower and to think what I'm going to say. Dad

says to stop, relax, not get excited, and take a fresh breath and start over when I stutter. In school my teacher tries to help by saying words for me when I start to stutter on them. And you want me to go ahead and have the block in a smoother way, an easier way. It's hard to do all these things and still remember what I have to say. I get mixed up. Then I stutter more and more and forget about everything I'm supposed to do.

There are also nonverbal ways to interrupt and distract speakers. A pupil tells how he feels when he gives an oral book report in class:

I wish my teacher would listen to me like she does to the other kids when they give reports. Whenever I stutter she looks as if I've done something wrong, not interested in what I'm saying. It makes me feel that my report isn't very good, that something's wrong with it. Then I stutter more, things get worse for both of us, and I either quit or give a punk report.

A fourth-grade stutterer paid his teacher the following compliment during a private conference in which he explained why reciting in her class was easier than it had been during his previous year at school:

It's easier to recite this year because when someone is reciting, the rest of the class does not butt in and try to answer. Last year it seemed that sometimes everybody was trying to speak at once and nobody was listening. It's always harder to talk when people aren't looking at me or paying attention. That's why I also stutter more when I ride in the back seat of a car and talk to people in the front seat.

Nonfluency When Speech Is Hurried and Overloaded

Every speaker has found that he tends to trip over his tongue if he speaks too fast. He knows, too, that he may become "jammed" if a number of thoughts are competing for expression at once. Under these conditions even the normal speaker tends to slur, misarticulate, repeat, prolong, or have speech reactions that resemble the symptoms of a primary stutterer; under similar conditions, a stutterer would be likely to have stuttering symptoms of greater frequency and intensity. In this school situation, reported by a stutterer, hurrying and overloading of speech occurred:

The thing I hate worst about giving book reports is the three-minute time limit that our teacher puts on them. We're graded on several things, and one of the important points is how close we can come to three minutes. If our talks are too short or too long, we're marked off. The teacher gives everyone in class a rating sheet for checking each other on how he speaks. It's hard for me to figure it so that I'll end up in three minutes, especially when I stutter and waste time having my long blocks. That makes me want to hurry and keep from having blocks, and that makes me have more blocks than ever.

Although a teacher may be justified in setting a time-limit for oral book reports and other speech topics, a range of two to four minutes would create less tension than would a narrowed limit of three minutes, strictly adhered to. Furthermore, for a stutterer or a cerebral-palsied speaker, whose speech rate may be necessarily reduced and whose fluency would be further reduced by hurry, it would be advisable to adjust his time-limits for speaking in accordance with the optimal rate which will enable him to have the greatest control over his speech.

There are many subtle and indirect ways to imply to a pupil that he should hurry his speaking. Pupils soon sense the crowded and compartmented program and scheduling imposed upon them and teachers. They soon learn, for instance, that a popular criterion of a "good reader" is a fast reader, one who can read the most paragraphs within the limited time. This pressure to hurry may build up toward the end of the reading period, with time running out, when audience interest in the story may wane as more and more readers have completed their turns, and if pupils become bored and restless in their eagerness to begin the next activity. Similar pressures of hurry and impatience may be created in conversation and in recitation if teachers are not alert and considerate. One kindergarten teacher revealed how the fluency of several pupils rose when she avoided asking them questions which demanded long answers:

> On Monday mornings, and especially on days following holidays like Christmas and Thanksgiving, I had had the habit of calling on each pupil to report on what they did over the holiday. Well, with thirty-three children in my room, it soon became evident that these broad questions were too much for everyone in the room to answer with satisfaction. After Christmas vacation, for example, I may invite each child to tell about only one gift he received from Santa Claus. In this way, each child has a more equal opportunity to talk, and there's no shameful comparison of what each child received for Christmas. Some of my pupils come from poor families and do not get much.

A child's nonfluency may be aggravated by a tendency to speak too rapidly—a tendency being transferred and maintained by influential speakers who talk too rapidly in conversation with the child. Children often speed up their rate in trying to keep up in conversation with parents, siblings, and even teachers and therapists who speak too fast. Although these adults may be aware of the child's excessive rate of speech and may ask and expect him to "slow down," they may not be aware of their own primary need to correct this same contagious habit in themselves. Unless parents, teachers, and therapists can discipline themselves and set an example of calm, unhurried, and improved speech, they have little right to expect the child to correct these same fostered habits. However, it is not easy for adults to alter their habituated rate of speech.

An overemphasis on speed in oral reading may lead a child to increase his rate of speech in recitation and conversation, affecting his organization of thought and his fluency. A supervisor of education for the elementary grades has declared: "I firmly believe that pupils need more time to think and to speak without being in a state of hurry and impatience. Too often our sessions of reading and recitations are being conducted in the hectic spirit and pace of a circus ring. It's not surprising that pupils become rattled, uncomfortable, read without meaningful expression, and give superficial recitations."

Nonfluency may result when children's speech is hurried and overloaded with tension under strong emotion and communicative pressure. A kindergarten teacher describes a situation of this kind:

> It started with Freddy's terrible fire experience in which his family was routed from their sleep one wintry night. They lost everything except their pajamas and suffered some burns, smoke inhalation, and cuts from a narrow escape through broken windows. But for several days after that fire, Fred seemed to be in shock. He would talk only about the fire. No other school matters would break his preoccupation. In class throughout the day, Freddy would bring up the horrible account of his experience. As a teacher, I had two main concerns over his talking about this fire. First, his story was upsetting the other children; second, his speech became so jumbled up with broken words and sentences during these two or three days that I feared he'd become a stutterer. However, supported by recommendations from our speech therapist and school psychologist, I gave Freddy more chances to get things off his chest. Within a week he had reconciled the troubling aspects of the situation, had lost the compulsive urge to talk about it, and had regained his former level of fluency. Besides letting him air his gnawing preoccupation, I also made a special effort to find interesting subjects and activities that would bring Freddy back into the realities of his present school life.

Nonfluency from Insufficient Experience, Learning, and Adjustment

Occasionally teachers and other adults will sympathetically react to a stuttering pupil by excusing him from speech, by encouraging him to avoid speech, or by restricting the number, types, and duration of his speech situations. As one teacher explained: "Knowing that stuttering is largely psychological and a matter of fear and tension, I am very careful to spare the stutterer the necessity to talk any more than I can help, for fear that he'll become more fearful and tense and get worse. I'm also afraid that the other children will notice it and start teasing or something."

A teacher with these fears is likely to transfer the same attitudes to the stutterer and his classmates, who otherwise might not develop them. A policy

which restricts speaking for a primary stutterer may also restrict his opportunity to cultivate the various adjustments and learnings which are needed
for fluency: confidence, favorable social attitudes toward conversation, and
development of the mental and physical skills for oral expression. For the
secondary stutterer, this sheltering policy may simply tell him that his teacher,
too, is aware and fearful of his stuttering. A secondary stutterer needs encouragement and practice in maintaining the ordinary skills of speech. If he is working
therapeutically to control his stuttering more effectively, any policy which
generally restricts his speaking will also restrict his chances to work directly
upon his stuttering.

By their efforts to create for pupils certain social adjustments to stuttering,
some teachers have unwittingly created in the stutterer the same maladjustments
which they tried to prevent. The following teacher explains how she fostered
rather than prevented social maladjustments for a third-grader who stutters:

> When I discovered that John stuttered and that several of the children were teasing
> him about it, I decided that I'd settle the issue once and for all. I picked a time
> when John was absent from school and really gave his classmates a lecture on how
> they should act toward his stuttering. Well, I found out that I had created new
> problems for John. Some of his classmates seemed to have become wary and
> uneasy toward him. John, too, appeared to sense this air of caution and seriousness
> when he spoke in school situations, even on the playground, where he had been
> one of the most active and popular children. In fact, after my talk to the class on
> its adjustment to John, I also felt more on guard around him whenever he spoke,
> and it's likely that my change of attitude was sensed and transmitted to the others,
> including John. Well, I learned a lesson from that experience. I should have
> consulted John in the beginning and let him help decide with me whether or not
> he could handle the social adjustments to his stuttering. After all, he was the one
> who had to make the adjustments to his problems whenever and wherever he
> found them.

The need for a stutterer to be as self-reliant as possible in speaking should
not lead us to expect him to meet and to handle all speech challenges by himself.
As teachers, we are in a position to select and to build speech situations so that
their levels of difficulty will be kept within the child's range of confidence
and ability. One primary stutterer, although he was generally shy and reluctant
to talk before class, was handled in the following way by his first-grade teacher:

> Silas wouldn't come up before the class and talk in show-and-tell like the rest of
> the pupils. Since he was very interested in playing baseball, I planned a little
> class demonstration in which he could take part without having to speak if he
> didn't want to. I told the class that I wanted to show how a ballplayer stood at the
> plate, holding a bat and ready to swing. I placed a sheet of paper on the floor for
> home plate, took a yardstick for a bat, and said that I needed someone who could
> show us how a batter would act. Hands went up, but not Silas'. I let one of the
> boys come up and position himself as a right-handed batter would grip the bat

and stand. I thanked him and let him take his seat. Then I told the class that some ballplayers were left-handed and that they stood differently. I asked for another boy to demonstrate that. Silas didn't raise his hand, but I asked him if he'd like to show us. He accepted, came up, went through his little act, was thanked, and took his seat. He also came out with the word *three* when I asked how many strikes a batter gets before he's out. And he said *four* when I called for the number of balls before a batter walks. Anyway, this little experience must have been important for him, because after that he began to talk and read before the class.

There are other ways by which teachers help to strengthen a pupil's skills and feeling for fluency and keep his speech aspirations in line with his speech abilities, so that his success-failure ratio in speaking will be favorable. Choral speaking is commonly used to give a child benefits from identifying and practicing with others who have better speech patterns than he has. For a stutterer, who usually becomes fluent while speaking in unison with others, choral speaking may help to replace his self-image and habits as a stutterer with those which permit him to associate fluency with himself. For a severe stutterer, whose speech is difficult and uncommunicative, practice in silent role-playing and charades may give him a successful start in associating himself with the possibility of communication and satisfactions from it—an important step even though that communication is not verbal. We often find that even the most severe stutterer becomes more fluent when he speaks in the characters of role-playing or when he speaks simultaneously while acting out a skit in charades.

Because even a severe stutterer usually sings without stuttering, he can gain some values from singing; benefits from participating vocally in a normal and satisfying manner, from feeling the flow and the momentum of oral production, even though singing is on a different communicative level from conversation. However, one third-grade teacher, who had observed how singing freed the tongues and inhibitions of shy and nonfluent children, conducted exercises in a calypso type of singing. Equipped with a homemade bongo drum, made by capping with plastic covers the opened ends of a coffee can, a child was given the chance to chant improvised tales of any sort, long or short, true or fantastic, in accompaniment to his drumbeat. This calypso-like exercise, halfsong and halfspeech, partly self and partly someone else, became a popular medium for creative and free expression. Every child needs some opportunity and practice in speaking when he is not being judged and held accountable for what he says and how he says it. As in creative art, there should be times when a pupil's written and oral expression of language should not be graded, judged, or made-to-order. A pupil will enjoy speaking with increased freedom and fluency in situations where audiences are merely respectful and appreciative, not judgmental in a restrictive and conforming sense. This democratic spirit is allowable in situations employing calypso-talk, creative dramatics, the spinning of tales and limericks, and talking through puppets.

Other Hazards to Fluency

We know that speech fluency of schoolchildren is affected by other factors, ones which teachers may overlook or find difficult to control. For example, parents have the main responsibility for a child's well-being, his amount of sleep, his nutrition, and his security at home. But if a child's parents do not fulfill these responsibilities, teachers and others must try to compensate for the deficiency.

Although programs for children of nursery and kindergarten ages generally provide nap periods and operate on a half-day basis, there are other fatigue-producing conditions which undermine mental and physical efficiency, including speech fluency. A kindergarten teacher has reported:

> My five-year-olds arrive at our consolidated school at 7:50 A.M. with the busloads of other older children. Some of them ride thirty-five miles from home, a tiring stop-and-go trip that takes an hour. At 11:30 the kindergartners are dismissed for the day and are sent home for lunch. This means a long and busy forenoon for some of them. At ten o'clock I give them a twenty-minute period for milk and a nap, but I still find that some get droopy before the morning is over. There's not much I can do about the school's operating schedule but I have been able to help the chronically tired children through their parents. Often a conference will disclose that the children are not getting enough sleep, that they are staying up too late to see TV programs. Proof of parental cooperation comes from seeing more vigor and learning ability in their children at school.

In another instance a second-grade teacher, suspecting that physical causes were contributing to listlessness in an apparent primary stutterer who never volunteered, referred the case to her school's nurse, who secured medical attention for the cause, a lack of minerals and vitamins. The result was a pickup in the child's general spirit and participation in activities, as well as in his fluency. His teacher afterwards commented: "If I hadn't noticed and checked the physical symptoms of this tired, puny little boy, I might have wrongly blamed stuttering for his reluctance to talk."

It is often observed that stutterers have "good days" and "bad days" in which their attitudes and fluency vary. If we knew the reasons for these fluctuations, we might find that some of their causes are products of such states as fatigue, illness, or general anxiety and excitement, or are reactions from meeting difficult or easy speech situations rather than an inevitable rhythm pattern or periodicity to be expected of stuttering. Whatever the causes of these "good" and "bad" periods, and whether or not we know what may be producing them, it is generally advisable to induce more speaking when fluency is higher than when it is in a slump. Yet, at these times, it is important not to let the stutterer know that his speech output is being reduced because of his increased stuttering. Otherwise, he may become more intolerant of stuttering and thereby suffer an increase of nonfluency.

Minority group children, such as Negroes and migrant workers of Spanish-American origin, too often will find that our schools are intolerant of their cultural, regional, or foreign-bred accents, vocabularies, and articulation patterns. If not enough consideration is given to their speech and language heritages and to the patterns to which they must conform in their present lives at home, in their neighbourhood, in the fields, etc., these schoolchildren may be subjected to speech restrictions which place unfair demands upon their personal rights and abilities as speakers. The following speech therapist reports one aspect of this problem:

> In my school district we have a minority group of Negro children, many of whom have recently moved up from the South with the characteristic language expressions and speech traits of the region. In my conference with the parents of these children, I also realized that the present home and neighborhood influences were often maintaining some of these speech and language patterns more effectively than we were altering them at school. Well, in investigating why a relatively high percentage of these children stuttered or were shy and insecure in speech situations, I found that they were unable to meet the double standards that were expected of them. Moreover, we were making them feel in school that they were uncultured and uneducated because they didn't talk like us, that their speech was "wrong," "bad," "faulty," and in need of speech correction when, perhaps, our only complaint was that they omitted the *r* in a word like *car*, or substituted the short vowel for the *er* in a word like *sister*. However, these pronunciations are normal in many parts of the English-speaking world. If we clearly realize this, we understand and accept them as such.
>
> In our school system, where the majority of us speak with the "midwestern *r*" and a "northern accent," I may give a Negro child, for example, the chance to adopt the speech patterns of our locality and culture, but I do so in the sense of teaching him a *second* language without making him feel that the language of his home and heritage is wrong and disrespected. I may point out that some of our greatest Americans, like Roosevelt and Kennedy, were understood and were judged as good speakers, even though they spoke with different *r*'s and accents than we teach in our community. Moreover, I find that if a child is offered a clear and free choice to learn and to use our "northern *r*" when it becomes an advantage for him to use it in school or in other speech situations, he will more readily and easily do so—without becoming shameful and tense in the process. I find, also, that most of our Negro children, before they graduate from high school, have learned to turn on or off advantageously either of their dual skills of talking in southern or northern style.

Most of us as children have squirmed and sputtered when obliged to think up something to say under the implied command, "Has the cat got your tongue?" How often do we demand of young children what we would not consider to be polite or reasonable to demand of older children or of adults? As one kindergarten teacher stated:

> I try to treat my children as I would want to be treated, the same as I'd treat

adults. It's not easy to do. Our treatment of children often follows a different standard, a double code of etiquette. But when I'm tempted, for example, to require pupils to put forth special displays of their abilities when their parents visit school, I remind myself how I felt as a child when I was put on the spot to entertain or to justify the pride of adults. Then, too, I try to give my children the feeling that our silent thoughts may be as important as our spoken ones and that we are entitled to have inviolate moments of silence as speakers and as listeners during our class discussions. Children should not be made to feel that their contribution in class depends upon how frequently they talk or how long they hold the floor. At times when there is too much competitive, spontaneous, and indiscriminate talking in class, I call for a period of quiet thinking before anyone resumes the discussion. I believe that we should train children to think and should give them more opportunities to do so. We develop a gift of gab that is too often measured only in verbal output. It's important for us to learn not only to endure silence but to make good use of it.

A wise teacher says:

When I start children to read and to recite orally, I try to make the situation natural, informal, and pleasant for them. Although there are situations later on in which pupils stand and face the class in giving a report or in reading a passage, I am careful to give them plenty of practice and confidence in just plain communicating. Later on we may add some of the disciplined skills that may be effective for the sophisticated public speaker. At times we place so much stress upon maintaining proper carriage, gestures, and eye contact with the audience that we make our pupils into miserable marionettes.

The general noise level in a classroom may also affect the speech fluency of pupils, as a teacher explains:

In my years of teaching in both public and parochial schools, I have become aware of how much teachers vary in their control of noise in their classrooms. I have known classrooms which have been kept uncomfortably quiet and classrooms which have been so noisy with uncontrolled daily hubbub that you can spot them the entire length of their halls. Then again, there are classrooms with frequent sounds of activities but where the sounds are meaningful and appropriate to the occasion. I know that children are bothered by noise. They and their parents have reported that they don't like certain teachers and their rooms because of the distraction and handicap which noise imposes upon study and school participation.

The speech behaviour of children may be disrupted by factors other than noise in the classroom. This is the complaint of one tenth-grade stutterer who found it difficult to volunteer in his class: "What makes it bad is that our history teacher tells us to ask questions but sometimes gets mad when we ask them. And when you answer his questions, you can't be sure whether you should speak out without being called on or whether you should wait until he sees your hand and calls on you. So I don't recite as much as I should. When I do, I'm uneasy and stutter more."

Another seventh-grade stutterer told a speech therapist about recitation difficulties: "I wish our teacher would keep the other kids from butting in when someone is reciting. You never know when you'll be able to finish what you want to say. It makes you feel like not saying anything. It makes me try to talk faster. I forget to work on my blocks; I stutter more and get disgusted about the whole thing and figure, 'What's the use!'"

Speech fluency may be hampered by stresses which are more subtle and indirect than those we have discussed. Children who frequently move from home to home, neighborhood to neighborhood, and from school to school suffer various effects from their unsettled lives. A speech therapist explains this mobility factor as follows: "I find that speech maladjustments are included in the educational difficulties often found in children who follow their parents all over the country, changing schools, breaking in new friends and adjusting to new teachers and to different methods and materials. Speech therapy for some of these migrants should be more a matter of general tutoring than anything else."

A perceptive teacher comments on the practice of favoring too much "togetherness" in children's activities on the playground: "I have come to the conclusion that children should be allowed to have some opportunities for escaping social stimulation, which surrounds them from the time they board the bus in the early morning until they step off at dusk. For some of them, recess is the only time for relaxation. Even our lunch periods are tightly packed with activity and noise. So when I see children going off at recess to play in solitary, I hesitate to regard it as abnormal, antisocial behavior which should be discouraged. It's lucky our playground is large enough to allow these brief respites."

A child's worries over problems at home may also cause disturbances which are tied in with school activities. A second-grade boy, whose stuttering and enuresis fluctuated with his school attendance, was worried over what his preschool brother would be doing to his prized possessions at home when he was at school. After his parents realized this cause of anxiety and supplied a personal cabinet for him with assurance that his collection of model airplanes and personal treasures would be safe while he left them, his dislike for school, his stuttering, and his enuresis began to clear.

The Role of the Speech Therapist

Throughout this chapter on stuttering we have emphasized that any complete speech correction program calls for observational conferences and joint remedial action by the therapist, teachers, and parents, but that the diagnosing and treatment should be integrated and directed primarily by the speech therapist. We have stated that speech therapists should be trained to assume this major responsibility to inform teachers and parents of the stutterer's special needs and to direct everyone in fulfilling these particular needs. However, if a speech therapist is not available, the classroom teacher must assume a reasonable added responsibility within her schedule to direct help for her pupil. Although the aim of this chapter has been to make the teacher as self-sufficient as possible in ways to help the child, we have also emphasized that there are duties which require a speech therapist.

The Therapist's Role with Primary Stutterers

Speech therapists who speak of their work with a primary stutterer as being more "indirect" than "direct" are usually implying two characteristics about therapy with him. First, they are emphasizing the fact that they are careful not to work directly upon the child's speech and nonfluency in ways which will create or accentuate the child's self-awareness and concern over his speaking and its nonfluency. Second, "indirect" work refers to the fact that therapy for a primary stutterer is often channeled "through" others, particularly parents and teachers, who are in influential positions to provide the child with more favorable opportunities, support, learning, and practice so that his fluency rather than nonfluency may be developed. The goals and the guidelines for the therapist in working directly with primary stutterers are largely the ones we have already outlined for teachers. The therapist's schedule, however, is likely to allow for more individualized contact with the child and with his parents in working toward these goals.

Before considering samples of how a speech therapist might work with a primary stutterer in both "direct" and "indirect" ways, we shall review the following goals and policies for work with primary stutterers:

To earn and maintain a good basic relationship with the child, his parents, and teachers. This point is of special importance for the therapist, who must not only gain the confidence and cooperation of the child but must also depend upon information and help through the child's parents, teachers, administrators, and others. Rapport, as we have stated earlier in this chapter, is not something that comes ready-made. We earn it through daily experience and contact with clients. We may fail to gain it; we may lose it too. *How* we gain and hold a favorable working relationship with others depends upon such human virtues as understanding, kindness, tolerance, honesty, helpfulness, humor, companionship, support, and other intangibles which are difficult to define in words. "Good" parents, teachers, and therapists are likely to have these traits.

To avoid or to reduce factors that may cause the child's nonfluency to become for him a matter of self-concern and avoidance. We have defined "primary stuttering" as being the initial stage of the nonfluency disorder, before the stutterer has become specifically aware or concerned over his nonfluencies as something to be shunned. We have repeatedly emphasized that the primary stutterer should be helped to avoid developing into the later stages, which are complicated by concerns, conflicts, and handicapping reactions that add to his problem. We have sampled some of the experiences in which a child's nonfluencies lead to predicaments which force him to feel that his nonfluencies are "bad," bothersome, and to be pitied and avoided.

To build the child's personal security, ego, confidence, self-respect, and social interests. A child develops these strengths and attributes through his total experience, which must allow for more satisfying success than for disappointing failure. To achieve this positive balance for the child, there must be a suitable tailoring of his environment to fit his present abilities, disabilities, and interests. He needs help to develop a sense of adequate social worth and group-belonging, to reconcile his strengths and weaknesses, and to develop constructive interests and activities.

To encourage and to provide the child with enough personally satisfying experience in which his fluency may be as high as possible. In this area of need, the therapist is guided by the same principles discussed in our preceding sections on the conditions and factors for teachers to consider. In therapy, teachers and therapists have much in common.

To build and to strengthen the primary stutterer's total skills needed for speech and communication, so that his oral language may function in an automatic sense. This goal calls for learning and habituation on the levels of articulation, vocabulary, syntax, and the prosodic features which pertain to accent, tonal inflection, and rate of speech. The therapist of a primary stutterer should know the fundamentals governing the learning and the teaching of speech and language at different levels of their development. Not only should the therapist be able to work with the child in these areas, but she should also be able to understand and to enlist similar work through parents and teachers.

To investigate the special factors which cause and maintain the child's nonfluency and to follow with remedial action. We have already indicated that teachers, too, need to be informed and vigilant concerning these causal factors, especially when there is no speech therapist to assume leadership in this trouble-shooting role. We were also reminded that referral requires a knowledge of *when*, *where*, and *how* to refer a client for help by others.

Keeping in mind the above-stated goals for primary stutterers, we shall now consider examples of specific methods and case reports to show how speech therapists have worked toward these goals. It will be evident that a therapist often works on more than one goal at a time: she will be giving a primary stutterer "direct" work as simultaneously she will be conducting a program of "indirect" help through the child's parents and teachers. The illustrations will warn us that therapists cannot afford to narrow their sights nor to overlook opportunities to help a primary stutterer.

The following more specific goals will give hints of what a speech therapist may do in "direct" and individualized therapy with a primary stutterer:

To prepare and to conduct speech situations with the child, situations in which conditions will permit a relatively high level of fluency for him. Materials and approaches may involve pictures, toys, games, strip films, puppets, and masks. Various devices and methods are used to stimulate and to permit more fluent speech on a spontaneous, automatic, or interjectional level; speech on a fictional or nonsense level; various types of speech with accompaniment; reading with controlled commentary; "monkey" talk with interspersed play; speaking with a tape recorder or megaphone; speaking with the use of masking noise; and controlled conversation facilitated by the aid of another child.

To strengthen the normally needed resistance or degree of immunity which primary stutterers must develop in the face of the fluency-disrupting "pressures" which normally occur in his speech life. The therapist may use the preceding materials and activities in ways to build adjustment to both general pressures and specific speech pressures which may be social, perceptual, physical, and linguistic. This therapeutic process, sometimes referred to as "desensitization" therapy, is not as novel and technical as it has sometimes been called. It may be described as a means of regulating a person's speech experiences so that he will have favorable opportunities to meet the challenging problems in his communicative world and so that he will also be assured of more success than failure in coping with these speech experiences. Since many of the ordinary pressures which challenge a child in his speech life involve his parents and home, the therapist must closely consider his family in this "desensitization" branch of therapy. The therapist should bring the child's parents into the therapy situation, to take an inventory of existing pressures and to observe how they affect his fluency. The therapist's "direct" work with the child includes her "direct" work with the parents— the latter work sometimes called "indirect" work with the child. A parent can helpfully work with the therapist in a cotherapist sense, learning to regulate pressures in conversation with the child in the actual therapy situation.

These actual case reports of therapy illustrate how work with a primary stutterer may become a combination of "direct" and "indirect" therapy, integrated and directed by the speech therapist. The following reports were written because the therapist had a large caseload and a schedule serving six schools so that she could not always arrange to give reports orally when they were needed for teachers and parents. Furthermore, written reports enabled her to share and to integrate the information for the several team members who helped this child. Finally, the therapist wished to file the information for future reference.

The following letter, written in answer to a first grade teacher's referral of a primary stutterer, is a report of the therapist's first half-hour diagnostic session with the child. Her investigation, centering around informal conversation using a strip film of animals, also included a classmate with normal speech, who was invited to attend this "movie" in order to insure that the stutterer did not feel he was being singled out by the "speech teacher" because of a speech problem. The letter aims to create a cooperative relationship with the teacher, to orient her with some of the basic principles in helping primary stutterers, and to begin the sharing of practical information concerning this case.

REPORT ON INITIAL EXAMINATION OF SPEECH

Date: Sept. 19, 1967

Child: Larry Stark

Dear Miss Swanson:

This preliminary report contains general information on early-stage stutterers and the policies which are suggested for Larry. It is being sent to you because you are in an important position to observe and to help Larry in matters which determine the trends in his speech and adjustment.

Larry had very few nonfluencies in his first session with me. His nonfluencies were simple repetitions of syllables, words, and speech sounds. In this situation he may have been more fluent than usual, due to the fact that he appeared to be secure and at ease, and no significant speech demands were forced upon him. The presence and participation of the classmate who accompanied him in this first little "movie of animals" was arranged to insure that Larry would not feel that an issue was being made of his way of speaking. Both boys were eager to converse and enjoyed the half-hour period. I was careful not to let either of them realize that speech was under examination. In fact, speech therapy generally should be "indirect" with a "primary" stutterer such as Larry, so as not to foster self-awareness and concern over speech and its nonfluency. With advanced or "secondary" stutterers we usually follow a "direct" and open approach.

I hope and believe that Larry will feel privileged and eager to work with me when I continue therapy with him. His classmate's favorable reaction to that first session of therapy should help to assure Larry that going out "for speech" is suitable for any child and certainly is nothing to be ashamed of.

From our first conference, I'm glad to learn that Larry is willing to take part in your class recitations, reading, etc. So long as speaking is enjoyable or satisfying to him, and so long as he feels that his speech is not a concern to others, his stuttering should not pass into the more serious secondary stages. He will need a conducive atmosphere while he gains added speech security through maturation and the learning of skills needed for normal speech—motor abilities, vocabulary, grammar, etc. Of course, a child's parents and his total home situation hold great responsibilities in maintaining a favorable environment for speech development. In some stutterers' backgrounds, we find that speech standards are too high, that immature speech is criticized, and that various conflicts undermine their personal security and put pressure upon speech.

It's good to see that stutterers in the early stage, where Larry appears to be, are referred for special help of the type we have started. Too often the policy is "Wait and see if they'll outgrow it"—a policy sometimes spoiled by the anxiety and harmful attempts of others to "help." However, the prognosis for a primary stutterer is good if necessary help is recognized and given early enough.

Barbara Lynchfield
Speech Therapist

P.S. A copy of this report is being sent to Larry's parents so that they may cooperate with us in therapy for him. This shared information will also help to prepare us for the joint conference I hope we can arrange with Larry's parents, perhaps at the next regular report-card conference period. I shall consult with you about these arrangements.

Although speech therapists with large caseloads cannot regularly send long reports like Miss Lynchfield's to the teachers and the parents of all cases, the foregoing letter reduced the costs in time and labor by serving the dual purpose of orienting both the teacher and the parents of this primary stutterer in preparation for their teamwork with the therapist.

Following three weeks of work with Larry, the speech therapist arranged a conference with Larry's teacher and parents. Larry's father, a prominent physician, attended the conference with his wife, despite his heavy professional work schedule. His cooperation is evidence that we, as teachers and therapists, should not assume that certain parents in esteemed or learned professions need not or will not come for our conferences over problems of school children. Speech therapists and other professionals in the public schools should avoid addressing their invitations or requests for parental conferences only to the child's mother, even though only a few of the fathers attend the parental conferences, with or without their wives.

In the conference attended by Larry's parents and his teacher, the speech therapist outlined the most probably inciting and maintaining factors in Larry's case and what remedial measures were being taken at school. The teacher explained how some of these measures were being followed in the classroom. Larry's parents revealed that he was "caught in the middle" in many situations, flanked on one side by an older brother and on the other side by younger twin brothers.

As a follow-up of the forty-five minute conference, the therapist sent the parents and the teacher copies of the recommendations, thereby insuring their further coordinated work in helping Larry:

October 4, 1967

Dear Dr. and Mrs. Stark:

The purpose of this letter is to offer information and suggestions which may help in your home-based work to correct Larry's stuttering problem. Some of the recommendations are "standard" ones, considerations which are generally applicable to any young stutterer in any home; some have been proposed specifically to fit Larry's needs, in the light of the information you contributed. However, since I do not know Larry and his home situations as well as you do, it will be your responsibility in the final analysis to determine what shall apply to Larry and how it shall be carried out. Therefore, please consider the following "home remedies" as being suggestive for you, Larry, and his home. They are partly suggestions which have accumulated from experiences with many other young stutterers and their home environments and from parents who have solved similar problems.

Anything you can do to build up Larry's self-pride, self-respect, and sense of self-worth and achievement will not only help to stabilize him and his speech but will also reduce his need to compete with your other children, as you said, for "status in the family." This position, of course, is not easy to achieve because Larry appears to be bracketed at the lower end of the family ladder by a lively and widely admired set of younger twin brothers and overshadowed at the upper level by an older brother who has achieved advanced privileges and achievements. In other words, there may be a special need to convince Larry that he is fully as important and as admired as is everyone else in his family. If so, devices and practices of the following nature may help to convince Larry of this fact:

1. Set up a "bulletin board" in the home where a display of school and home achievements of all the children may be given equal recognition and admiration by parents, visitors, etc. With this skill in art, Larry may have more items to post in this display of his school achievements and may, therefore, have a good chance to "shine" in this opportunity.

2. Give added expressions of your individual affection and companionship shown to each child, while being careful, of course, not to arouse jealousy in the others. Each child needs enjoyable time to be spent individually with each parent. A boy of Larry's age may be in special need of experiences which he can feel are for him and Dad. And little experiences of an everyday nature, such as sharing help on a special home chore or an errand, may be more encouraging to a boy than to take him along to see a circus or a ballgame.

3. Sometimes it proves helpful to create "islands" of security within a home, where each child can exercise individuality in work and in play and where excessive stimulation and interference from the family may be avoided. Also, it is important to provide each child with means for safeguarding his rights of possession by supplying, for example, a personal desk or a set of safe drawers for each person's belongings. In Larry's situation you may find that it will be easier to train and to manage the twins, too, if they are equipped with such physical "props" to help define and to remind them of boundaries.

4. When the younger twins receive comparatively too much of the limelight from admiring and "gushy" visitors, tactfully include commendable remarks about the older boys if they are present. Of course, in situations when visitors indulge in "polite" talk which is embarrassingly personal about a child, he should not be forced to participate.

5. Share as much as possible in the main interests of each child. For instance, your time spent in group reading of story books having mutual interest to Larry and the twins should have several values. Read in a clear and leisurely manner, pausing occasionally to make interesting comments about the story and its pictures, allowing each child equal freedom to interject his comments. Besides receiving auditory patterns of correct and fluent speech from you, Larry will gain personal and social satisfactions in that group situation. In addition, the twins will be influenced to correct the articulatory errors that you reported in their speech.

6. Your report of Larry's being in the "middle" of the sibling picture, and of the improvement noted in his stuttering when his older brother was sent to scout camp last summer, is suggestive of the type of factors which affect stuttering in a young child. You also stated that for this reason you are planning to take the eldest son with you next summer on an extended trip to Europe, leaving Larry and the twins home alone with a housekeeper and "baby-sitter." I presume you have considered that the effects on Larry may not be the same if *you* take his brother on vacation. Although his elder brother

will be removed from the competitive home scene, you will be gone too, taking that chosen brother on what Larry may regard as an enviable trip. Being an eldest child in the remaining part of the family at home might not mean enough to Larry unless enough is done in preparing him, the twins, and others for the experience, to insure them plenty of satisfying home experiences in your absence. It may be advisable to arrange a definitely planned home schedule during your absence. The "baby-sitter" given another title and qualified to take over your responsibilities could be assigned games with them. Perhaps Larry would profit from having a favorite pal lined up to come to spend weekends with him. In fact, it would be safer to give this person access to this same information and counseling that we are trying to evolve and follow for Larry.

As you know, parents sometimes overlook or neglect the need to *prepare* a child for an experience which is likely to be new, exciting, or upsetting, such as the first experience of a funeral, lightning and thunder, surgery, staying in a hospital, attending a horror movie, a wrestling match, a summer camp for children, the arrival of a new baby, and even his first haircut.

You realize also that Larry should not be made directly conscious of *how* he speaks, through corrections, speech advice, or even praise of his speech performance. Parents, relatives, housekeepers, "baby-sitter," etc., should not reveal their concern over his speech by nonverbal means either. Some of these tell-tale negative reactions occur when we glance away or glance at his mouth during stuttering, show worried facial expressions, and let his stuttering divert our attention and communication with him. At times our exaggerated attempts to disregard a child's stuttering will make him feel that we are not interested in what he has to say to us.

If you notice that Larry has more difficulty when tired, excited, ill, etc., tactfully avoid imposing heavy demands upon his speech at these times. Generally let him set his own speech pace.

Of course, we should keep our interruptions in conversation as infrequent as possible, and we should not try to "help" by finishing statements when nonfluency strikes a child. He should be unhurried and should feel that he has a good chance of finishing any sentence he starts. A calm and unhurried conversational manner by parents will tend to foster a similar manner in children.

Avoid the tendency to ask Larry questions which are likely to require long and involved answers. Also, word your questions so that they may be readily understood and answered satisfactorily in a short and specific way, if he desires.

For example, greeting a tense child returning from an active day at school with the broad question, "Well, what did you do in school today?" may be bidding for nonfluency in him. We adults get a mild taste of this feeling of being disorganized or inadequate when we're confronted with that vague greeting, "Whadya know?"

Try to be ready to pay attention to Larry in conversation so that he won't be burdened with the necessity of repeating what he says. Generally more difficulty occurs when a person must repeat himself.

Parents of young stutterers should regularly get together privately to compare notes on their child's problem and progress and to plan their cooperative roles in procedures for future correction.

If this letter has seemed presumptive in some of its suggestions, it is because I do not fully know Larry's situation at home but am following the principle that nothing should be taken for granted when a young stutterers' welfare may be at stake.

Please feel free to call on me for any reason. Although Larry's problem has not yet reached serious stages, I certainly want to attend to any details which will help him to develop more normal fluency rather than more nonfluency and the complications which could develop.

Sincerely,

Barbara Lynchfield
Speech Therapist

P.S. In accordance with our agreement at the conference, a copy of this letter is being sent to Larry's teacher, Mrs. Martinson, who has similar needs for this information in our team approach to improve Larry's speech.

A speech therapist sent the following report to a classroom teacher who had been overly critical of the nonfluency shown in two of her second-grade pupils whom she had referred for speech examination:

REPORT ON INITIAL SPEECH EXAMINATION

Date: Sept. 18, 1967

Pupils: Wilbur Matson
　　　　Charles Post

Dear Mrs. Parsons:

Although my observations of Wilbur and Charles were made in a testing situation which was informal and enjoyable for them, where they felt relatively at ease and free of pressures which tend to aggravate nonfluency and stuttering, there were enough factors present to test their fluency.

In contrast to the symptoms which characterize a full-fledged stutterer, these boys did *not* show the following traits:

　　1. *Reluctance to talk.* Fortunately, both of the boys had a reasonable degree of willingness to enter into conversation, to answer questions, and to read for me.

　　2. *Personal awareness and social concern over speech difficulty.* Fortunately, neither boy reacted in any way which would indicate that speaking is a special problem to him. Neither showed any fear, shame, or anxiety concerning speech itself.

　　3. *Force and unusual tension at the moment of nonfluencies.* Fortunately, both boys had relatively few nonfluencies, and these were easy, short, and simple, without forceful effort and abnormal movements.

　　4. *Complexity of nonfluencies in other respects.* Fortunately, neither boy showed that his "primary" type of simple repetitions of sounds, syllables, words, and phrases had become overlaid with facial contortions, abnormal breathing reactions, gestures, a changed rate of speech, altered pitch, etc. In other words, their nonfluencies resembled those which are found in varying degrees in all children of this age and even in adults. Repetitions ranged from few to moderate in frequency, depending upon the emotional and communicative pressures of the moment. They also showed the normal tendency of having relatively more repetitions of phrases, words, and syllables than of single sounds, and rarely did they have prolongations of sounds.

　　I did get the impression that Wilbur has a rather sensitive nature. At one point, when the discussion became crowded and when one of the four boys who were brought into the test situation became overly competitive in interrupting and monopolizing the conversation, Wilbur appeared rebuffed, had some tears, and temporarily withdrew from the conversation.

As I previously stated, the informal and easy speech situation of this examination does not give a complete basis for evaluating the limits of the boys' speech skills, their attitudes, and adjustments. Therefore, it will be important to have your continued evaluations of them in terms of the above-listed points, which discriminate primary "stutterers" from genuine secondary-type stutterers. If you find definite contrasts to my observations, please keep notes on them for our information and follow-up.

However, I do not feel that either of these boys has reached a point which warrants out-of-class individual work in therapy. You and their future teachers, and their parents, are likely to be in the best positions to help them in ways which you may well know, such as:

1. By not making an issue of their nonfluency.

2. By building their general security, personal respect, and satisfactions from achievements of all sorts, especially in speech communication.

3. By trying to avoid or to reduce the conditions which cause and increase their nonfluency, such as imposing hurry or time-limits upon their recitation and reading; trying to "help" by saying their blocked words; creating a build-up of too much anticipation and excitement in recitation; calling on them for communication which is likely to be threatening or unsure in their minds; asking them questions which are likely to require long, involved, and disorganized replies; giving them specific advice or "pointers" on how to talk without stuttering, etc.

I shall arrange a conference with the parents of each of these boys in order to check on their home situations and to insure that their parents are on the right track.

On behalf of Wilbur and Charles, I thank you for your interest and action in these matters.

Sincerely,

Grant Starbuck
Speech Therapist

P.S. I am enclosing two copies of this report so that you may file a copy in each of the boys' folders. I've written this initial report as a joint one, to save time and work which would be duplicated in giving separate reports, since the present information and recommendations apply to both boys. If future reports on either boy are needed, they will be separate.

It is apparent that the complex and time-consuming role of the speech therapist in helping primary stutterers often requires a series of conferences with parents and teachers and the preparation of written instructions and reports. If a public school therapist has a required caseload of seventy-five or more clients, it is difficult or impossible for her to give many primary stutterers the full attention that they deserve. Our preceding discussion of the extent of a therapist's direct work with a primary stutterer, as well as with his teacher, parents, and others, indicates that more time is needed to work on the problem of primary stuttering than on cases of ordinary misarticulation, which comprises most of the problems in a caseload. Nevertheless, the importance of working to correct stuttering in its early stages, before it becomes fixed into relatively incurable lifetime handicaps, fully justifies our spending this extra time and work with primary stutterers and other cases in special need of team-work with teachers, parents, nurses, doctors, psychologists, counselors, etc. If speech therapists are required to serve an excessive number of cases, they may tend to neglect special problems which require supervision and coordination of this teamwork.

The Therapist's Role with Secondary Stutterers

For stutterers who have advanced to secondary stages, therapy is both "indirect" and "direct." But until the therapist has examined the child and has reason to believe that he is a "secondary" stutterer, therapy for him should proceed cautiously, on the assumption that he may be "primary," still unaware, unconcerned, and nonreactive with respect to his speech nonfluency. Even after the client is found to be "secondary," therapy continues to respect the same basic goals and principles that encourage fluent speech in anyone, stutterer and nonstutterer alike. The difference in therapy for the secondary stutterer arises from the fact that he is already self-aware, concerned, and reactive toward the abnormality and handicap of his stuttering.

For the secondary stutterer the therapy must be factual and honest. It must determine and respectfully acknowledge how he feels toward his stuttering and what he is doing because of these feelings, help him to correct his misconceptions, relieve tensions over speech, and eliminate reactions which handicap his communication, often complicated by involuntary habits which can cause him to feel helpless and hopeless about speaking. Therefore, therapy for the secondary stutterer often requires difficult and qualified work in the area of mental hygiene, with some direct psychotherapy to weaken or change the attitudes which feed undesirable reactions and create the bulk of his handicap.

A speech therapist's "direct" work with a secondary stutterer should be individualized according to the factors and behavioral patterns which fit each stutterer. One must guard against a tendency to categorize and generalize concerning a stutterer's needs and treatment. Because of the fact that the speech therapist's direct work with secondary stutterers is individualized and specialized in its mechanics, we shall not attempt to detail it. Instead, parents and teachers who work with a stutterer should keep in close contact with the speech therapist, to learn her specific goals and approaches for his unique case. By so doing, teachers and parents can help the therapist by supplying information needed for therapy. They can help by learning what to expect and what not to expect of each stutterer as he proceeds under his therapist's direction; they can give him encouragement and opportunities for therapeutic practices.

The following exchange of reports presents examples of thoughts and procedures which enter into the referral, examination, and therapy procedures for a second-grade pupil who has become a secondary type of stutterer.

REFERRAL FOR SPEECH EXAMINATION

Date: Feb. 2, 1967

Pupil: Stanley Pratt

Dear Mr. Whelan:

Stanley Pratt, who transferred into our school two weeks ago, has shown symptoms of stuttering. Because he missed your screening survey of my pupils at the beginning of the year, and because his problem appears to need special attention, I am referring him to you.

I have made the following observations of Stanley's classroom behavior during the past two weeks:

Stanley enjoys sharing with the class in all activities except when they involve lengthy speaking. He does not have trouble in reading, but in recitation and in conversation with me he has difficulty. He uses many accessory body movements to help release the blocks. At times, he voices his inability to speak fluently—with such comments as *Oh*.

The children in the room have not criticized or ridiculed Stanley or his speech, as far as I can detect.

Stanley has an urge to tell "stories" about his father. Last Friday he shared a ball with the group, saying that his father had given it to him. He kept the ball in his desk, taking it out to play at recess time. Later it came out that that ball belonged to the school and that he had found it on the playground the previous day.

Within the past few days Stanley has spent most of the recess time affectionately holding my hand. He is constantly striving for attention within the room, often annoying the other children. He prefers to stay after school at night, helping me in the room rather than going home. After leaving school, he frequently goes other places rather than home. It could be that his home situation needs improvement too.

Sincerely,

Alvina Stine
Teacher, Grade Two

The speech therapist promptly responded to the teacher's request for help by arranging a visit to her classroom to observe this pupil's speech behavior in regular classroom situations. Following this preliminary observation of the child, the therapist scheduled an individual examination in order to check on behavioral items which could not be tested in the group setting of the classroom. The following report of the therapist's findings was sent to the child's teacher:

INITIAL REPORT OF SPEECH EXAMINATION

Date: Feb. 8, 1967

Pupil: Stanley Pratt

Dear Mrs. Stine:

This report will cover my first two observational periods with Stanley: the scheduled visit to your classroom and the diagnostic period which I arranged to have with him alone.

While Stanley was talking in the classroom, I noticed several speech symptoms and reactions which definitely indicated that he has advanced beyond the primary stage of stuttering. He is obviously aware of his speech deviations and has begun to adopt ways to avoid and minimize his nonfluency. Some of his apparent devices are to pause or to inhale deeply before starting a word on which he anticipates stuttering. And he usually did stutter after these pauses or inhalations. I noticed also that he spent force and accessory body movements to break blocks, as you stated in your referral letter.

Approximately one-half of his nonfluencies were silent prolongations—postures of the initial speech-sounds of words, with a suppression of voice. Other nonfluencies were repetitions of sounds, syllables, words, and phrases. There is also evidence that he is adopting unnatural inflection patterns, a special rate of talking, and inconsistent ways to approach blocks, such as saying "ah" or "oh" during the pauses before tackling them. The nature of his blocks, too, suggests that Stanley's stuttering is of a secondary type— proof that he is well aware of it as a problem and is trying to do things to help himself.

Despite the foregoing symptoms that reveal that Stanley has advanced beyond the primary stages of stuttering, I was glad to see that in that classroom situation there were no signs or immediate causes of social maladjustment. He was willing to talk in class even though his stuttering was a personal problem from the standpoint of his speech mechanics. He did not hesitate to volunteer speech. He appeared to say what he set out to say, without abbreviating or altering his language because of stuttering. Although the children appeared to notice his stuttering, they did not react in ways that would provoke more stuttering and social maladjustment. Their calm, matter-of-fact acceptance of Stan and his speech is undoubtedly a reflection of the same wholesome adjustment that they see in your attitudes and actions toward him.

In my private diagnostic session with Stanley, I found that he has developed definite feelings about his speech problem. He explained how people have tried to help him and how he has tried to help himself. However, he did not express any blame or resentment toward others and their attempts to help. He seemed to be glad to know that I was a speech teacher who would help him talk more easily.

In accordance with your observations of Stanley, I also noticed the unusually strong tendency to bid for recognition and companionship. His willingness to be scheduled with me for therapy may be due partly to this social need. In my arranged conference with Stanley's parents, I plan to explore this apparent lack of emotional or social security which, of course, may be an important factor in his stuttering, and I shall work upon it.

Stanley will be scheduled for therapy on Tuesday and Thursday from 10:30 to 11:00, starting February 21. If these times create conflicts for you, I shall make different arrangements.

I appreciate your referral of Stanley's speech problem to me and shall keep you informed of our therapy developments. This case appears to be one in which progress will depend upon cooperative efforts by parents, teacher, and therapist.

Sincerely,

Charles Whelan
Speech Therapist

After a month of therapy, which included a conference with Stanley's parents, the speech therapist sent the following report to his teacher:

THERAPY REPORT # 1

Date: March 23, 1967

Pupil: Stanley Pratt

Dear Mrs. Stine:

This report is a summary of therapy with Stanley since it began on February 21. It also contains some recommendations, which are becoming more evident as understanding and work on this case continue.

First, I shall give the main points concerning my first conference with Stan's parents. They showed interest in his stuttering and therapy. I briefly outlined the subject of the disorder and referred them to some specific books and pamphlets to study and relate to Stan's situation. But I also plan to arrange monthly conferences with them and to offer specific information on ways they can help. For example, Mr. Pratt admitted that he doesn't spend enough time with Stan, who idolizes his father and tags after him whenever he can. We planned a move whereby the father will share Stan's strong interest in airplanes: to provide the boy with some model-building kits; to get and share some illustrated library books on planes which the father flew in World War II; and to make Stan feel that his father really respects and enjoys this and other mutual companionships with his son who, as you know, is the only child in the family.

The parents' information concerning Stan's stuttering and their attempts to help him gave me a good opportunity to counsel them on how to react to his stuttering, how Stan should react to his stuttering, and how I shall be working to teach him to speak and to handle stuttering more freely and cleanly—without resorting to the handicapping avoidances and devices which the parents admitted they were telling him to use when he encountered stuttering or its fear. They were relieved to learn what they should do and what they should not do. For instance, both parents had been enforcing a well-meant policy of reminding Stan to "Stop, take a deep breath, and start over" whenever he stuttered. They now realize that their urging him to "Try to speak more carefully" might have caused him to become more anxious and tense and to expend more force and struggle in encountering his stuttering blocks. I explained that our goals for Stanley would be to make him less impatient and less intolerant of his stuttering, for him to study it and work upon stuttering as a student in science would—as an interesting phenomenon of behavior that may be improved through readjustment and learning. I also pointed out to the parents that unless they too adopted this view of Stan's stuttering, he would find it difficult to do so.

My direct work with Stan this past month has centered around the above-mentioned goals which were explained to the parents. In the first place, Stan has shown relief from the chance I have given him to express his frank feelings about stuttering and to tell of troublesome speech experiences. Apparently he has had personal thoughts about his stuttering but too often has had to keep them to himself. Some of his thoughts are realistic; some are misconceptions, such as the beliefs that something was wrong with his tongue and that stuttering was inevitable. He has shown relief after learning that he can have control over his stuttering in ways that reduce its abnormality and penalty.

He expresses greater confidence in talking and in meeting prospects of stuttering. Consequently, he has fewer moments of stuttering, with less need to employ his new skills.

In my conference with you the other day, I demonstrated how Stan is controlling his moments of stuttering and suggested that you find opportune ways to compliment and remind him of his "smoother," "nicer" way of stuttering. In our compliments about his progress, we must be careful, of course, not to make him feel that he should work *directly* toward having *fewer moments* of stuttering. He should be kept reminded that reduced stuttering will come as rewards from his work with it, not against it. Otherwise, Stan may resort to his old policy of trying to avoid stuttering at all, a policy which leads to more and more stuttering and its complications.

I shall arrange a conference with Stan's parents concerning this information and their cooperative roles with us in these matters.

Sincerely,

Charles Whelan
Speech Therapist

The foregoing reports have given some hints on how a speech therapist may work directly and indirectly on a case of secondary stuttering. It is important to remember that therapy, like the teaching of reading, involves a combination of factors and principles and that individuals differ in how their particular combinations of needs are most effectively met. The therapist usually proceeds through trial and error, following her most educated guesses, testing the results as objectively as possible, and realizing that success and credit for results depend upon a joint endeavor by the client, the therapist, his teacher, parents, and others. As in the teaching of reading, the therapist and the teacher serve largely as catalysts, providers of opportunities and materials, stage-setters, supporters, and suppliers of the special aids that may be needed. And as in the teaching of reading, parents lay the foundation and give help along the way. But, as in reading, the child is the one who must gain the inspiration, who somehow must master the patterns of adjustment and skill, and who must enjoy the rewards.

Additional information on the nature and treatment of stuttering is available from books by such authorities as Van Riper,[4] Johnson,[5] Robinson,[6] Luper and Mulder,[7] and others.

References

1. C. Van Riper, *Speech Correction: Principles and Methods.* Englewood Cliffs, N.J.: Prentice-Hall, Inc., 1963.

2. W. Johnson (ed.), *Stuttering in Children and Adults.* Minneapolis: University of Minnesota Press, 1955.

3. C. S. Bluemel, *The Riddle of Stuttering.* Danville, Ill.: The Interstate Publishing Co., 1957.

4. Van Riper, *Speech Correction: Principles and Methods.*

5. W. Johnson, *Stuttering and What You Can Do About It.* Garden City, N.Y.: Dolphin Books, 1961.

6. Frank B. Robinson, *Introduction to Stuttering.* Englewood Cliffs, N.J.; Prentice-Hall, Inc., 1964.

7. H. L. Luper and R. L. Mulder, *Stuttering Therapy for Children.* Englewood Cliffs, N.J.: Prentice-Hall, Inc., 1964.

Questions

1. To what extent must speech therapists and classroom teachers cooperate for best results?

2. Which is more important: recognition of the positive factors which encourage fluency, or knowledge of conditions which deny fluency?

3. Is stammering the same as stuttering?

4. Define *overt* and *covert* stuttering.

5. What stages of development are usual in stuttering?

6. Describe the stage of development of a stutterer you know.

7. Name three reactions which may precede the moment of blockage. What reactions may occur during the moment of block?

8. What are some causes of poor fluency?

9. What classroom pressures may damage fluency?

10. Is there a connection between left-handedness and stuttering?

11. Is stuttering hereditary?

12. Contrast the stutterer's opportunities for help in school twenty years ago and now.

13. If you had been Jimmy's first teacher, how would you have handled him?

14. Describe the value of group dynamics in speech therapy.

15. How may stuttering affect personality? Physical health? Social traits?

16. Explain: "Handicaps from stuttering spread in cancerous ways."

17. Why is honesty the best policy in dealing with stutterers?

18. Does the presence of a school therapist guarantee adequate supervision of stutterers?

19. What are the danger signs indicating that a child's nonfluencies are developing into stuttering?

20. What is the parents' responsibility in the diagnosis of stuttering?

21. What behavior indicates transition into the secondary stage of stuttering?

22. What are the effects on the stutterer of his avoiding speech because of his stuttering?

23. What excuses do parents and teachers make for not referring suspected cases of stuttering?

24. What are some danger signs in the child which indicate the need for referral?

25. Is there significance in the recognition of the danger signs by the child's associates?

26. Where is speech therapy available at: (1) the local level; (2) the county level; (3) the state level; (4) the university level; (5) national level?

27. What is the responsibility of the speech therapist for information on how to refer problems for aid?

28. Is diagnosis as important as therapy?

29. Is speech therapy an exact science? Explain.

30. How would you discuss a stutterer's problem with a father like Carl's?

31. What personality traits are especially valuable in a speech therapist?

32. Discuss the dangers in the indiscriminate application of procedures and sequences to individual cases.

33. How would you try to persuade an unwilling stutterer to speak in class?

34. Define "direct" and "indirect" goals.

35. Suppose you are working with two stutterers. With one, your personalities clash. With the other, you work smoothly together. On which stutterer would you tend to concentrate your efforts and to spend more time?

36. What is "indirect" therapy?

37. How would you protect a primary stutterer from speech anxieties?

38. Is stuttering the result of abnormal pressures?

39. Describe some controllable school situations which discourage speech fluency.

40. In what way is mastery of grammar a challenge to fluency?

41. What may be the effect on fluency of the teacher's failure to observe adult listening etiquette with children?

42. Describe some audience reactions which penalize speech.

43. How would you counsel a stutterer to accept teasing and laughing about his defect?

44. How can the teacher avoid pressures to hurry speech?

45. How can a lack of opportunity to get something off his chest harm a person's speech fluency?

46. Why must teachers work *with* the stutterer, not *for* and *without* him?

47. A stutterer usually becomes fluent while speaking in unison with others. What does this fact reveal about the handicap?

48. What physical conditions may discourage speech?

49. How may conflicting language standards affect fluency in minority group children?

50. How may noise level in the classroom affect fluency?

51. What goals and policies will earn the therapist a good relationship with child, parents, and classroom teachers?

52. Describe the methods by which the therapist may realize his goals and policies for primary stutterers.

53. How do referral, examination, and therapy practices differ for secondary types of stutterers?

54. "The therapist usually proceeds through trial and error." Is speech therapy likely to develop into a more exact science?

Suggested Subjects for Term Papers

1. As a speech therapist, how would you rate and advise the following class-room teachers on their attitudes and methods of dealing with stutterers?
   a. "Oh, I just dread having Wilbur in class next fall! Stuttering makes me so nervous!"
   b. "Well, of course, I give him higher grades than he probably deserves. He knows it, I'm sure, but at least I'm going to act civilized to a poor stutterer."
   c. "Yes, that's my little stutterer, mounting drawings for me. Shh. Don't let him hear us talking about him. This way, staying after school, he escapes that darn bully Bob from the sixth grade too!"
   d. "Heavens, yes! If I didn't finish saying what poor Lanny is trying to get out, we'd all die of boredom!"
   e. "Children, we have a celebrity with us. Did you read in the *Times* that Joe won *first prize* in handling his cocker spaniel at the Kennel Club meet Saturday?"
   f. "Just how can *he* be in plays and such! He won't be speaking a word

when all the rest have their lines said. And he just stands there like a sore thumb!"

    g. "I beg to differ! We are all creatures of habit, Miss Jones! If Bobby gets the habit of never talking in class, that's surely worse for him. Break the ice, I say! Force him to begin talking!"

2. Write an article on: "Is Stuttering Funny?" Try sending it to national magazines.
3. Summarize research on neurological aspects of stuttering.
4. Interview ten parents and write up their views on the causes of stuttering and how they would handle a child who stutters.
5. Interview ten teachers and write up their views on the causes of stuttering and how they would handle a stutterer in the classroom.

nine

Helping the Child
with a Hearing Problem

To even the casual layman it is obvious that hearing is essential for speech. An examination of the normal development of speech from infancy indicates that hearing is a primary and continuing factor in the acquisition, use, and maintenance of spoken language. When speech or language problems occur, a qualified evaluation of hearing is one of the first recommended steps in their diagnosis. Therefore, speech correction generally requires that speech pathologists and audiologists cooperate closely in speech and hearing centers. The consideration given to hearing in the diagnosis and treatment of speech disorders is also revealed by the fact that audiologists, speech pathologists, and speech therapists share in the membership, qualifications, and activities of their joint national organization, the American Speech and Hearing Association. The training of speech therapists in university centers would not be complete without requiring some foundational courses and practice in the diagnosis and treatment of hearing problems as they relate to speech.

Hearing problems are often misinterpreted: many are overlooked or misunderstood while they seriously affect a person in various insidious ways. It has been estimated that from 5 to 7 per cent of the three million or more schoolchildren in the United States suffer some hearing impairment which handicaps communication and adjustment and which retards a pupil's school progress by one grade in eight. The hearing problems of many of these children will go unnoticed because some states do not yet have compulsory programs for testing hearing. Testing is not uniformly valid or thorough with follow-up services for children who are tested and found to be defective. Because there has always been a serious shortage of special teachers, classes, and schools for the severely handicapped cases of deafness or hearing loss, most children with hearing problems attend regular classrooms and are handled by regular teachers. This inclusion of children with hearing problems within regular classrooms requires not only that all teachers should be aided by speech therapists and others but also that they deserve some basic training in the recognition and treatment of hearing problems in their classrooms.

The Hearing Process and Its
Related Problems

Hearing, which has been called a "glorified sense of touch," involves a highly specialized and complicated process whereby sound vibrations are successfully transmitted through the outer, middle, and inner mechanisms of the ear and finally are sent along neural circuits which are linked with brain centers where the incited patterns of stimuli are perceptually interpreted as the meaningful patterns which represent our spoken language, for example. Three types of sound-wave transmissions occur in this process: the acoustical entry of air-waves into the outer ear; a conversion of the airborne patterns of energy into mechanical vibrations, which are conducted via the membranes and bones of the middle ear; then the action by fluid-waves within the inner ear where the hair-cells of the sensory organ of hearing are stimulated, mysteriously converting the mechanical patterns of stimulation into the neural patterns of excitation that are transmitted to the brain and are meaningfully interpreted. Disorders may occur at different points along this highly specialized pathway.

The following types of hearing problems will be discussed with reference to this process of hearing.

CONDUCTIVE HEARING LOSSES

Conductive losses in hearing occur when there is a poor transmission of the sound energy patterns to the sense organ in the inner ear. This type of hearing problem may be caused by impacted wax or foreign objects which obstruct the passage of airborne vibrations through the outer ear canal to the eardrum, which in turn transmits the energy of the sound waves to the chain of tiny bones in the middle ear. Or the further conduction of the sound vibrations may be impaired by imperfections of the eardrum or by an abnormal presence of fluid within the middle ear chamber or by disease or damage to the delicate bones which mechanically conduct the sound stimuli patterns from the vibrating eardrum to the flexible membrane of the oval window, the boundary of the inner ear. Although the conduction of sound waves continues beyond this oval window into the fluid system which surrounds and activates the inner ear's nerve-connected organs of hearing and equilibrium, "conductive" losses of hearing will arbitrarily refer to impairments of conduction up to the oval window boundary of the inner ear.

Hearing losses which are purely of the conductive type are characterized in several ways. They cause a reduction in the person's hearing acuity of airborne sounds, although hearing by bone conduction, through the skull or mastoid structure, is not impaired because in hearing through bone conduction the vibrations of sound are not dependent upon clear passage through the outer and middle ear. Moreover, in conductive losses, the person's loss of acuity is not as great as it may be in losses which result from damage to the nerve structures of hearing. In losses which are solely conductive, the perceptual impairment is commonly characterized by a lowered level of the sound's loudness or quantity but without any loss of quality and without distortion of the auditory patterns. Therefore, the conductive type of deafness may be determined by audiometric tests which measure the extent and profile pattern of the sound losses and rate the person's ability to hear through air conduction in comparison with that from bone conduction. In addition, otological examination determines not only the nature and location of the conductive loss within the outer or middle parts of the ear but may often provide surgery or medical treatment to correct losses which are of the conductive type. However, medical or surgical corrections of sensory-neural impairment are generally impossible.

SENSORY–NEURAL IMPAIRMENT OF
HEARING

In this type of hearing problem, there is damage or deterioration of the organ of hearing within the inner ear or of its auditory nerve composed of thousands of highly specialized delicate neurological structures. Losses of the sensory-neural type may occur in all degrees of severity, ranging from a slight reduction of perceptual ability to a profound or sometimes total failure to hear. Usually, however, there is some residual hearing even in cases of profound hearing losses. Residual hearing, however slight it may be, is an important factor in rehabilitation.

Unlike the relatively uniform pattern of loss in the conductive type of hearing disorders, the typical audiogram of sensory-neural impairments shows an irregular pattern of losses along the range of sound frequencies which are heard. A pupil with sensory-neural impairment may hear speech in a distorted fashion because he may hear some phonemes clearly and loudly enough while other speech sounds are heard faintly or not at all. Such a condition may be difficult and even impossible to fit with a hearing aid. For the determination and handling of sensory-neural problems of hearing, it is also important to consult qualified audiologists, otologists, and speech pathologists.

Sensory-neural deafness or hearing losses may be caused by such infectious diseases as measles, scarlet fever, influenza, meningitis, pneumonia, whooping cough, diphtheria, and Ménière's disease. At the third month of embryological development, the ear, eye, and nervous system are especially vulnerable to viruses in such infectious diseases as German measles, mumps, and influenza. Damage to the delicate sensory organ of hearing or to its nerve circuits may result from noise or brain injury. Hearing loss may, therefore, be associated with cerebral palsy. Hearing may degenerate from the toxic effects of certain drugs and poisons and from Rh incompatibility. Finally, in the elderly person there is a sensory-neural deterioration from the process of aging. However, with all these various sensory-neural factors, the degrees and patterns of hearing impairment are highly individualistic. No two persons with sensory-neural impairments show identical audiograms and handicaps to speech and other forms of behavior.

MIXED CONDUCTIVE AND SENSORY–NEURAL IMPAIRMENT

A hearing problem of the "mixed" type with both a conductive loss and a sensory-neural loss may affect a pupil with a congenitally based impairment of hearing and added hearing loss from such conductive factors as ear infections which rupture his eardrums or damage the conductive mechanism of his middle ear. A person's threshold of acuity may be lowered by more than one causal factor within the same type of impairment. For instance, a sensory-neural type of hearing loss resulting from noise trauma or aging may later complicate the original problem of congenital damage to the neural structures of hearing. Or a schoolchild's conductive loss from perforated eardrums may be heightened by impacted wax in the outer ear or by infectious or noninfectious fluids in the middle ear. The fact that problems may become worse should remind parents, teachers, therapists, and others that a pupil with a hearing impairment should be carefully supervised so that other preventable complications do not add to his original hearing problem.

OTHER TYPES OF HEARING IMPAIRMENTS

Davis and Silverman[1] describe other types of hearing impairments which do not fit under the more common categories of conductive and sensory-neural problems already discussed in this chapter. Under the label *central dysacusis*, they include hearing disorders which lie somewhere in the central nervous system beyond the inner ear and its auditory nerve. The higher nerve centers of hearing may be affected by brain diseases and tumors, cerebral damage from hemorrhages, thromboses, embolisms, skull fractures, and birth injuries. Hearing disorders caused by cortical damage may take various forms. In *verbal dysacusis*, commonly called *receptive aphasia*, the person has clear acuity of the sounds of speech but he cannot hear the sounds as meaningful speech.

While most cases of deafness result from organic faults, some are functional or psychogenic with symptoms of personality aberrations or of emotional conflicts which may lead to hysteria, with resulting conversions or malingering in the sensory areas of hearing, sight, and other behavioral functions. This type of hearing disorder is relatively rare in children, however.

The diagnosis of functional deafness should not be attempted by laymen. It requires a team approach by qualified professionals—the audiologist, otologist, psychologist, and psychiatrist.

How Hearing Impairments
Affect Pupils

Although impaired hearing causes many problems for the schoolchild, parents, teachers, and others often do not understand that the hearing impairment is the primary cause of those difficulties. We may readily accept statistical reports that hearing problems lead to school retardation, faulty speech articulation, abnormal voice patterns, difficulties in language acquisition, social maladjustments, personality problems, etc. But when we come across a particular case of impaired hearing, such as a pupil with a moderate degree of conductive loss, we may blame his inattention and poor performance in the classroom upon "immaturity," "laziness," "mental retardation," and so on.

In the following samples of how hearing disorders may affect pupils, it should be remembered that there is no truly typical case of a hearing problem. Physiologically, psychologically, and socially, each case is unique with respect to the pattern and extent of the disorder. We cannot fully predict or judge a pupil's hearing handicap by merely consulting his audiogram. The uniqueness of each case's handicap from a hearing defect becomes more evident as we gather information on the case from a variety of contributing sources.

The following high school student tells how his moderate binaural loss of hearing interfered with his academic achievement and social life:

My hearing loss developed before I was in the fifth grade. When my hearing was first tested, we lived in a poorly supported school district. My family couldn't afford to give us eight children the medical and dental care we needed. I remember having lots of bad earaches in my childhood. After days of steady aching, my ears would start running, and then I'd feel better. Those earaches were caused by infections which destroyed my eardrums and the middle part of my ears. But before I learned that my eardrums were perforated and that I shouldn't get water in my ears, I went swimming. During swimming season I had earaches all the time. Now I can swim without trouble because I wear earplugs.

I was big for my age, and teachers usually seated me in the back of the classrooms. It was hard enough for me to hear some of the teachers even when I was close to them, but when I had to sit way in the back of the room, I usually gave up trying to understand what teachers said. It was harder to understand my classmates' recitations from back there too. I depended a lot on lip reading, and when they spoke softly with their backs turned to me, I was completely lost. I was often scolded for not paying attention when I didn't reply to a question or could not repeat an answer someone else had given. But I tried to let on that I was interested in things, even though I didn't know what was going on. I know that most of the teachers thought I was dumb, and some of the kids told me I was dumb. I thought I was dumb too. The teachers and my parents also scolded me for being lazy.

Later, we moved to this city, where we had much better schools. But I found that some of my old problems followed me here. Some of the teachers still put me in the back of the room. And when I got into the upper grades and high school, I preferred to be seated in the back for other reasons. I felt less conspicuous there. I had a hard time to hear some teachers because they didn't talk loud enough or because they had the habit of talking while they were turned toward the blackboard or something. My social life was not too good either, partly because I'm a Negro and the school was run mostly for whites. But I had a few close friends who understood that I had trouble hearing, and they helped me fit into their conversation.

In my junior year of high school, a new speech therapist came to our school. He found out that I was hard of hearing and had several conferences with me to talk over my problem and tell me how the problem might be helped. I liked him because he was honest with me. He talked me into trying out a hearing aid, explaining that he could arrange to get me an aid without cost through a state agency—an aid that wouldn't be conspicuous either. I agreed to give it a try. I wish I had had an aid sooner. I hadn't realized how much I was missing in class and outside of class too. My grades have improved this past year, and I have more friends. Even the teachers seem to respect me more. This hearing aid should make a big difference in the jobs I can handle.

The next college student, who suffered severe sensory-neural damage from German measles before her birth, tells of her hearing problems in school and how she has overcome some of her handicaps:

My hearing loss has been so extensive that it was noticed soon after I was born. Fortunately, we lived in a community which supports a modern speech and hearing center where residents of the surrounding counties may get excellent professional diagnoses, advice, and rehabilitative services. My parents received counseling and demonstrations on how to teach me to compensate for my inability to hear. The center gave me preschool speech therapy and practice in lip reading. They also gave my parents instructions in how to help me speak and lip-read better. My hearing loss was too great to justify getting a hearing aid for me to wear regularly, but the speech therapist did use amplification devices in some of the training she gave me in speech and lip reading.

I was also fortunate to be in a school system which has a special school where teachers trained in the education of the deaf, blind, and physically crippled children continued with the special help which had begun at the speech and hearing center during my preschool years. In addition to all the special services and facilities, this special school teaches a well-balanced curriculum of regular public school subjects. In fact, this special school aims as soon as possible to transfer its pupils into the city's regular schools to continue education with normal children in their classrooms. I was transferred into my neighborhood school when I reached the sixth grade.

In looking back over my school years, I don't think I've been generally handicapped in my school or private life. Oh, there have been activities I couldn't do, but I think I've made up for those difficulties in other ways. I've had to work harder by doing more reading and writing than other pupils have had to do. Consequently, my language skills, except for speech, are graded higher than average. Socially, I've not been handicapped. I've always had plenty of good friends. My parents have followed the policy of letting me have the same responsibilities and experiences which girls with normal hearing have. That's important. I've the chance to find out for myself what I can do and what I can't do. At times I've surprised myself by learning how to do things despite my deafness. I really think that for the most part my deafness has given me a life with many extra challenges and that most of them have been met. I expect to get married and have a happy family life. With my type of deafness, there's no danger of passing it along to my children. My faulty speech may be a handicap in training a child to talk, but I'll find ways to avoid that danger and to compensate for my speech deficiency.

The next youth, who dropped out of school in the ninth grade, has a different story:

No, I wouldn't go back to school for anything. When you can't hear what goes on in school, why should you? I had meningitis when I was four. Since that time I've had a hard time to hear anything unless it's really loud, like a siren or thunder. And the things I hear don't sound the way they should, I guess. My grades have been poor in school, but I think the teachers have passed me along just to get me out of their way more than anything.

Everyone pretty much left me alone. I'm not bad at lip reading, except when people don't look at me when they talk. It's really easier for me to understand strangers before they know I'm deaf. After people find out I'm deaf, they sometimes stop talking natural and even stop talking with me at all. It burns me up to have people getting bothered and feeling sorry for me. That's why some of the teachers have left me alone.

Helping the Hard-of-Hearing Pupil

Although a classroom teacher may not be a specialist in the education of deaf and hard-of-hearing children, she may help these children in many direct and indirect ways. The hearing problems must be recognized, and at times the classroom teacher is in position to be the first person to recognize it. An adequate diagnosis of the problem must be made and a flexible plan of treatment formulated and followed. Consequently, the classroom teacher must be equipped with information about the various symptoms which may indicate hearing impairments. She must know the procedures for referral and sometimes must be the one to take the initiative in insuring that an adequate diagnosis is obtained for the pupil. The teacher should have a basic understanding of the results and recommendations of the audiological examination. Finally, the teacher must fulfill the pupil's special needs while also attending to his general educational program.

To meet these requirements, a teacher must know the special policies, techniques, and equipment for handling the pupil with a hearing problem. She must have the ingenuity to adapt all of this specialization within her regular role in the school's total program. It is obvious that a regular classroom teacher faces many challenges and deserves all possible assistance when a hard-of-hearing child is included in a regular curriculum with a full class of pupils with normal hearing. Because of the fact that a pupil's hearing problem usually requires the cooperative support of parents and others, the teacher may become the central figure in this team approach to the problem. Acting cooperatively with such team members as the audiologist and speech therapist, the teacher is often in the best position to offer parents information and guidance in the policies and procedures at school and at home.

There are several practical reasons for a regular classroom teacher's obligation to assume the added special responsibilities which confront her when a deaf or hard-of-hearing pupil is included in her class with other pupils who have normal hearing. A grade or school with only one or two children with hearing problems has too few cases to justify the formation of a special class or school with special teachers for handling them. Moreover, there has always been a severe shortage of special teachers for deaf and hard-of-hearing persons. Another limiting factor is the added expense, due to the small classes, special equipment, and the specially trained teachers which would be ideally needed for these pupils. Therefore the majority of pupils with hearing problems, other than cases of profound deafness, are being taught by regular teachers in classes with normal children. Obviously, these special needs of pupils with hearing problems place extra burdens upon the dedicated teacher. Consequently, it should be emphasized again that whenever a classroom teacher includes a pupil with a hearing problem within her program, she should be given all possible support by audiologists, speech therapists, psychologists, parents, school counselors, school nurses, and others whose services may be indicated.

Recognizing Problems of
Hearing in the Classroom

The following list of symptoms should be regarded with caution. A particular symptom of behavior *may* or *may not* be an indicator of a hearing problem. Many of the listed symptoms may be associated with conditions other than hearing disorders. A pupil's inattention or failure to respond in class may be an indication of normality under certain circumstances. Certainly it is advisable to be acquainted with as many indicators as possible, in order to be equipped and alert to recognize a group or syndrome of symptoms which collectively add their weight to the likelihood that a hearing problem exists. Some symptoms of behavior are more indicative of hearing impairments than are others. A review of the following list of possible indicators from time to time is insurance against overlooking hearing problems which are sometimes disguised by compensatory reactions or abilities, asocial behavior, and other personal reactions which distract attention from the true nature of the problem's cause. Yet the problem may be a serious one, in need of further diagnosis. It is also practical to remember that children of elementary school age should normally hear better than adults. Judging young children too loosely according to adult standards may result in overlooking slight defects of hearing which may grow worse if they are not corrected.

FAULTY SPEECH AND VOICE

The question of a pupil's hearing should be considered whenever his voice patterns and articulation are found to be abnormal, as in severe misarticulation, the omission of speech sounds, the tendency to speak with odd inflections, a monotone, or a voice which is too loud or too soft. The hearing-handicapped child is likely to have difficulties with the multiple meanings of common words, the proper usage of verb tense, and the exceptions in forming the plurals of nouns.

ABNORMAL RESPONSES TO SPEECH AND OTHER SOUNDS

Deafness has been discovered in early infancy by noting the infant's failure to turn toward sound stimuli or to startle from loud and sudden noises. The failure to respond correctly, or to react at all, to a question or other sound stimulus may also indicate that a child does not hear correctly. A child's perceptual difficulty in understanding speech through hearing may be greater than it appears—because of his reliance upon lip reading. A child with a hearing defect may indicate his problem by being an unusually close watcher of speakers' lips. Under the effort and strain of trying to understand speech, he may frown or become restless and irritated. He may have the habit of asking people to repeat what they say when he does not understand them, unless he has withdrawn because of the penalty from their impatience and irritation over this difficulty. In that case, he may avoid speech and may even become a "loner," choosing to play in activities where physical actions predominate and where social interactions do not demand speech and hearing.

ACADEMIC DIFFICULTY

The hearing-impaired pupil usually is rated as an underachiever. Pupils with severe but undetected hearing losses may be wrongly judged as mentally defective because of their poor record in classwork. However, some of these children may confuse this misconception of them by their ability in arithmetic, laboratory projects, art, or in other situations where motor learning and performance are more possible. In addition to his lowered academic grades, the pupil with a hearing loss is often branded as lazy, listless, inattentive, indecisive, lacking in self-confidence, restless, a daydreamer, a procrastinator, or unhappy with school. Some of these traits exhibited in the classroom may lead the teacher to overlook the underlying factor of faulty hearing and to classify the hard-of-hearing child as being primarily and principally a "behavior problem."

PERSONALITY AND SOCIAL TRAITS

When impaired hearing interferes with a pupil's communication, he is likely to experience frustration, feelings of failure, anxiety, fear, discouragement, unhappiness, shyness, aggression, belligerence, withdrawal, suspicion, etc.

ASSOCIATED PHYSICAL SYMPTOMS

When a pupil complains of earache or shows ear discharge from middle-ear infection, his teacher should promptly refer the problem to the school nurse or parents for medical attention. At times the pupil will show his earaches by nonverbal means. He may hold his hand over the painful ear, rub it, or complain about loud sounds which aggravate the pain. As one experienced teacher reported:

> I know of one first-grader who suffered through three weeks of bad earache before his teacher, school nurse, and parents finally learned of it. However, during these miserable weeks he had perplexed his teacher by whimpering whenever the piano was played in the daily music periods. Of course, his continued earache made him inattentive and restless in all school activities, but the cause of his trouble was not suspected until the teacher finally asked him why he didn't like music. He admitted then that he had an earache and had been reluctant to tell anyone about it for fear that he'd have to go to a doctor and have shots.

The pupil who is hard of hearing or deaf may show other peculiar patterns of physical action. Some deaf children shuffle their feet while walking because of an inability to hear the scraping of their footsteps. Some develop odd or offensive mannerisms while eating, sipping, sneezing, clearing the throat, blowing the nose, etc.

Referral and Diagnosis

Every classroom teacher should expect the school records of each pupil to show evidence of an adequate hearing examination. If his hearing has not been evaluated and recorded, his classroom teacher shares the responsibility of obtaining an audiometric examination. Cooperative assistance in securing hearing tests for pupils should be expected from the principal, speech therapist, school nurse, and others. The school's speech therapist should also be relied upon for consultation in the interpretation and application of information from hearing tests.

In her parental contacts too, the teacher is often a go-between in giving information and support in matters of hearing conservation, perceptual training at home, the use of hearing aids, and in providing good practice in lip reading. In addition, the teacher is directly responsible for the pupil's adequate total adjustment and learning in school so that he may develop normally with a minimum of handicap from his hearing problem.

CONSERVATION OF HEARING

It should be stressed again that the early detection of a hearing problem is the first requisite in insuring that the problem is corrected or that it does not become complicated and even incurable from neglect. Classroom teachers should work closely with audiologists, otologists, and pediatricians, who initiate the medical measures to conserve hearing and also depend upon follow-up support from teachers, parents, and others. An otologist listed the following ways in which teachers have cooperated in his medical programs to conserve hearing:

> Although a hearing conversation program is primarily a medical responsibility, a good share of the credit for its success comes from schoolteachers. Most of our clients are schoolchildren under the daily care of teachers who are more watchful and informed about hearing problems than are many of the children's parents. The initial spotting of problems often comes from teachers. They note signs of infection or of hearing loss. From the standpoint of conversation, many teachers and speech therapists teach pupils good practices of aural hygiene, such as not to poke anything into the ear to remove wax or to relieve itching and how to blow the nose gently and without creating excessive nasal pressure which forces infectious discharges up the Eustachian tube into the middle ear. Pupils should be taught to avoid excessive noise and to inform their parents when earaches or other complaints occur.
>
> Parents and teachers have an important responsibility to protect children who have suffered permanent perforations of eardrums, from injury or disease, or when children have had mastoidectomy, fenestration, or eardrum operations which have left avenues for further complications from outside infection, exposure to cold wind, etc. In these cases, we must guard against such dangers as swimming, by the use of earplugs and nose clips. Occasionally we still find children with ear injury which reportedly was caused by parents and others who punish by boxing the ears. Before corporal punishment was outlawed in our public schools, some teachers were known to rupture ears in this way too.

THE PRESCRIPTION AND USE OF
HEARING AIDS

Only qualified otologists or audiologists should determine the need for a hearing aid and the type of aid best suited in each case of loss. Sometimes a desk-type of aid, instead of a personal one, may be prescribed for a schoolchild.

An unwarranted or ill-fitted aid, or a lack of training in the use of an aid, may even add to the person's hearing problems as well as cause considerable unnecessary expense. Many complaints come from poorly prescribed hearing aids or from poorly serviced aids sold through unqualified or unlicensed dealers, salesmen, drugstores, and mail-order houses. In the field of hearing disorders, as in all other areas of human ailments, it is important to protect the handicapped from quackery and commercial exploitation.

PERSONAL AND SOCIAL ACCEPTANCE

OF THE HEARING AID

A pupil's satisfactory use of a hearing aid may also depend upon the help he gets from his teacher in its use, care, and social acceptance in the classroom. The following classroom teacher explains how she has cooperated with audiologists and speech therapists in helping pupils with hearing aids.

> In my fourteen years of teaching in the elementary grades, I have had ten pupils who have worn hearing aids. In my experience with them I have learned that it pays to consult and cooperate with speech therapists in our school because speech problems often accompany the hearing problems.
>
> One of my basic problems with a pupil who wears a hearing aid is to make and keep him willing to wear the device, despite its inconveniences and the negative social reactions which it sometimes provokes. The personal and social acceptance of a pupil's aid rests primarily upon how advantageously he uses it. He must be convinced that it pays for him to wear that aid. The speech therapist usually gives him training in speech discriminations within communicative situations designed to convince the pupil that the aid really improves his understanding of speech. If a child's hearing loss has caused speech misarticulations, he may also be shown that his speech improves from the sharper self-monitoring which his aid provides. Ordinarily one does not convince a child of his improvement by just telling him that his speech is better with the aid than without it. He needs practical experiential situations in which he hears for himself that the device aids his speech and reception. For instance, it may be helpful for the pupil and others to make tape-recorded comparisons of his speech, with and without the aid. In this way, the benefits of amplification can be convincingly proved not only for him but for other persons whose judgments he values. In my classroom I have redesigned various speech and listening situations so that the pupil and his classmates sense the value he receives from his aid. For example, in a class exercise on spelling, I may have the children listen and write out the sentence which I dictate, containing a specified word and its meaning. After they have finished writing each dictated sentence, I write the sentence on the board to give them a check on their performance. I may demonstrate the value of the pupil's hearing aid in this class by having him hear and write the first half of the list of sentences without the benefit of his aid, then do the second half while using it. To make the value of this aid more impressive, I may ask everyone in class to listen to my sentences while I speak to his back from the rear of the room. In this way, obviously none can rely upon visual cues from lip reading to make up for losses in hearing. All of the children enjoy

these listening exercises. The classmates of the pupil with the hearing aid are also respectfully impressed with the values he demonstrates from using the instrument in this situation. It places their judgments on a level of performances which they can understand and share.

One of our speech therapists conducted a classroom lesson which I felt was exceptionally valuable for several reasons. He visited each elementary classroom in which he learned there was a pupil with a hearing aid and conducted an interesting demonstration of old and new types of hearing aids, from the ear trumpets and big cumbersome aids of the past to the little and attractive modern aids which are concealed within the frames of eyeglasses, worn behind the ear, and even some that are worn entirely within the ear. He compared hearing aids with eyeglasses, developing his lesson in such a way that the children were given a respectful and positive feeling toward all such corrective devices. He also compared hearing aids with a telephone, which the children have commonly used to hear speech that otherwise would be too far off and faint for them to hear. He let the children satisfy their curiosities by hearing through the ear trumpet, compared with a modern desk-type aid fitted with a headset which each child could easily put on. In the course of this educational lesson, the therapist included constructive facts about the aid being worn by the pupil in our room. The pupil was usually invited to contribute with information on certain aspects of his hearing aid.

I am convinced that if every parent and teacher would regard hearing aids wich as much objectivity and acceptance as they ordinarily give to eyeglasses when vision needs correction, children and their classmates would treat hearing aids as they treat glasses.

TRAINING IN THE USE AND
MAINTENANCE OF THE AID

A hearing aid is a delicate electronic instrument, engineered with precision for a highly specialized function. Therefore, in order to gain the outputs for which the instrument is intended, the user of a hearing aid must learn to operate it correctly and to assume responsibility for its careful maintenance. Teachers, too, should know the general principles and mechanics of an aid. A hearing aid, like a telephone, has a microphone and a receiver; like a battery-powered transistor radio, it has an off-on switch, a volume control, and sometimes a tone control. Teachers should realize that hearing aids with weak batteries or corroded contact points will lose power until reception diminishes or fails. Poor reception also occurs from wax or water in the opening of the eartip or from a worn or broken cord.

Teachers and the hearing aid wearer should understand the conditions which may cause and correct the feedback phenomenon heard as an annoying squeal or whistle from the receiver in the eartip of the aid. Some of the common causes of this feedback squeal are readily correctable by the user if he or his teacher is aware of them. There may be a leakage of sound from an eartip which is not snugly placed in the ear, causing a reamplification of the escaped sound, until it progressively builds up and overloads into the squeal. Squeal results more readily when the volume of reception is turned too high. Squeal in a two-part aid may occur if the case holding the mike is worn too close to the receiver in the ear—a condition which may be corrected by placing the microphone farther from the receiver. Feedback squeal may also be externally caused by an excess of sound which is reflected from a wall surface near which the pupil is positioned. Unless teachers are alert to the occurrence, causes, and remedies of feedback squeal, a pupil who is unable to diagnose and correct this troublesome phenomenon may lose confidence in his aid and may even turn it off or conveniently lose the aid.

Pupils should be taught not to wear hearing aids in rough-and-tumble play. The wearer must learn to tolerate loud unavoidable noises which are amplified along with speech and other sounds. In conversation with a hearing aid user, teachers and classmates should speak naturally and at normal volume. In average conversation with a person who is closely dependent upon his hearing aid and lip reading, a teacher should cooperate by stationing herself at the best conversational distance for lip reading—usually between three and six feet. Likewise, a pupil in a classroom should feel free to place himself wherever he can best hear and see in the learning situation at hand. However, in the early grades some classmates may need special briefing to understand why a handicapped pupil who is dependent upon special aids and lip reading should be given extra privileges to insure his equal opportunity to learn.

Classroom teachers should rely upon speech and hearing therapists for assistance in helping a pupil to gain as much value as possible from his hearing aid. If the pupil's hearing loss has impaired his articulation or learning of perceptual patterns, the speech and hearing therapist may give him individualized auditory training in the finer discriminations needed for speech and its comprehension. Speech therapists should also give instructions in the use and care of the hearing instrument. Working cooperatively with the pupil's classroom teacher and parents, the therapist may also prevent or correct emotional maladjustments which may become associated with the hearing problem and the use of the aid.

MAKING FULL USE OF RESIDUAL
HEARING

Generally, even in the most severe cases of hearing loss or deafness, there is some residual hearing. This remnant of hearing may exist even though hearing aids are being fully utilized. However slight or partial his residual hearing may be, with or without electronic aids, it is important that the handicapped person be given full opportunity to use and compensate for this partial hearing. Parents, teachers, and others are generally advised to "talk, talk, and talk" to the "deaf" person as they naturally would to a person with normal hearing. This advice applies even though the person is profoundly deafened and has obvious difficulty in understanding or answering spoken language. In our teaching of speech to the severely handicapped child, our patterns of voice, articulation, rate, rhythm, and language should be expressed naturally, correctly, and clearly, giving attention also to the listener's visual perception of what we say. The effective teacher of speech and language for the deaf is one who not only naturally uses good habits of speech but who may also deliberately adjust to special patterns of stimulation which may be specially required for certain handicapped persons. Perhaps a teacher learns that a certain pupil with a profound loss but without a hearing aid may hear speech best when she speaks somewhat louder than normally, at a rate which is slower than she habitually uses, and with special efforts to give the pupil added visual cues from lip reading. It is often best to invite the trial and judgment of the handicapped person, because he may well be in the most authoritative position to determine what patterns of our stimulation are best suited to his perceptual ability.

LIP READING

Lip reading has been synonymously termed *speech reading* or *speech perception*, because in the visual perception of speech there is much more to be "read" than the postures and movements of lips. Facial expressions and body gestures also convey language. For instance, if a deaf person is viewing the warning command "Oh, no! You shouldn't go!" he may not gain much from merely watching the speaker's lips. However, he may fill in more meaning from the natural expressions of the eyes, movements of the eyebrows, head, and limbs. One deaf person stated this fact when he advised:

> Many people don't seem to realize that they speak with their whole bodies. When they speak to me and try hard to make me understand, they seem to act as if speech is meant to come only through the lips. Consequently, they overwork their lips, and that makes speech harder than ever for me to interpret. If they'd just be natural and talk as they ordinarily should talk, we deaf people would have a better chance to "read" them. It's easier to speech-read speakers who are well adjusted, who have normal feelings and appreciations in their conversations, and who are not inhibited about showing these feelings naturally, from head to foot, while they talk. In fact, when I am "reading" a person, I focus mostly on his eyes, but I can still watch his lips, tongue, head, shoulders, hands, trunk, and general movements. Although there are some gestures which people seem to have universally learned as a part of their native language, each speaker seems to have developed some mannerisms which are peculiar to him. After I become well acquainted with a person, I find that his individualisms are worthy of notice. They are informative and help to make speech reading more picturesque and challenging.

There are many direct and indirect ways to facilitate a pupil's lip reading. Some of the indirect aids, such as equipping the pupil with a good language foundation, are of more importance than are the direct measures to train him in the technical skills for reading lips. Also, if a child is not given sufficient incentives for understanding spoken language, efforts to train him in the skills of lip reading will fail. The following list of factors which favor lip reading does not intend to show their relative importance or their order for attainment. While all the factors are important, they are not equally required by every lip reader. Therefore, when we work to improve a child's lip reading, we should do it analytically on an individual basis, also realizing that the profile of his needs is in a dynamic state of change. It is also revealing and important to remember that a person does not necessarily require instruction by a professional in order to become an expert at lip reading. It is possible for deaf children of preschool age to be so skilled at reading lips that their deafness is unsuspected. However, when one finds a child who has this "natural" ability, it is usually evident that his parents, siblings, or other laymen have followed the same practices which professional teachers of the deaf advocate and follow.

Language training: a good foundation. If a pupil is to be skilled at lip reading, he must have a better-than-average vocabulary and grasp of grammatical structure. Whatever applies to the development of good language for the normal child is required even more by the child with a hearing problem. The lip reader's intuitive ability to fill in the invisible gaps of spoken language hinges largely upon his ability to make extra use of words, his knowledge of synonyms, and his ability to deduce from the fragments of sentences which are viewed. His vocabulary must be kept up to date so that he will understand rather than be perplexed by slang, idioms, or colloquialisms. He must learn the informal as well as the formal patterns of language.

To achieve these extra abilities in language, the lip reader will require maximum use of his intact senses of sight, touch, taste, and smell in association with his learning of language. One teacher of the deaf gave the following advice to parents of deaf children:

> In teaching vocabulary to the deaf child, there is a special need to convey meanings through pictures and other visual aids, demonstrations, and physical actions. As for the normal child, this language teaching for the deaf should begin in early infancy through first-hand experiences which contribute their bits of information to the language meanings which parents and others teach. The hearing-handicapped child needs repeated and imaginative experiences from a variety of angles before he can compare, abstract, generalize, and use language as a child with normal hearing does. The deaf person may need some special experiencing before he learns that the word *sweet*, for instance, may refer not only to a variety of taste characteristics which apply to sugar, candy, sweet pickles, unsalted foods, etc., but also to an auditory quality of a certain type of music or of a smooth-running motor. Visually, the term *sweet* may refer to a shapely or attractive face or figure, dress, or a good-natured manner; while on a more abstract level, *sweet* may signify a pleasant experience, gratification, or agreeableness. Although reading and the use of the dictionary helps the deaf child extend his concept of this word, he may still need the visual and tactile experiences of learning the

characteristics of "sweet music" and a "sweet-running machine." Language learning should be experience-based for every child, but for the deaf or hard-of-hearing child it should be built into his reality even more.

Because of the discrepancies which exist between spoken language and the written or printed symbols of that spoken language, the lip reader who cannot hear has difficulty in knowing the pronunciations of many words with nonphonetic spellings. The following college student, who has been profoundly deaf since birth, expresses this difficulty which arises in lip reading when he does not know the pronunciation of words being spoken:

> Although I am considered an expert in lip reading and have gained a good command of printed language, I often have difficulty in bridging the gap between the regular reading and the lip reading of certain words. It is much easier to lip-read words I have learned to speak—even though my articulation of these words may not be perfect. When I began to read printed language, I learned many words but could not tell from some of their spellings how they would be viewed on people's lips. This confused me in lip reading. For instance, I learned correctly to read printed words containing *ough*, such as *tough*, *dough*, *bough*, *trough*, and *through*, but was mixed up when I saw these words on people's lips until I learned how the vowels in these words should be differently spoken. Of course, when I had reason to wonder about the pronunciation of spellings, I could look them up in a dictionary, but a person who cannot hear does not always readily suspect that a spelling is not spoken as it appears.

By closely coordinating the written and oral forms of language, classroom teachers may reduce such a difficulty as that expressed by the foregoing lip reader. An excellent teacher of language in a school for the deaf indicated how lip reading was closely integrated with reading instruction, writing, and spelling:

> We help our pupils in lip reading by correlating the written with the oral patterns of language. We are especially watchful of irregular language patterns in reading materials which are new to pupils. We have the policies of marking the pronunciations of new printed words and of saying them so that pupils will recognize them later in lip reading. We have observed that lip reading of language improves when it is taught through the use of the Initial Teaching Alphabet, popularly known as I.T.A. Later, we carefully teach the pupils the diacritical marks corresponding with the I.T.A. symbols in order that the pupils may independently use dictionaries to determine pronunciations in preparation for lip reading these irregular words.

Making Use of Residual Hearing in Lip Reading. Lip reading may be significantly aided by cues from the various degrees of partial hearing which usually exist even in the most severe cases of deafness. This help from combining hearing with seeing is proved even when residual hearing is so slight that only fragments of the speech sounds are brought within the lip reader's perception, even by powerful amplification. A person who attended a school for the deaf gave the following credit to his limited use of a group-type of hearing aid with which each of his classrooms was permanently equipped:

> I am too deaf to get enough help to justify wearing a personal hearing aid in my everyday life, but when I was a pupil in school, I found that the powerful headset aid at each desk did help me to learn lip reading. When my teachers were reading instructions, I could hear most of the vowels in their speech, and even some consonants, but I couldn't understand anything they said when I closed my eyes. My scores in lip reading tests were definitely higher when I had the chance to use my little bits of hearing too.

Because of the valuable cues a lip reader may receive from residual hearing, classroom teachers should carefully consider the factor of noise and a pupil's position in the classroom relative to the sources of the noises which interfere. A pupil who sits near a loud blower or door may have his hearing, and especially residual hearing, completely masked by noises from inside or outside the classroom.

Pupils who depend upon lip reading to compensate for their hearing losses should generally be given "roving seats"—the permission to leave their seats and to shift to temporary positions in the room where the teacher or other pupils may be conducting demonstrations and using speech. Another purpose of the "roving seat" is to encourage the hearing-handicapped pupil to make extra use of encyclopedias and other sources of information which he may have missed in oral instruction. The pupil who relies upon lip reading in class recitations should also be allowed to turn around in his seat in order to view the recitations of classmates. When these special privileges are granted, other classmates should be given a clear and frank explanation for them, without creating any feelings of apology for the hearing problem.

Physical Conditions in the Classroom. There are other classroom conditions which have important bearing on a pupil's ability to lip-read his teacher and classmates. Yet we occasionally find neglected pupils who are dependent upon lip reading and are seated in the distant fringes of classrooms where they are unable to see or to attend to what their teachers say or do.

Generally, there are at least three factors to consider in the lip reader's classroom location. He should be near the teacher or other speakers who are being lip-read, where the lighting will neither cast shadows upon the speakers nor compel the pupil to face a tiring and obstructing glare of light. Distance is another important factor for viewing. Because a distance of six feet is often suggested as a good average distance for lip reading, a front seat in the classroom is usually recommended for the pupil. Furthermore, the best location allows a full and clear view of the speaker's face. A deaf college student gave the following suggestions concerning placement of pupils who lip-read in the classroom:

In my experience with many teachers in all types of classrooms, I've usually found that a front seat directly facing the teacher's desk is the best for lip reading. That's where the teacher usually does most of her talking. And when she steps back to write on the blackboard, I'm still close enough to get a good view of her face. None of my teachers have placed me in really bad positions. Most of them have let me pick the desk I prefer. My teachers have conferred with my parents and speech therapists in these matters too.

Another deaf pupil, who was not as fortunate with classroom seating arrangements, had this to say:

I remember three bad periods of lip reading in my twelve years of school. Once I was put over to one side of the room, where I had to face the light from the windows. I couldn't see the teacher's face very well. It bothered me mostly on sunny days. Besides, there were two kids sitting in front of me who were horsing around most of the time. My attention was on them more than on the teacher. It takes concentration when you lip read.

I remember in the third grade when the teacher put me in front of her desk, in the middle of the front row. It was easy to read her while she was there, but when she later moved her desk over to the side, right beside the windows, I couldn't see her face clearly at all. My mother told her that I was having trouble, and so I was moved over to the windows in front of her. I also remember that she told the kids why my seat was changed. I was glad she told them, because otherwise they'd think I was a teacher's pet and would resent it.

Another teacher was hard to lip-read because she was in the habit of moving around when she talked to the class. Half of the time she was turned sideways or away from me when she talked. My grades were not so good that year.

Speech Habits, Mannerisms, and Policies of the Teacher. Much of the responsibility for a pupil's success in speech reading should be assumed by the speaker being "read." The following list of suggestions has been compiled from various counselings to parents, teachers and others concerning personal habits which make them more easily "read":

Talk naturally. Don't exaggerate your speech by trying to articulate over-precisely. Talk with your voice. Don't whisper or merely mouth your words.

Don't talk too fast or at an unnaturally slow rate either.

Check and eliminate any of your mannerisms which may distract the lip reader or obscure your articulation, such as talking with a deadpan expression, talking through clenched teeth or with continuous smiling, using excessive head movements or irrelevant gestures, or obstructing the view of your mouth with hands, papers, books, etc.

Get in the habit of facing the lip reader while speaking to him. Don't speak while you walk or write on the blackboard.

Speak in full and correct sentences. If the lip reader does not understand you after perhaps one repetition of your first statement, rephrase it so that he may get the essential thought of the sentence from a different wording, the change of a modifier, clause, or phrase.

When you are speaking to a lip reader who is seated, try to keep your mouth near the level of his eyes. Either sit at your desk or stand about eight feet from the pupil so that he will not be required to look from below.

While reading to the lip reader, hold your book so that it will neither obscure your mouth nor cause you to tilt your face downward. This practice is helpful also for children with normal hearing.

Supplement your oral instructions with visual aids, such as maps, outlines, sketches, models, etc., so that the lip reader and others who miss parts of what you say may fill in with information from these visual aids.

Encourage the hearing-impaired pupil and his classmates to repeat directions for the benefit of everyone. By asking the handicapped child to repeat important directions, you may learn whether or not he understood your oral directions.

It may help a pupil in reading your lips if you use a moderate amount of lipstick. However, avoid distracting jewelry, such as dangling earrings.

Give thought to your facial expressions while you are being lip-read. It is unpleasant for a person to lip-read a face which shows impatience, irritation, embarrassment, anxiety, etc. Eyes are driven away from such unpleasant sights.

Before launching into a class discussion of a subject, introduce it in some way so that the pupil with a hearing handicap will know what you are talking about. It would help him become oriented to the subject if you'd outline your topic on the board or demonstrate in other concrete ways what you speak about. If the discussion contains new vocabulary, it would also be helpful if you would list and define these key words before they are used in your talk. All pupils would benefit from these good teaching practices.

Accept your pupil's hearing impairment in a matter of fact way and never apologize for it.

Help the pupil get tutoring in subjects which are suffering from his lack of hearing.

Encourage and allow the hearing-handicapped pupil to participate in speaking and singing even though his vocal skills are below par.

Parental Cooperation

It is especially important for parents to give early and continued cooperative help with hearing problems. Parents should realize that hearing serves important functions which begin at birth. Parents should be acquainted with the common symptoms of behavior which may indicate that an infant has a hearing loss or has complications which may lead to a hearing problem. Furthermore, parents should know where and how to get valid hearing tests, which have been developed even for infants less than one year of age. Parents of a hearing-handicapped child should realize that the preschool period, from birth to four years of age, is the most optimal period for developing a person's lip-reading ability and other compensatory adjustments to a hearing loss. If training is neglected during these early years, it may be difficult to revive later.

Audiologists, otologists, teachers, speech therapists, school nurses, and other school counselors share the responsibility of insuring that parents get valid information and services for hearing-impaired children. The following organizations can provide valuable information to parents:

The Alexander Graham Bell Association for the Deaf, 1535 35th Street, N.W., Washington 7, D.C.

The American Hearing Society, 919 18th Street, N.W., Washington 6, D.C.

The American Speech and Hearing Association, 1001 Connecticut Avenue, N.W., Washington 6, D.C.

John Tracy Clinic, 806 West Adams Boulevard, Los Angeles 7, California.

The John Tracy Clinic, for instance, offers a correspondence course which has given worldwide aid to thousands of parents of young deaf children. Other modern schools and agencies for the aurally handicapped are giving increased attention to the roles of parents and the home in the education and rehabilitation of deaf children. Progressive schools for deaf or blind children have either lowered the admission age for pupils' residence in them or have offered preschool workshops and counseling for parents.

References

1. Hallowell Davis and S. Richard Silverman, *Hearing and Deafness*. New York: Holt, Rinehart and Winston, Inc., 1960.

Questions

1. Why should speech pathologists and audiologists work in close cooperation?

2. What is the significance of the serious shortage of special teachers for the hearing-handicapped?

3. In terms of onset, how are hearing problems classified?

4. What are functional causes of hearing problems?

5. Explain: hearing has been called a "glorified sense of touch."

6. What are the types of sound-wave transmission in the process of hearing?

7. Describe conductive hearing loss.

8. In what way is bone conduction useful in hearing problems?

9. Define residual hearing and its significance in hearing problems.

10. What infectious diseases may damage hearing?

11. Explain how a person's hearing may be lowered by more than one factor in the same type of impairment.

12. Define: *central dysacusis*, *verbal dysacusis*, and *receptive aphasia*.

13. How do hearing impairments affect pupils?

14. How may the classroom teacher help hard-of-hearing pupils?

15. How does hearing loss affect academic standing?

16. List the signs which may indicate that a pupil has a hearing loss.

17. Explain the duty of parents and teachers in problems of physical impairment leading to hearing difficulties.

18. What is the aim of an adequate referral and diagnostic program for hearing examination?

19. Why is the classroom teacher a key member of the team aiding hearing cases?

20. In what ways may teachers cooperate in hearing conservation programs?

21. Why is language training important for hearing-impaired pupils?

22. Discuss lip reading as a factor in hearing problems.

23. How may lip reading be made most effective?

24. What controllable physical conditions in the classroom affect pupils with hearing handicaps?

25. What effect may the teacher's speech habits, mannerisms, and policies have upon a pupil's ability to lip-read?

26. Where may parents secure help for the hearing problems of their children?

Suggested Subjects for Term Papers

1. On a dozen occasions, plug your ears effectively enough to prevent your hearing most voices. At what stage do you resort to attempting lip reading? Record your moods, impulses, and reactions to the behavior of the persons who speak.

2. Devise a game which would appeal to hard-of-hearing children and include them in play with children of normal hearing.

3. Visit several grade school classes and note (1) how the pupils' hearing ability affects their behavior and learning; (2) how teachers' voices rate in projection quality for ease of hearing by the pupils.

4. Consult *Readers' Guide to Periodical Literature* and report on a half-dozen articles discussing impaired hearing problems.

Index